# Crucial Decisions at the Beginning of Life

## Parents' experiences of treatment withdrawal from infants

In association with
Peter W Fowlie, Robert Hume, Ian A Laing,
David J Lloyd and Andrew J Lyon

Foreword by

David Harvey

Radcliffe Medical Press

Radcliffe Medical Press Ltd
18 Marcham Road, Abingdon, Oxon OX14 1AA

British Library Cataloguing in Publication Data

A catalogue record for this book is available from the British Library.

ISBN 1 85775 479 4

Typeset by Aarontype Limited, Easton, Bristol
Printed and bound by TJ International Ltd, Padstow, Cornwall

# Contents

# Foreword

The last few decades have shown remarkable advances in neonatal care. Babies now survive at gestational ages which were once thought to be incompatible with life. Unfortunately, this has a cost. Treatment with ventilation may last many weeks or months and is often very stressful for the parents, and also for the nursing and medical staff involved in their care. When a baby dies, very sensitive support is needed for the parents. Their perceptions may be very different from those of their relatives and professional advisors. A mother once told me of her feelings after some relatives had attempted to console her because she had three other children. She said, 'I had not lost 25% of my children, but 100% of one child'.

Sometimes, it becomes clear that the treatment is doing more harm than good or even is fruitless in merely prolonging death. The skills of the doctors and nurses are needed more than ever at such times. They need to achieve consensus and to involve the parents in the difficult process of decision making.

This is an important book and I am very pleased to have been asked to write the foreword. It recounts the experiences of families whose babies died or were involved in the withdrawal of medical treatment. The interviews were undertaken after the families were identified in three neonatal intensive care units in Scotland. A lot of hard work has gone into the project and the discussions with the parents lasted many hours. What the parents have to say is very revealing and demonstrates how easy it is to make mistakes in their care. Their comments are instructive and will help us in the care of other families. Great care should be taken to use the right name and gender when talking about the baby. It is important to pay attention to detail in helping the parents to find the right hospital and department. As far as possible, named staff should not be changed, so that the parents do not have to give the medical history yet again and do not have to repeat the delicate process of building up relationships.

One thing which comes through very clearly is the desire of parents to be involved in the care of their babies and to take part in the important decisions which have to be taken. It is encouraging to read of the appreciation of the parents for the individual time given by the staff. To realise that it is recognised and valued makes it all worth while.

We must aim to give faultless care, but need to recognise that we often fall short of our aim. At least, we can do our best not to make things worse. The parents who recounted the events in these interviews are excellent teachers in showing us where it is easy to go wrong.

David Harvey
Professor of Paediatrics and Neonatal Medicine
Imperial College School of Medicine
Division of Paediatrics, Obstetrics and Gynaecology
Queen Charlotte's and Chelsea Hospital, London
*January 2001*

# About the authors

**Dr Hazel McHaffie** is a Research Fellow in the Institute of Medical Ethics at the University of Edinburgh and Deputy Director of Research in the Institute of Medical Ethics. She has spent over six years exploring the experience of treatment withdrawal from infants through in-depth interviews with doctors, neonatal nurses and patients.

**Dr Peter Fowlie, Professor Robert Hume, Dr Ian Lang, Dr David Lloyd** and **Dr Andrew Lyon** are all consultant neonatologists in busy Neonatal Intensive Care Units. They were anxious to improve the care offered to these families, and willingly involved their Units in the research programme to that end.

# A tribute

The death of a child is one of the most devastating and profound losses anyone can suffer. We can bear testament to the depth of pain that the parents of dying infants endure. However, despite their grief, every one of the 108 courageous mothers and fathers who participated in our study contributed valuable insights into the experience of treatment withdrawal and death. They wept in the telling. As a result of their experiences they are now changed people. As a consequence of being with them in their sorrow, and coming to understand their pain better, we too are changed.

However, these parents did not agree to participate in the research for their own ends. A more powerful motivation than personal gain was an altruistic one. Again and again they acknowledged that if someone else could benefit as a result of their telling, then they were prepared to put themselves through the trauma of remembering. Some good would then have come out of their tragedy. In unfolding their stories they were reaching out to others who, in the future, would share their suffering. They were also anxious to touch those who would never know this loss, but who value too lightly the normal experience of having babies.

It has been both an enormous privilege and a humbling experience to meet these families and listen to their stories. We can never hope to express our gratitude to them adequately, but we offer this report as a mark of our respect and admiration. Our thanks will be best expressed in the use we make of what they gave us, and we have absolute assurance that practice has already changed to take account of their messages. This report will enable others both in this country and elsewhere to increase their sensitivity too. The parents have not told their stories in vain.

# Acknowledgements

My biggest debt by far is to the parents who gave so generously of themselves. I felt welcomed wherever I went, from the Shetland Islands to the Borders. Their trust and commitment, which kept them talking often into the small hours of the night, was heart-warming. Going back to see them one year on was like visiting old friends. Whatever is good in this report is thanks to them.

The Chief Scientist Office at the Scottish Executive showed their commitment to improving care for these vulnerable families by funding the project in its entirety. I am grateful for their support.

No researcher could ask for a better team of co-researchers. Dr Peter Fowlie, Professor Robert Hume, Dr Ian Laing, Dr David Lloyd and Dr Andrew Lyon ensured that their Units remained committed to the project, that families were referred to me, that numbers were as good as we could get them, that reporting was effective and that practice was changed. I particularly thank them for scrutinising so many articles for publication and drafts of this book at a time when they had so many other responsibilities. Dr Peter Fowlie and Mr Rob Bercovitch carefully and methodically listened to a percentage of the interviews to ensure that coding was accurate and that parents' views were being heard and interpreted reliably. The co-operation, friendship and encouragement of the whole team were invaluable.

This field of study is emotionally exacting, and support is essential. With their wide experience and excellent listening skills, Professor Alex Campbell and Dr Colin Walker were ideal supporters and advisers. They made themselves available when I needed to share the burden, and they offered wise counsel during data collection and again at the stage of publication. I always came away from meetings with them refreshed. My colleague, Dr Kenneth Boyd, was unfailingly supportive. His belief in my capacity to cope and in the value of the work, coupled with his ongoing interest and constant friendship, has fostered an ideal working environment.

Clinical colleagues in the study Units supported the endeavour by referring families. They knew that their own practice was under scrutiny, and I appreciated their willingness to co-operate. Consultants practising in the Units at the time in addition to the co-researchers were Professor

N McIntosh, Dr P Midgley, Dr G Menon, Dr B Stenson, Dr J S Forsyth, Dr W Tarnow-Mordi, Dr A Mehta, Dr P Booth and Dr P Duffty. My thanks go to all of those who participated.

The Institute of Medical Ethics Working Party supported this idea with enthusiasm, and provided useful philosophical input, which has influenced the final chapter of this report. In particular, Dr Tony Hope, Professor Roger Higgs, Dr Michael Parker, Dr John McMillan, Professor Richard West, Dr Richard Ashcroft, Very Rev. Edward Shotter and Dr Jane Smith debated the issues at length.

There were times when the vagaries of my computer threatened to over-whelm me, but the computing staff in the University and the Royal Infirm-ary adjusted it to cope with the demands I made on it, and eased me through several crises with patience and good humour. Dr Ian Atkinson took on the task of transforming my lists and tables into figures, and Dr Richard Bingham and Ms Beth Egan gave invaluable assistance when things took an unexpected turn.

Bearing pain on the level required for an in-depth enquiry such as this takes its toll. My family were as ever endlessly supportive. David bore my constant absences and preoccupation with his usual calm fortitude. He, together with Rosalyn, Matthew, Jonathan and Camille, provided com-fort, encouragement and distraction when it was most needed. Abigail became my weekly therapy.

I am indebted to them all.

Hazel E McHaffie
*January 2001*

All royalties from the sale of this book go to the Diana Princess of Wales Children's Hospice and Home in Kalafong, Pretoria.

# Notes for the reader

Decision making on behalf of neonates is a complex subject with many facets. For greater clarity the report has been divided into phases, each of which is an entity in itself, drawing its own conclusions. However, to take any part of the experience out of its lived context is to diminish it, and appreciation of the full enormity of the experience for the families whom we studied can only be obtained from the more comprehensive coverage provided by the whole. References to other works are given for those who wish to pursue further study of these issues, but we have refrained from in-depth reviews in order not to detract from the powerful messages given by these special families.

Throughout this volume the term *withdrawing treatment* is used to denote the stopping of aggressive or invasive procedures, but not to indicate the withholding of basic comfort measures or caring. These were provided for all babies without exception.

For the purposes of clarity, to avoid cumbersome alternatives and to protect identities, the pronoun *she* is used for midwives and neonatal nurses (the majority of whom were women), and *he* is used for the doctors (almost all of whom were men).

If a surgeon reports an unusual case in a medical journal, showing photographs of what he achieved, to a great extent it becomes the surgeon's story. The patient is not named and his eyes are usually blanked out to protect him from identification. By removing identifying features from this report in order to respect and protect our respondents, there was some danger of eclipsing their experience by telling the whole as if it were something outside and beyond them, something which essentially belonged to the research team. From the outset we were conscious of this risk. However, the individual stories of real families touched us deeply. Respecting their confidences and protecting their identities is part of the ethics of good research, but this is very much their story, and the strength of this study's findings and recommendations is a measure of the integrity and power of their narratives.

For every one of these families the present was not what the past was supposed to lead up to. They were shocked and sometimes bewildered by events. Relating their stories helped them to bring some order to the ensuing chaos. No attempt was made to distance the facts from the emotions. 'The challenge of encountering the chaos narrative is how not to steer the storyteller away from her feelings . . . The challenge is to *hear*.'[1] To some extent, in pain as great as this, only part of the story can be told. 'Ultimately, chaos is told in the silences that speech cannot penetrate or illuminate. . . . Chaos is what can never be told; it is the hole in the telling.' In order to capture those untold depths, on occasion adjectives and emotions are used which are normally not to be found in the objective researcher's dictionary.

The study set out to gain insight into the parents' own experiences and perceptions of treatment limitation. They tell their own stories powerfully, with obvious sincerity and commitment to the truth. Without implying any doubt, however, it must be recognised that these are uncorroborated accounts; no attempt was made to clarify their stories by referring to the staff involved. For most families the two parents provided their own internal checks of details, but even there it is possible that their perceptions might not have matched those of the other participants in their drama. We make no claims beyond this being a faithful account of the parental perspective. This was how they remembered and understood the events.

Again and again the parents emphasised their appreciation of the service provided in the three study Neonatal Units. They were anxious that their comments should reflect this point, and were at times loath to identify perceived deficiencies, fearing that they might distort the reality. To minimise the risk of any such distortion, attention is here drawn to the overall excellence of the compassionate care that the parents reported receiving. In highlighting scope for improvement, this book aims simply to provide insights for clinicians to enable them to be even more sensitive to the experiences of the consumers of the future. It was to this end that the clinicians so readily agreed to research into their practices, and that the parents so generously re-lived their intensely painful experiences.

In places there is an element of repetition. Not all readers will tackle this volume in one sitting; some will refer to single chapters. To take account of this we have tried to make each chapter an entity in itself. Where points recur again and again over the different stages of the process, the parents are themselves emphasising the crucial importance of these factors to them.

We are aware that in discussing these painful issues we run the risk of treading on 'other people's secret sorrows.'[2] If we do inadvertently step unwarily in this way we apologise sincerely.

# List of figures

# List of tables

# CHAPTER 1

# Introduction

Developments in medical knowledge, technology and skill have dramatically improved the chances of survival of small and sick infants. So much is now possible and so much is attempted that, in modern practice, 'nature' is rarely left to take its course. As results improve and the impossible becomes possible, the possible becomes the expected, and the war against death acquires its own momentum. Expectations rise and pressure mounts on the medical team to deliver. It is important to pause periodically and reflect on current practice. Invasive and aggressive interventions carry their own burdens and costs. Who is paying the price? Who are its 'accidental victims?'[3] Are we listening to the perspectives of those who speak for them? Do we even know what they think? Not to do so would be irresponsible and unethical.

## Treatment limitation

It has been said that 'The acid test for any society that claims to be civilised is whether it really protects the life and promotes the wellbeing of its most vulnerable citizens.'[4] Numbered among the most vulnerable must be the very young – babies who cannot protect their own interests. Since classical antiquity the practice of exposing or killing infants has been countenanced in some cultures.[5] In pagan societies, human value was seen to be acquired rather than something inherent in a child – acquired through the development of intelligence or by acceptance into a particular society – and thus there was no compelling reason to preserve the life of an infant who failed to conform to the basic criteria demanded of members of that society. It appears to have been only with an early Christian revulsion against all acts of pagan brutality or immorality, and a belief that humans are formed in the image of God, that the principle of the inherent value of human life came into being,[6] although the practice of selectively killing infants has continued to some extent in many cultures.[7,8]

Whilst the idea of killing babies may be abhorrent in our Western civilisation, selective non-treatment is both professionally approved[9,10] and widely practised.[11-13] Indeed, in some of the studies reported, as many as three-quarters of deaths in intensive-care units were found to be associated with withholding or withdrawal of treatment,[11,13] which is seen as a necessary and compassionate response to the limits of modern medicine. However, these are not easy decisions to make. For one thing, powerful emotions are competing and a technological imperative as well as a parental desire for a live child make it difficult to stop. Then, too, the choice is sometimes between two unpalatable alternatives – death now or the possibility of future severe impairments, a poor quality of life or intractable suffering in the months or years ahead. In addition, it is not possible to make a *substituted judgement* for babies, as no one can know what they personally would choose if they had the capacity to do so. Instead, decisions are based on other people's notions of what constitutes the child's *best interest*.

# Who should decide?

From the medical point of view, three main factors have been found to influence the decision to stop, namely the imminence of death, the futility of treatment and the quality of life.[11-13] The first two rely on professional assessments of the medical facts. But quality of life is a more 'polymorphous collage.'[14] It embraces ideas of the capacity to function in normal everyday life, intellectual capabilities, the ability to relate to others or communicate, the potential to appreciate with the senses, and satisfaction with life. All of these things are difficult to quantify, especially for a neonate. Furthermore, children who would objectively rate low on some of these factors can lead happy lives. An infant who has known no other kind of life might assess his own existence as fulfilled and worthwhile, whereas an observer might rate it quite differently. It is impossible to assess the value of an 'inner life' for another person.

Despite the difficulties, however, in real life decisions do have to be made. Who should make them? The task has been widely seen to be best shared by a number of people. The necessity to involve the medical team is self-evident – they are the ones with expert knowledge and a duty of care to the child. But professional frameworks designed to guide clinicians also advocate involving parents in the decision-making process.[9,10,15,16] Furthermore, empirical evidence exists that doctors and nurses in clinical practice agree that parents should be involved.[12,17,18] There is, then, a general consensus that parents and healthcare professionals involved with the baby share a commitment to make a wise decision on behalf of the infant.

Together they form a 'moral community,'[19] and together they take responsibility for examining the issues and the alternatives, making the decisions and living with the consequences. These are weighty decisions, and the issues are rarely clear-cut. Judgements must be made, and inevitably mistakes will sometimes be made, but to date no one has been able to find a better solution than the agonised decisions of those who are most intimately involved with the child.

However, although there is widespread agreement that this should be a shared commitment, the balance of responsibility has not been spelled out. Arguments have been put forward that parents should decide,[20–26] while others have cautioned against giving them this responsibility.[8,27–29] A recent in-depth study of opinions within Neonatal Intensive Care Units (NICUs) found that only 3% of doctors and 6% of nurses felt that parents should take responsibility for the actual decision.[12] How much does the decision depend on medical assessment and how much is it, or should it be, influenced by other factors?

Clearly quality of life is an extremely elusive thing to assess,[30] but it would appear that the family themselves might have a view on what constitutes a good quality of life for their child and what would impose an intolerable burden on them all. Their standards, expectations and aspirations might differ from those of the medical team. In addition, although it is generally accepted that the wider interests of society and of costs are secondary considerations which should never overrule the best interests of the individual baby,[12,31] the infant's interests cannot be altogether divorced from those of the family. These lives are intertwined, and what impinges on the one may affect the other. Children with severe impairments will place significant demands on their family. Parents' feelings towards a child may be affected if the baby is kept alive against their better judgement; their own lives may be irrevocably altered if the child either lives or dies. Objectively it could be argued that only they can determine the limits which should be set in the case of their own child.

# What the parents themselves think

In 1994, in the state of Michigan, USA, Traci Messenger went into premature labour at 25 weeks' gestation. She had had two previous Caesarean sections, and this third operation resulted in delivery of a 780 g baby boy. The parents had explicitly stated that they wanted no extraordinary efforts made for this child but, despite his poor condition, he was resuscitated. When the child's father, Dr Gregory Messenger, a dermatologist, protested, the neonatologist said that she wanted to conduct tests and try certain treatment options before deciding about termination of life support. The parents then requested that they be left alone with their son. Dr Messenger personally disconnected the ventilator and placed the baby in his mother's arms. Some 5 to 10 minutes later he opened the door and informed the staff that the child had died. This case went to court with Dr Messenger accused of manslaughter, but the jury were sympathetic to his position and he was eventually found neither grossly negligent nor in breach of his legal duty to provide proper medical care for his son.[32] Cases such as this convey powerful messages about parental wishes, communication and hierarchies. However, they make bad exemplars. We need to listen to the voice of many parents from different backgrounds and in different circumstances to know more precisely what their opinions are.

A wealth of literature exists on parents' perceptions. Some of it has revealed something of the pain and tension that accompany the experience of having imperilled children and of decision making.[17,21,33–38] Some of it looks more specifically at the parents' role in decision making. A plethora of studies of parents has limited their scope to those facing non-life-threatening decisions.[39,40] Many of these studies have been conducted in the USA with parents who are on the periphery of decision making.[17,35] Inherent in many of the reported studies are methodological problems relating to the range of losses (miscarriages, stillbirths, neonatal and cot deaths), the time intervals since the death (from 20 years to a few months), selection from non-representative populations (support groups, middle classes, NICUs with specific policies and practices), and questionable interpretations by researchers who are unfamiliar with the world of neonatology.

In summary, it is evident that we still know far more about how other people think decisions *should* be made than about how they actually *are* made.[17] Our own attempt to fill this gap is itself subject to limitations, although all members of the team of researchers were clinically experienced in neonatal care, and the study was designed in such a way as to overcome many of the methodological issues which have bedevilled earlier efforts. As Holm has said, 'In empirical research there is a great temptation to seek greater clarity than the subject-matter admits of.'[41] We have tried to resist this temptation. We make no extravagant claims, but we believe that the perceptions of the parents whom we studied illuminate understanding of both the clinical issues and the philosophical questions which relate to decision-making in NICUs.

# CHAPTER 2

# Parental grief

Before describing our own work in this area, it is necessary to set a context in order to capture something of the enormity of parental grief. Whenever parents contemplate withholding or withdrawing treatment, they must face the death of their child. What do we know of such a loss?

The death of a baby is experienced differently in different cultures.[42] In some cultures, children are not recognised as real people until they reach a certain age. In areas of high infant mortality, women delay personalising their children and forming an attachment to them until they are more certain that they will survive. Mourning for certain babies is expressly forbidden among some races. However, in our Western culture the loss of a child is regarded as a highly significant and devastating event.

A huge literature exists on perinatal death, grief and mourning. Many people have tried to synthesise what is known,[43–49] but these academic and theoretical reviews can do little justice to the experience as parents feel it. We too can only set a scene for the reality which the parents will describe.

## A profound loss

Research findings have consistently concluded that bereavement following the death of a child is 'intense, complicated and long-lasting.'[50] Centuries of literature on parental grief show many references to parents' belief that no amount of eloquence could possibly convey the depth of blackness they experienced when their children died.[42,51] Nor can those who have not experienced that level of anguish imagine its searing pain.[51,52] As one bereaved mother put it: 'On a scale of one to ten, when your child dies, it's always a ten.'[51] The loss is a combination of 'an outrage',[53] 'a fundamental insult ... worse than unfair – it's almost obscene,'[54] and 'one of the most disturbing, shocking, unacceptable events that can occur.'[53] It strikes deeply at the 'foundations of life.'[55] The world 'that was once experienced as secure and ordered becomes unjust, unfair, anomic and out of control.'[48]

# Features of parental loss

## Unnatural order

There are a number of features which make the loss of a child uniquely difficult to deal with. The first and perhaps most obvious one is its unnatural order. 'It is a death out of season . . . an outrage against the natural order of things, disrupting our sense of purpose, of future promise, of our progeny continuing after our death.'[53] Not only is this so, but the parent must also live with the burden of survivor guilt.

## Loss of future

It is often said that 'When your parent dies you lose your past. When your child dies you lose your future.' When we lose an older person the grief we experience is part of the actual memories we have of that person and our relationship with them. We are mourning a past. But when the deceased is a baby, the grief is for the loss of a future and the dreams and aspirations that are bound up in that child.[56]  Special parental feelings – of being needed or being depended upon, admired and appreciated, of being a unique source of love – will never now be experienced with this child. Significant parts of the self, which are invested in one's child, are also lost along with that sense of continuity or 'immortality', which is bound up in reproduction.

## Failure to protect

The parental role is a protective one. When a child dies, this represents the ultimate failure in protection and may precipitate powerful feelings of guilt.[57,58] If the death has genetic or unexplained medical components, there may be a sense of personal guilt and biological responsibility.

## Loss of role

If the baby is a first child, the parents lose something of their identity as parents with dependants and a family structure. Their role as caretaker and provider is lost, and the way in which they expected to be filling their days is now not what they find themselves doing. Even if there are other existing children, the balance within the family is disturbed and the role is changed from what was anticipated.

## Unseen loss

If few people saw or knew the child there is a sense of both unreality and isolation. The parents themselves may find it difficult to believe that they had a child. Others may not acknowledge or appreciate the depth of their loss. As has been said, the absence is inconspicuous[42] – 'there is a birthday no one remembers'.[51] When so much around them seems to deny the reality of their experience and their sorrow, parents may sometimes need to be given permission to grieve.[51]

## Emotions

As a result of all of these losses and anxieties, on top of the other manifestations of grief that are shared by all bereaved people, the parent faces intense guilt associated with inappropriate and unrealistic expectations and a sense of personal failure, anger at the loss of meaning and the unnaturalness of the death, an intense pain of separation arising from the unique closeness of a parent to a child, a search for meaning to try to make sense of the death, problems with inadequate support and unrealistic expectations aggravated by society's problems with child death, and upsurges of grief over the years as the parent envisages and laments milestones which the child would have reached throughout his or her life.[59] The injustice of this happening may generate feelings of anger.[56,60] An initial feeling of numbness may be protective in the early hours, but it soon passes and the reality impinges in all of its force as the parents recognise that the situation is true and will go on being true.

If two parents are both grieving for the same child, there are added complications. Masculine ways of grieving are typically 'less overtly expressive of distress and depression' than those found among females.[61] Men tend typically to identify and take specific courses of action, be active in their approach to grief resolution, minimise their emotional reaction and employ intellectual rationalisation, while women have a greater need for sharing, listening and reminiscing.[59] Mothers have been found to experience a more prolonged period of sadness or depression than fathers.[60,62–64] Bereaved mothers in essence have been found to be more loss oriented than fathers,[61] with men tending to be more problem orientated or restoration orientated, although people may oscillate between the two in reality.[61] Although the traditionally female approach rather than the male one is regarded as representative of the skills and behaviours consistent with successful mourning, it is necessary for each parent to grant the other 'a wide latitude in their mourning.'[59]

Attempts to achieve a new equilibrium in a world which has changed profoundly, bring a change in the equilibrium within the parents' relationship.[57] The differences in their ways of coping can strain their own relationship and raise questions about the depth of love that a partner felt for the child or feels for the other. For example, when men get on with day-to-day living and do not overtly express distress, women can perceive this as an absence of grief. Communication problems, unexpressed emotion, inappropriate explosions of emotion, unrealistic demands, sexual difficulties and unanswerable questions may impose additional strains. The literature on the effect of the death of a child on the parents seems to be divided.[65–67]

# Effect of death

The shared trauma of losing their child may bring parents closer,[65] and an initial 'honeymoon' phase has been identified.[68] However, some researchers have found that this may be followed by a subsequent deterioration in the relationship,[68,69] while others have found that the shared sorrow may strengthen the couple's relationship.[59,70]

Whatever the long-term effect, the couple may well experience difficulties in dealing with their partner's reactions, which feel so alien to their own. Bereaved fathers have expressed both irritation with the mother's intense and prolonged grieving, and frustration at their own inability to lessen their grief.[71] Bereaved mothers, on the other hand have expressed anger about the apparent inability of their male partners to share in their intense grieving,[71] although in time each may come to realise that they were simply adopting different coping styles.

Other effects of this profoundly distressing experience are also felt and are on-going. The parents will never experience the world in quite the same way after the loss – it becomes a 'watershed event'[42] in their lives. Fundamental certainties have been challenged and a certain innocent expectation has been lost. Periodically and often unexpectedly chance comments, songs, plays, events, dates or specific items invoke bitter-sweet memories and trigger bouts of acute distress. As one bereaved father put it: 'They speak with forked tongue, words of joyful pride and words of sorrow. ... Everything is charged with the potential of a reminder. There's no forgetting.'[72] Given the immensity of their grief and the complexities we have outlined above, it can be a daunting task to try to help and support parents in their grieving.

# Helping bereaved parents

In the nineteenth century, in the consolation literature the child was depicted in the haziest of terms. Today 'every crumb of detail is offered up as proof of the child's existence – the photo, the lock of hair, the footprint, the sonograph. A name is given, a child is created, and a child is mourned.'[51] The necessity for remembering the baby as a real individual with specific characteristics is accepted. Countless books have been written on the grieving process and on ways to help parents who are experiencing such loss.[73–80]

We shall explore the different needs and preferences of parents in more detail later, but perhaps the most important thing to remember in any endeavour is that each death is unique, and a certain 'solitude of suffering' accompanies that uniqueness.[72]

> Grief cannot be measured or compared. Grief is like a fingerprint, composed of identifiable universal characteristics and yet uniquely individual.[81]

Parents have worried that neonatal medicine has outstripped compassion.[21,34] When the decision is made to withdraw treatment, is it a compounding factor in bereavement? Earlier studies have suggested that it does not adversely affect the grieving process of parents.[62,82] Whether this is the case, whether it is possible to support such parents in their sorrowing, whether the event does adversely affect relationships, and whether emotions are different when there has been such a decision, are all issues which will be explored in the following chapters.

# The study method

As we have seen, the death of a child is an immeasurably sad experience, and great sensitivity is required when obtaining information on this topic. At each stage of the research process the interests of the parents themselves were of paramount concern.

## Overall design

The overall design was that of a descriptive survey. In-depth face-to-face interviews were chosen as the most effective means of investigating parents' lived experience and opinions, allowing the researcher to be sensitive and supportive during data collection.

## Aims

These were to explore parents' perceptions of:

- the experience of treatment being withdrawn or withheld from their baby
- the actual decision making
- follow-up care.

## Setting

The three Regional Neonatal Referral Centres in the East of Scotland, situated in Aberdeen, Dundee and Edinburgh, were selected as the study Units. These three Units cover a range of populations drawn from island as well as mainland families – rural and urban, local as well as those referred in from a distance, and all social classes. Five neonatologists (two each in Dundee and Edinburgh and one in Aberdeen) were co-researchers in this study. They liaised with the principal researcher and with their consultant colleagues to facilitate recruitment.

# Ethics Committee approval

Ethics Committee approval for the three study Units was obtained by these neonatologists.

# Selection of the sample

The sample was drawn from all parents of babies for whom there had been discussion of treatment limitation. It was a scientifically selected sample rather than a self-selected one. Parents were eligible for inclusion in the study if:

• the baby died in one of the three study Units
• the baby was allowed home to die, but the parents attended the same hospital/clinician for bereavement follow-up
• treatment was withdrawn but the infant did not die
• the parents elected not to have treatment withdrawn, even though this option was discussed.

Calculation of possible numbers was based on the figure of approximately 95 deaths per annum reported for the three study Units. It was estimated that 50 to 80 families would meet these inclusion criteria in the 12 calendar months of recruitment. In reality, deaths during the study period were considerably fewer than predicted, and recruitment had to be extended for a second year in order to obtain adequate numbers. During the two-year period, 3398 babies were admitted to the three study Units, of whom 116 died. Of these, 81 families met the eligibility criteria for the study, and 59 families (73%) were recruited. Important differences in eligibility and recruiting patterns were seen between the study Units, so figures are given for each separately (*see* Figure 3.1). Notably, Unit 1 recruited the majority of the parents and had the highest percentage of eligible families, but also the highest percentage lost to the enquiry. Unit 3 had the highest percentage of families who were ineligible for the study.

Two consultants declined to participate, so the families in their care were lost to the study. Since these parents had no opportunity to take part, they have been classed as ineligible. Of the eligible families, a total of 22 were lost to the enquiry – 11 families declined to participate and 11 were not told about the study. The reasons why the 11 families were not

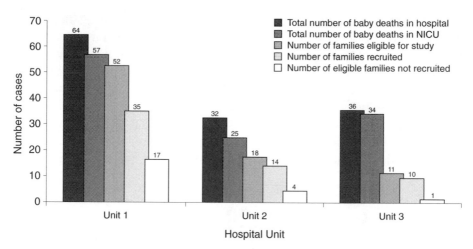

**Figure 3.1:** Number of baby deaths during the study period and of families recruited in each study Unit.

asked were that they declined all follow-up ($n = 6$), they could not be contacted by the hospital ($n = 2$), they were considered unsuitable for recruiting ($n = 1$) or unknown reason ($n = 2$).

Of the 11 sets of parents who declined to participate, three did so at the time of being asked by the consultant for permission to forward their particulars. Eight families initially agreed to have their particulars sent to the principal researcher. Of these, two asked that they should be left to contact her subsequently rather than the other way round, but neither of them did so. Three further families were uncontactable by phone and unresponsive to written communication. Two were expecting another baby and did not want to be upset by recalling the earlier tragedy, preferring to look forward rather than back. One couple was busy becoming established in a new environment and did not want to be deflected from that.

# Tools

Semi-structured interview schedules were designed expressly for this enquiry by the principal researcher (HMcH) in consultation with one co-researcher (PWF), who at that time was not a consultant, and with the study's scientific advisers. The consultants who were co-researchers on the project, and who were providing a service to the participating families and referring parents to HMcH, were kept unaware of the exact content of the schedules in order to minimise the influence of the research on their practice. Two different schedules were needed for the two points of enquiry – 3 and 13 months after the death of the baby.

Specific tools to measure feelings and attitudes were considered, but were rejected for several reasons. Experience with the families of sick infants has shown that, given the opportunity, they are very able to talk and express their emotions freely. Indeed, parents find it therapeutic to share the experience with a sympathetic listener.[83–85] Many studies use psychological scales to measure feelings and well-being, but research has indicated that simply asking people about feelings such as depression is not only a 'reliable and remarkably accurate' test, but also eliminates the false conclusions that are sometimes drawn from highly sophisticated measuring tools.[86]

# Areas under investigation

Although the principal focus was decision making about the withholding of treatment, areas under investigation included parental perceptions of the following:

- the way in which bad news was conveyed
- the timing of the decision making
- the parents' own involvement in the decision making
- the management of events
- factors which helped or which were unhelpful
- relationships with staff in the Unit and healthcare professionals outside it
- relationships with their partner, family and friends
- grief resolution over time
- suggestions for the improvement of service provision before, during and after the decision making and death.

# Procedure
## Setting up the study

Early in the project, the principal researcher visited each of the Units to discuss with co-researchers and their colleagues a study procedure which would be convenient for their Unit. The overall process was the same, but there were small differences in each to fit in with individual preferences, division of labour within Units and the protection of confidences and individuals. In one Unit, parents were asked to give signed consent to their details being forwarded to HMcH. Area Medical Committees were alerted to the fact that this study was ongoing in two areas. Written procedures were drawn up and sent to all consultants, nominated senior registrars and senior nursing staff in each Unit prior to the commencement of recruitment.

# Referring families

In all of the study Units it is policy to offer parents a follow-up visit. Consultants reported that this was usually approximately 6 weeks after the death of an infant. A decision was made to arrange first interviews for 3 months after the death of the baby. When parents attended their first follow-up visit the consultant would tell them about the study being carried out by an independent organisation. It was agreed that the neonatologists would emphasise the 'outside' nature of the enquiry in order to ensure that parents recognised that it was an independent, scientific study, and to encourage them to be frank and critical. The consultants then sought consent from the parents to have their name, address and telephone number, together with the baby's gestation, date of birth and death, passed to the principal researcher. If the parents were willing to be approached, the consultants gave them one of HMcH's visiting cards. Their basic information was then recorded on a duplicate form designed for this specific purpose, with one copy being sent in confidence to HMcH and the other attached to the baby's notes.

A total of 12 doctors referred families to HMcH. Four of them referred only one set of parents. Five consultants referred two, three, four, five and six families, respectively. Two others referred nine sets of parents and one consultant referred 17 sets of parents.

# Recruiting the parents

On receipt of the form, HMcH then wrote to the parents telling them about the research and inviting them to participate, using a personalised copy of a standard letter. If the parents were on the telephone, about one week after they had received this letter HMcH rang them. They were given an opportunity to discuss the study further and to discuss the implications of being involved, before being asked if they were willing to take part. If they consented, a time and place for the first interview were arranged for a date approximately 3 months after the baby's death, or as soon thereafter as was convenient to the family. Details of the arrangement were confirmed in a letter one week before the interview was scheduled to take place. If the parents were not contactable by telephone, additional letters were sent with forms for parents to indicate their preferred setting, time and place for interview.

At the end of the first interview, the parents were reminded that there was an opportunity to be involved in a second interview 13 months after the death of the baby. Their consent was not sought at this stage, but permission was asked for the researcher to contact them again nearer that time. It seemed likely that the anniversary of the baby's death would be a poignant and significant time for families. However, the effect of receiving a card or letter at this time was unknown. The decision was therefore made to delay approaching the parents for the second interview until one week after this date. A letter was then sent to them asking if they would be willing to participate a second time. Thereafter a similar procedure was adopted as for first interviews.

## Conducting interviews

All of the interviews were conducted by the principal researcher herself. At the commencement of the interview she reinforced the fact that information which the parents supplied would not be fed back to clinicians in its raw form, but that the collective, anonymised results would be made available to them. To encourage honest appraisal, she repeated that the staff were keen to know about weaknesses as well as strengths in current service provision, and that such knowledge would be used to inform future practice, thereby improving practice for future families. Written consent was obtained before interviewing began.

It was considered important to give respondents the opportunity for support during a painful re-living of events. Couples could elect to be interviewed together, and for the first interview 44 out of 59 (75%) couples participated together for the whole session; for the second interview 40 out of 50 (80%) did so. In three cases, although the mother was the principal interviewee, the father provided a few responses at the end of the session, and in one instance the father answered a limited number of questions about his opinions by telephone a couple of days after the mother had been interviewed. Three single mothers elected to have other people remain in the room. In one case this was the mother's own mother, in the second instance both her mother and her sister, and in the third a cousin.

In ten families (17%) only the mother was involved in the study, and in one first interview the father was the sole contributor, although he consulted his wife on a couple of factual points. This gave a total of 107 parents participating in first interviews, and 90 parents at the 13-month point. For the purposes of analysis, and where their perceptions converged, the parents of each baby are sometimes taken as a single item, but where they expressed different views their individual opinions are reported separately. On matters of crucial importance related to decision making, each parent's individual views are considered.

There was a notable eagerness on the part of fathers to take part and, when work patterns changed or threatened to preclude the father's participation, some couples changed appointments in order to ensure that he was there. In one case a father was unexpectedly called to work immediately before the scheduled interview; he made his contribution by telephone subsequently. Several mothers expressed some surprise at their partner's in-depth responses, as they were not normally given to expressing their emotions. Two mothers said that they were astonished that their partners had even stayed in the room, and were even more amazed that they had spoken. However, the fathers contributed valuable insights.

It is possible that the presence of their partner might have influenced a parent's responses, but experience demonstrated that having dual interviews gave each parent the chance to reflect while their partner talked, and also the opportunity to correct erroneous information. If their memories differed, they discussed the facts and usually established what had actually happened. If no agreement was reached, the difference in perception was noted so that the results were not distorted. The experience of being interviewed together was regarded as very beneficial by many families, who volunteered that they had discovered things about their partner's experiences and feelings which had been hitherto unknown.

The parents' own young children were present for part or all of 14 first interviews. Sometimes the youngsters appeared to provide welcome relief for the parents from the intensity of the discussion and the powerful emotions generated, as they were forced to take a break or to respond to insistent demands for attention. However, if the children were lively and engaged in play with the interviewer this created some difficulties, as it felt incongruous to be cheerfully responsive with them in the middle of harrowing stories of pain and distress from the parents.

Permission was sought to tape-record all of the interviews in order to enable the researcher to concentrate on listening to the parents, and to be sensitive to non-verbal cues and powerful expressions of emotion. The recordings also allowed checks to be made for accuracy of coding and interpretation. None of the parents objected, and all of them readily gave permission for their verbatim quotes to be used to illustrate the reporting of the data.

Parents could choose the setting for their interviews. Most of them elected to stay in their own homes and the interviewer visited the houses of 55 of the 59 families (93%). Two mothers chose to go to the researcher's office for privacy, and a third one asked to have her second interview there in preference to a rather overcrowded home environment. Two couples decided to return to the study hospital for the interview, and quiet rooms were provided for this purpose. One couple said that they were very emotionally disturbed by events but still wanted to participate. Initially the father asked if he could be interviewed by telephone to protect his wife from the trauma of reliving the experience. When it came to a second interview, however, they requested a home interview, in which both participated.

Many families requested evening or weekend interviews to enable working fathers to participate. First interviews lasted for anything from 1 hour
to 5.25 hours (mean 2.75 hours; mode 3 hours), with 12 interviews extending well into the night or the early hours of the morning. Second interviews were shorter, ranging from 0.5 to 4.5 hours (mean 1.9 hours; mode
1.5 hours).

The stories which were recounted varied in their coherence and logical
telling. All of them were very moving, and the parents' courage was
impressive. No one opted out once interviewing had begun, even though
the majority of the parents became distressed and expressed strong emotion during their recounting. The interview schedules were used as a guide
to ensure that questions were not overlooked, but parents were encouraged to describe the events in their own way, keeping the account as
chronological as possible. Inevitably they jumped about in the narration.
Very occasionally it seemed inappropriate to return to an earlier point for
clarification of a detail, as the flow of the respondent's story would be
broken and their sense of mastery of the situation jeopardised. To interrupt
them in this way would have been inconsistent with the overall approach
of compassionate respect for their experiences, perceptions and priorities.
In such circumstances some data were lost. However, in most instances it
was possible to clarify points while still preserving the integrity of their
story and respecting their emotional responses. Wherever it was expedient
they were asked to fill in such gaps.

# Maintaining contact

The success of follow-up work depends to some extent on maintaining contact with respondents. A letter of thanks was sent to the respondents after
each interview. In this, and also at the end of each interview, parents were
asked to let the researcher know if they moved house. With parents sharing such intimate data a relationship developed with the interviewer
which made it important to stay in touch for other reasons. Contact was
renewed on the first birthdays of survivors of multiple births, at Christmas
time, and when parents notified the researcher of the birth of subsequent
babies. Except where families moved away without providing their new
address, all parents were sent a copy of the study findings.

# Ensuring subsequent support

It was recognised from the outset that resurrecting the powerful emotion
surrounding the life and death of their babies would be painful, and that

the parents might subsequently be in need of some form of additional support. In two Units, on the advice of the consultants, parents were reminded that Unit staff were available to them. In the third Unit, a list of potential sources of support was drawn up by Unit staff and given to parents on leaving the hospital. HMcH ensured that the parents had a copy before she left their homes and, if they did not, she arranged for one to be sent.

## Notifying general practitioners

The parents' GPs were sent a letter telling them that their patients had agreed to participate in the study, and inviting them to make contact with either the researcher or the neonatologist in the relevant study Unit if they wished for further information about the investigation. In the event, only two GPs did so. One strongly recommended that the family should not be included because of their circumstances. However, this letter arrived the day after the first interview. This couple was not approached for the second interview.

# Support for the interviewer

It was anticipated that intensive listening to many bereaved parents would be a stressful occupation. To be overburdened by such emotions would be counter-productive to good interviewing, so in order to prevent the build-up of such tensions, ongoing support for the interviewer was built into the design of the project. This took the form of *ad hoc* informal sessions with two retired neonatologists who could understand the medical complexities relating to sick infants and the methodological niceties of an investigation of this sensitive nature. They were thus able not only to provide psychological support to the interviewer, but also to discuss some of the issues raised by the research.

# Deviations from the protocol

## Recruiting

We had anticipated that a small number of parents, if offered discontinuation of intensive therapy, would elect to have treatment continued and that the babies would survive. Following such families would provide useful comparative data. In the event, no babies survived, so this group was not represented.

# Timing of interviews

In reality, the first follow-up bereavement visit to the neonatologist did not always take place at 6–8 weeks after the baby's death. Thirty-four families (58%) were interviewed at 3 months. First interviews were delayed for the remaining 25 families (42%). Seven of these took place within 1 month of the scheduled time, largely because it was impossible to find a mutually acceptable date for interview at short notice. Eighteen interviews were not carried out until considerably later. In four cases this was 9–12 months after the death of the baby. A detailed breakdown of timing is shown in Figure 3.2.

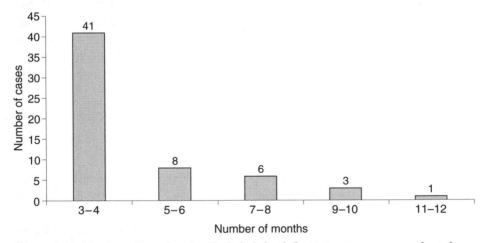

**Figure 3.2:** Number of months after the baby's death first interviews were conducted.

In only one case was the delay due to anything other than a late referral by the consultant to the researcher. In this instance, the parents were so busy that it was difficult to find a mutually convenient time for the interview. The reasons for deferred hospital follow-up varied, and included unexplained delays in appointment times, unavailability of test results, parents of multiple births being overlooked as bereaved families because they had surviving babies in the Unit, and the parents themselves not being ready to attend for follow-up so soon after the death. For research purposes, periodic checks of numbers were made and outstanding eligible families were detected.

It is impossible to say whether data collected at these later points will differ significantly from data collected on the same topics from the same parents at 3 months. However, internal checks would indicate that memories of the events are clear and accurate more than a year on, but that reactions to the events can change over time. Analysis has therefore taken account of the differing time periods and, where relevant, families have been split into time-bands. If first interviews were close to the time for second interviews, parents were given the opportunity to take part in one composite interview incorporating questions from both interviews, but only one family chose this option.

# Coding and analysis

Data were coded on to a computer using a framework designed for this purpose. The database was constructed around predetermined variables which gave an overall shape or skeleton to the research. The large range of responses was accommodated by adding each new idea to an unlimited value label list for each variable. The data were then analysed using the Statistical Package for the Social Sciences for the Apple Mac Version 6.1. By this means it was possible to retain control over the information obtained, and at the same time to include every aspect of the qualitative dimensions of the parents' accounts.

To ensure scientific rigour, a percentage of the tapes were checked for accuracy of coding and interpretation. In both cases the person responsible for checking was asked to select the tapes himself by number to ensure that selection was unbiased. HMcH recorded a total of 161 hours of first-interview data and 89 hours of second-interview material (a total of 250 hours). A practising neonatologist (PWF) checked 12% of the first-interview tapes. He listened to 20.5 hours of taped interviews, and found one error in a total of 1661 coded values. In addition, he picked up 18 minor points which might have been added. None of these was thought to be a significant point by either HMcH or PWF; they had been omitted because the items were already well documented. Nevertheless, they were added to the database. There were no discrepancies in the interpretation of the data by the two researchers.

A further 10% of the tapes (all different interviews from the ones to which PWF listened) were checked by a student in medical ethics (RB) for accuracy of coding and analysis of content. He listened to 14.67 hours of taped interviews. From a total of 1171 coded values, he found three errors which were corrected. He also noted two additional minor points which might be included in the analysis, and these were added to the database. The interpretations of RB matched those of HMcH.

An error rating of 0.14% confirmed a high degree of accuracy using this system of coding complex information, and demonstrated that three people coming from different backgrounds heard and interpreted what parents said in the same way.

# Timeframe

Recruitment began on 1 September 1996 and spanned two calendar years. Data collection for the first interviews ended in January 1999 and that for second interviews ended in November 1999.

# Ethical considerations

As well as the steps already reported, every effort was made throughout to protect the identity of respondents. Each family was given a number, and specific identifying information was removed from reported data.

# Limitations

Not all of the eligible parents consented to participate, and it is therefore possible that the sample was biased. Self-deselection is a 'perennial problem in research on sensitive and emotionally distressing topics such as parental bereavement.'[47] One large Australian study found that unmarried mothers from the lower social classes were significantly less likely to participate,[87] and some families from this group were certainly lost to the current study.

A very small number of parents were not invited to participate because the consultants felt that it was inappropriate to ask them. It is conceivable that clinicians might screen out those who would give adverse reports of their management. There is no evidence to support such a suspicion, and indeed a few consultants discussed particularly troubling cases with the principal researcher and took specific action in a positive effort to include these families.

Only two families (3%) who consented to take part changed their minds and withdrew before the first interview. In both cases the mothers said that they were reluctant to go over the events again as they were trying to move on. Nine sets of parents who took part in a first interview did not take part in a second interview, giving a response rate of 84% at the 13-month follow-up interview. Of these, five families could not be traced because they had failed to notify the researcher of changes in their contact addresses, although one couple subsequently wrote to the researcher to tell her of a subsequent tragedy (a cot death). Two mothers felt that they could not face talking about the events again. One of these women was involved in a court case and admitted that she was finding it harrowing endlessly going over the details. One family repeatedly failed to turn up for appointments which they had themselves set up with the researcher. The remaining family had many problems and their GP advised against contacting them again. However, these attrition rates are very low compared to those of other follow-up studies of bereaved parents. Videka-Sherman had only 17% of her sample participating at the second time point.[88] Dyregrov and Matthiesen started off with a low response rate of 51% 1 month after the death, and this dropped to 34% at the 13-month point of investigation.[89]

Clearly 'one-off' interviews with individuals provide single-snapshot pictures and may not reflect their feelings on different occasions. In order to obtain some measure of change over time a second interview was arranged, but it was not possible to say with any certainty how representative either of these days was of the total experience of the parents.

The purpose of the study was to gain insights into parents' experiences in order to help future families. However, many respondents volunteered that the research interviews had been therapeutic for them. They therefore constituted an intervention which is not normally available to such families. Consequently, data collected at the second point of enquiry must be interpreted in the light of this knowledge.

In each Unit the consultants who were providing the service were aware of the aims of the project. Knowing that their actions were under scrutiny could have influenced the care given. This matter was discussed at length prior to data collection, but it was felt that the research enterprise was not an attempt to monitor individual consultants' abilities. Rather, it was designed to identify strengths and weaknesses from the parents' point of view. If awareness of the study had a beneficial effect on practice, this could only be advantageous for the respondents.

# Discussion

Attention has been drawn to the 'chasm which separates bereaved parents from individuals who have not experienced this intensity of grief.'[90] The researcher entered the lives of the respondent families as an 'outsider.' A degree of detachment was essential in a prolonged study in such a highly charged field. As Knapp observed, the experience is analogous to being a 'war correspondent,' capable of presenting accurate information but remaining a non-participant in the 'war' itself.[56] However, having spent in excess of 250 hours listening to intense and harrowing accounts of parents' experiences and emotions, and many times that number of hours listening to the recordings of these interviews, the researcher came to understand more nearly what the parents feel. This awareness has influenced both the analysis of the data and the interpretation of the results.

The emotionally painful nature of the material under discussion required a sensitive approach. There is abundant evidence that in such circumstances parents feel a need to talk,[91–93] and that sharing their story with a sympathetic listener is a therapeutic experience.[84,85,92–94] A 'conversational' approach to interviewing,[95] as well as a 'narrative technique,'[96] was clearly an appropriate choice of method by which to obtain relevant and insightful data. These families talked for many hours at a sitting, not infrequently well into the night, which demonstrates their willingness to share their thoughts and emotions. Once started, none of them withdrew. Almost all of the families agreed to a second interview. Most of those who moved house ensured that the researcher knew where they could be contacted again. A considerable number volunteered to be approached at any point if they could contribute further. These factors would suggest that they were at ease with the way in which the study was conducted.

Unless interviewees feel that they are respected and that their vulnerability is of concern to the interviewer, they will be inhibited about providing personal or sensitive information.[97] Every effort was made to foster an environment which reassured parents that the interviewer was trustworthy, discreet and cared greatly for their well-being, and a 'research alliance'[98] was created with the participants which was founded on compassion, trust and collaboration. The depths of the parents' insights indicate that they felt supported. Qualitative interviews are always to a greater or lesser extent reactive. Both the attitude and the personality of the interviewer and the reflective and recollecting capacity of the interviewee shape the exchange, and the relationship between the two will influence the quality of the data generated.[90,99] We leave the quality of the information obtained in this study to speak for itself.

As well as having tapped into the lived experiences of so many parents, we have capitalised on a wealth of clinical knowledge within our research team. Five practising neonatologists formed a core part of that team, two retired neonatologists were our scientific advisers, and the principal researcher herself has had many years of experience of hands-on care of neonates. We believe that, as a result, the study was firmly rooted in clinical reality. In Zussman's study of adult intensive care, one doctor commented as follows:

> I generally do not read the medical philosophical things because I think most of them are garbage. ... My major complaint on this is that we have people who are writing very interesting and educated sounding expositions on philosophical aspects of medical care and ... very rarely are these people actually involved in the day-to-day practice of medicine.[100]

Such an accusation cannot be levelled at the present enquiry. Our collective hands-on experiences have shaped our interpretation of the findings and their possible consequences for practice. They resonate with everyday practice, and our recommendations are not impossible to implement. Even the research process itself highlighted to us a potential deficit in clinical care, namely that parents may be overlooked for bereavement care if they have surviving children still in the Unit, or if their baby is cared for in more than one Unit.

As with all research projects conducted out in the natural world, inevitably the study had its limitations. It has been said that 'all field researchers make decisions guided not only by canons of methodological adequacy but by considerations of politics, pragmatism, ethics and etiquette.'[17] Deviations from the protocol were occasionally expedient, but it is not our impression that the integrity of the research has been compromised as a result.

This report focuses on the parents' uncorroborated perceptions. We made no attempt to verify their stories, and their accounts stand alone. They were reflecting back over time and, although every effort was made to check for signs of internal integrity, their recollections may on occasion have been subject to distortions of recall. Nevertheless, the general sense conveyed both by the literature and by experience is that when it comes to serious news about a child, parental recollection remains vivid and accurate.

# Conclusion

Whatever its shortcomings, we believe that this report is a faithful representation of 108 parents' experiences, and that its findings illuminate practice where decisions about withdrawal of treatment from imperilled neonates have to be made.

# CHAPTER 4

# The respondent families

At the point of the first interview 59 sets of parents (58 mothers and 49 fathers) participated in the enquiry. Follow-up data at 13 months after the baby's death were obtained from 50 families (50 mothers and 40 fathers). In Appendix 1 certain basic data are listed for those parents who were eligible for inclusion in this study but who did not participate. This allows the reader to make a judgement about the representativeness of the sample parents. Proportionately more teenagers, primigravidae and mothers who were not in paid employment were to be found in the non-respondent group. The following information relates to the parents who did take part.

## Distribution

More than half (35 out of 59; 59%) of the families were recruited from Unit 1, 14 families (24%) were recruited from Unit 2 and 10 families (17%) from Unit 3. They lived in a range of settings throughout the East of Scotland, with urban, rural and island populations all represented.

Three couples came from countries outside the UK and from cultures with different approaches and practices with regard to dying babies. In one of these cases the mother had only limited English, but where she was unable to express herself, her husband (who was fluent) interpreted as necessary.

## Marital status

Forty-one couples (69%) were married. A further 13 couples (22%) were cohabiting, with two of these living together only intermittently, and one couple only cohabiting since the baby's death. An additional couple (2%) were currently living apart but planned to move in together in the near future. The remaining four mothers (7%) were single; three were not in touch with the baby's father at all, and one made contact occasionally.

# Ages

The majority of the parents were in their thirties or older (mothers: 35/59, 60%; fathers: 36/54, 67%). A detailed breakdown of the data is given in Figure 4.1.

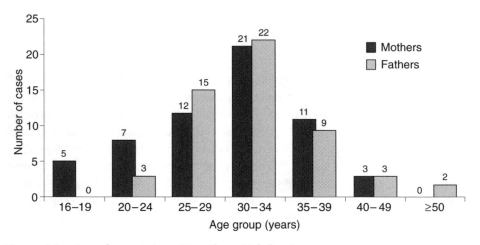

**Figure 4.1:**   Age of parents ($n = 59$ mothers, 54 fathers).

# Occupations

## The fathers

Of the 55 men for whom data were available, 52 (95%) were employed, with one of these taking occasional work but also acting as house-husband. Three were unemployed at the time of the first interview, two having only recently lost their jobs.

Occupations of the parents were varied and spanned all social group-ings. Given the idiosyncratic nature of many of the occupations, they will not be itemised individually lest identities become apparent. Instead, a crude description of the categories will demonstrate the range. Ana-lysts, businessmen, chefs, civil servants, consultants, drivers, electricians, engineers, factory workers, healthcare professionals, labourers, lawyers, managers, mechanics, members of the armed forces, musicians, offshore workers, plant operators, policemen, research scientists, supervisors, surveyors, technicians and workers with the disabled and underprivileged were all represented by the fathers in this study. No attempt has been made to group them into social classes, as it was apparent that occupation alone did not necessarily indicate the background, living standards or attitudes of individual parents.

## The mothers

Of the 59 mothers, 32 (54%) were actively working in paid employment at the time of the first interview, and a further six (10%) were returning to work in the near future. Ten (17%) were still on maternity leave. One mother had tried going back to work, only to find that she was not yet ready for the transition. Eleven (19%) did not work outside the home.

All social classes were represented. The mothers were employed as bankers, cleaners, computer operators and specialists, cooks, doctors, estate agents, factory workers, financiers, home helps, lecturers, nurses, receptionists, secretaries and bookkeepers, personnel workers, shop assistants, social workers, stewardesses, teachers, technicians and waitresses.

## Parity

For 18 of the mothers (31%) this was their first pregnancy. The remaining 41 mothers (69%) had had from one to five other pregnancies (*see* Figure 4.2).

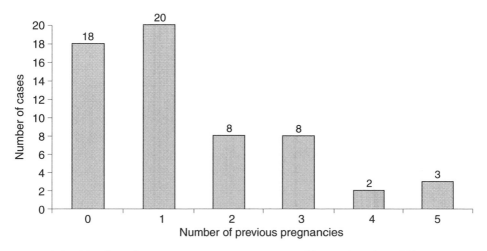

**Figure 4.2:**    Number of previous pregnancies experienced by mothers ($n = 59$).

# Obstetric history

Twenty-four mothers (41%) had suffered previous obstetric loss, 22 (37%) of which were early losses through miscarriage, termination of pregnancies, ectopics or blighted ova. Five (8%) had lost preterm infants at between 22 and 26 weeks. Six of the mothers had lost from three to five previous pregnancies.

Half of the mothers (30; 51%) had live children aged between 1 and 18 years (mean age 5 years). Of these, 24 mothers had either one child ($n = 20$) or two children ($n = 4$) with their present partner, with ages ranging from 1 to 14 years (mean age 4 years). Eleven mothers and 11 fathers reported pregnancies with other partners. In the case of 15 couples (25%) there were living children resulting from other liaisons by one ($n = 12$) or both ($n = 3$) partners; in 12 families it was just one partner who had such other children, and in three families both partners did. Eight mothers had living children from previous relationships, ranging in age from 2 to 18 years (mean age 8 years), and 10 fathers had children by other partners, ranging in age from 5 to 26 years (mean age 13 years).

Just under one-fifth of the couples (11, 19%) had a history of infertility, with both male and female problems represented. Some provided moving accounts of stressful and expensive treatment which had spanned many years. Six of the women had been on Clomid. Two of the subfertile men spontaneously talked about the stress of the discovery and the limited support they personally had received following the diagnosis.

# This pregnancy

In 36 cases (61%) this was a planned pregnancy. The remaining 23 sets of parents (39%) reported varying responses to the discovery. Eight mothers said that they were shocked initially, and two had contemplated terminating the pregnancies but found that they could not do so. In one of these cases pressure to abort had been exerted by a family member, and the mother found it distressing to recall this event now that the child had died.

There were eight multiple pregnancies – five sets of twins and three sets of triplets or quads. From these pregnancies 16 live babies were born, of whom 11 babies were eligible for inclusion in the study. For four sets of the twins, treatment withdrawal was discussed for only one baby – in two cases the other baby was stillborn, and in two cases the other twin survived. In the case of the fifth family, treatment limitation was discussed for both children. For the multiple births of three or more, there were survivors in two out of three of the families.

# Distances from study hospitals

The babies were all at some point in one or more of the study hospitals, and the parents had varying distances to travel in order to be with them. For island-dwelling parents, travelling was invariably complicated and involved 2 hours' flying time or a 14-hour boat trip in addition to the long distances they covered by road, sometimes in difficult weather conditions. It took the interviewer anything up to three days to accomplish the journeys (both ways) that these families had faced at a time of great stress. For parents who lived on the mainland of Scotland, the distances they travelled to the study Unit ranged from half a mile to 130 miles (mean distance 16 miles, mode 2 miles).

One mother was herself sent directly to a hospital 60 miles away before her baby was born because there were no Intensive Care cots available in the hospital closest to her home. Six women were initially in local hospitals and were later transferred to the study hospital prior to delivery so that they could receive specialist attention and intensive care could be available for their babies immediately after birth. This move meant that they were dislocated from their families and support networks to some extent before the problems with the baby presented. In one instance a mother was moved twice. She came from an island home so was transferred for delivery to the nearest regional centre on the mainland, which took several hours to reach. Following the birth, a specific problem was diagnosed in the baby, so she and the child were both then referred to another specialist centre a further 130 miles away. When the baby subsequently died, the parents faced a journey of many hours and much inconvenience to return home with the child's body.

# Travel to the NICU

Travel to the Unit was relatively straightforward for most parents who owned a car of their own (40 families, 68%), although two mothers and one father were dependent on their partners to drive them, and in their absence had to travel on public transport. Five families (8%) were transported by family or friends. One set of parents used the bus for the first six weeks, but then acquired their own car. The remaining family took a taxi. For some parents having the baby in the Unit involved repeated journeys back and forth, but for 12 sets of parents (20%) there was just one trip, because they did not leave the hospital while the baby was alive.

# The delivery

Almost half of the women (27, 46%) had Caesarean Sections (CS), and 17 of these women also laboured (*see* Figure 4.3).

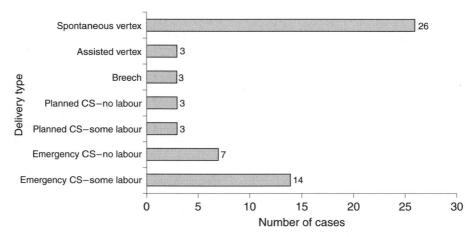

**Figure 4.3:**   Type of delivery (*n* = 59).

# The babies
## Gender

In total, 33 of the 62 babies (53%) were male and 29 (47%) were female.

## Gestation and weight

More than half of the 62 babies (34, 55%) were born at 28 weeks' gestation or below, nine of these (15%) being less than 24 weeks. Ten babies (16%) were more than 40 weeks. The mean gestation was 32 weeks and the median was 28 weeks. A detailed breakdown of the data is shown in Figure 4.4.

Just over half of the babies (32, 52%) weighed 1000 g or less at birth, with three weighing 500 g or less (*see* Figure 4.5).

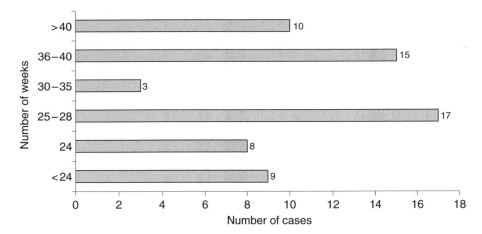

**Figure 4.4:**   Number of weeks gestation (*n* = 62).

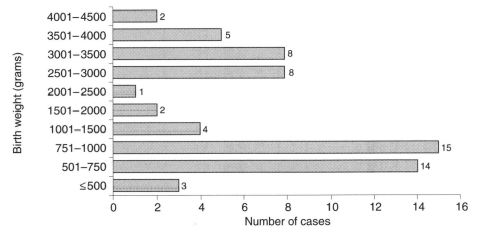

**Figure 4.5:**   Birth weight (*n* = 62).

# Categories of babies

The babies were divided into clinical categories for the purpose of analysis (*see* Figure 4.6). It should be noted that, of the 36 infants who were born preterm, five also had congenital anomalies and two were asphyxiated. Hence the total numbers exceed 62.

Some conditions or circumstances were extremely rare, and the shock of the discovery or the sequence of events had a profound impact on the parents. It would have been interesting to discuss these circumstances, but to do so would be to jeopardise the anonymity of families. To that end, groupings have been kept deliberately broad. However, where confidentiality can be maintained, some elaboration will be included in the body of the text in order faithfully to report and illuminate understanding of the parents' experiences.

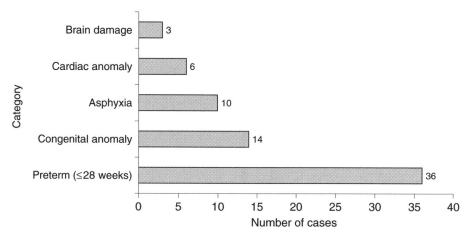

**Figure 4.6:** Clinical categories of babies ($n = 62$).

# Time of death

The comparative length of time the babies lived is shown in Figure 4.7. The majority of them (38, 61%) died within the first week of life. Of these

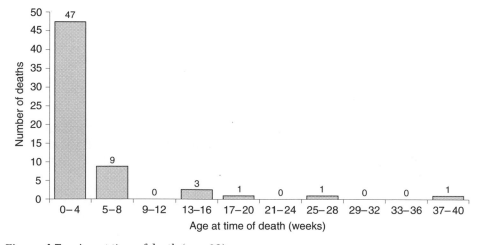

**Figure 4.7:** Age at time of death ($n = 62$).

23 babies lived less than two full days. However, six babies (10%) lived for more than three months, and one of these lived for almost nine months.

# Conclusion

We consider these families to be representative of those to be found in NICUs in the UK on all variables except ethnic origin. The East of Scotland has relatively few families from ethnic minorities.

# CHAPTER 5

# Pregnancy and birth

It is important to set experiences within an overall context. For some of these respondent families, the pregnancy had been uncomplicated and tragedy struck suddenly. For a few, there were weeks of anxiety or crucial decisions to be made before the birth. For others, the birth itself involved traumas which influenced later developments. Before we look at what went wrong and what decisions were made, we shall discuss the events which led up to that time. These events have been subdivided into those which pre-dated the onset of labour, and those which included labour, delivery and the immediate period following the birth, because this was the way in which they were demarcated in the parents' thinking and accounts.

## PREGNANCY UP TO THE ONSET OF LABOUR

## Complications of pregnancy

Apart from the normal minor ailments associated with pregnancy, as many as 51 of the 59 mothers (86%) reported more serious complications of some kind during the pregnancy. These are listed below in descending order of frequency of occurrence.

### Preterm labour

Pregnancy was interrupted prematurely for nearly half of the women (27, 46%). In only one case did this prove to be false labour. In five instances they had presented initially with premature rupture of membranes. For one mother this followed amniocentesis. Some of these women managed to continue with the pregnancy for a number of weeks (up to 9 weeks longer), but this was at considerable personal cost.

## Haemorrhage

One-third of the women (19, 32%) had bled antenatally at some stage but the pregnancy continued. Two mothers were hospitalised because they were found to have a placenta praevia. In one other case a placenta started to separate prematurely. Three women suffered complete abruptions accompanied by severe pain.

## Maternal illness

Eleven women reported illnesses, unrelated to the pregnancy, which had caused them considerable problems. Three had surgical operations, and in all cases their babies were born soon after the surgery. Others reported conditions such as cholecystitis, lung disease, pneumonia and a variety of infections.

## Congenital anomaly

In all of the five cases in which parents were given an antenatal diagnosis of a congenital anomaly, the abnormalities proved to be serious. Two of the mothers developed hydramnios, in one case necessitating weekly draining of amniotic fluid. However, whilst her partner was full of foreboding from the outset, one of these mothers remained convinced that it would be something minor. One other mother was given a test result indicating a raised alpha-fetoprotein (AFP) level, but this subsequently proved to be a false alarm.

## Raised blood pressure

Of the five mothers with elevated blood pressure, two reported developing pregnancy-induced hypertension.

## Reduced fetal movement

Three mothers experienced reduced fetal movement.

## Abnormal cardiotocograph (CTG)

CTGs were abnormal for two mothers.

## Incompetent cervix

Both of the women with cervical sutures had them inserted during their pregnancy.

## Additional factors

Three families had moved house during the pregnancy, two of them coming to Scotland from foreign countries. One of these mothers reported that she had been moving heavy furniture immediately prior to going into preterm labour. Two other women had had falls shortly before labour commenced.

# Warning of coming problems

Just over one-third of the sets of parents (21, 36%) could recall no discussion with a professional person during pregnancy about the possibility of things going wrong. For the remaining 38 families (64%) there had been some mention, even if on occasion it was only brief, giving them an inkling of what might happen. Twenty-one of these families reported having such a discussion on more than one occasion.

When these discussions took place, in 17 cases (45% of the 38 families) both parents were together, whilst a further 10 couples (26%) were on occasion together but sometimes not when discussion of possible difficulties took place. In some instances this involved telling the mother because she was on site before the father could be located. In other instances, in the parents' perceptions, the staff had judged that the mother was in no fit state to be given bad news, and it was left to the father to cope with it alone until either he or the doctors judged it expedient to tell her.

Thirteen of the 33 women who delivered prematurely recalled having some discussion with the medical staff of the risks relating to prematurity. Of the 20 sets of parents who had babies with congenital anomalies, six remembered engaging in some discussion about the possibility of an abnormality and/or its implications. None of the parents were aware of receiving any warning about the dangers of asphyxia or brain damage. Thus a large proportion (40, 68%) felt that they were unprepared for the problems which actually presented.

# Information givers

Information was commonly given by obstetric staff at this point, but seven of the 59 families (12%) recalled paediatric staff being involved when potential difficulties were discussed. Three of these cases related to fetuses with known congenital abnormalities detected by scans. Two involved twin pregnancies and two others threatening or actual preterm labours. Some of the parents, however, were unable to identify the staff who talked with them, and nine said that it was just 'different people' – some of these individuals might well have been paediatricans. Not all of the couples with diagnosed multiple pregnancies remembered seeing paediatricians before the birth.

# Responses

Parents' responses varied according to their own perceptions and attitudes. For example, one mother said that she was the dominant partner in the couple, her husband being the 'more sensitive one.' When the news was not good, she 'sent him home' for a shower and a sleep while she coped alone. Another mother reported that she reacted by deliberately getting close to the fetus she might lose, whereas her partner strove to keep his distance from it so that the loss would be less devastating. One young father who was faced with an important decision antenatally felt that the doctor disapproved of his unmarried status and did not involve him in the discussion fully because of it, whereas the mother was inevitably the centre of the discussion. He felt sidelined and criticised as a result, and he did not believe that the doctor took any notice of his wishes. The mother, on the other hand, very much wanted his input, but understood the effect of a rather 'bullying' approach (as they perceived it) on her boyfriend, leaving her increasingly vulnerable to pressure from the staff at a time when she felt powerless to resist it on her own.

Two couples said that they did not react to the news in any way; in one case the parents were no strangers to obstetric disasters and had been sceptical when early scans had appeared to indicate that everything was proceeding normally. Being given news of another problem pregnancy seemed much more believable. Others who had had problems were guarded in their approach to this pregnancy.

> In retrospect I'm glad I had the [previous] miscarriage because it meant that I didn't really get as involved with [this] pregnancy as I would have done, I think. I kept myself emotionally back from it a bit, which I think has helped in the long run. It sounds a horrible thing to say. But it never occurred to me up until that point that anything could go wrong. So the second time I was much more wary. I wasn't buying clothes and planning . . . I was trying to keep myself at arm's length from it all.
> (P25: mother of preterm baby with asphyxia)

Three sets of parents heard what was said but believed that the problem would be resolvable or correctable after birth. However, four others expressed doubts about the accuracy of the information being imparted: two of them just did not believe what they were hearing, while the other two heard it but decided to leave well alone and not intervene in any way, hoping that things would resolve themselves with time.

> During the whole [experience of premature labour] right up till [the baby] was born the way we described it: you're just standing on the edge of a cliff, an abyss and you're just about to fall into this abyss and

you've got absolutely no idea what's going to happen ... so actually we weren't that concerned because there was a fatalistic opinion that what will be will be. We were soldiering on day by day. There was probably quite a lot of false optimism as well. People were trying not to make it serious – keep your legs crossed and all this kind of stuff. It'll be OK and all that. And you just keep up with all that banter.

(P25: father of preterm baby with asphyxia)

# Satisfaction with management

For a variety of reasons not all parents were able to say whether they were satisfied with the way in which information was given during pregnancy, and it was inappropriate to pursue the point with others. Some of them were too engrossed in recounting the ongoing developments to be taken back in time with impunity. Some were dismissive of early experiences, putting emphasis on events after delivery rather than before it. As a result, information is available from only 29 of the 38 families who recalled early discussion. Of these 29 families, 11 (38%) were satisfied with the way in which this was handled, 12 families (41%) were unhappy, and a further 6 families (21%) had some reservations.

# Improvements

Twenty-three sets of parents were able to put into words ways in which this part of the experience could have been improved. Together they provided many suggestions, although it has to be recognised that they were speaking retrospectively, knowing that things had gone tragically wrong and their babies had died. As a small number pointed out, it is impossible to know whether these factors would have remained with them if the outcome had been a happy one.

## Listening to the mother

The biggest single factor related to the need to listen to the mother when she had noted worrying symptoms ($n = 6$ parents), and to detect deviations from the norm more accurately and earlier ($n = 4$ parents), to allow earlier intervention ($n = 6$ parents). Parents were frustrated when staff appeared to ignore their cries for help and the onset of appropriate treatment was delayed.

# Adequate monitoring

Where there had been early signs of trouble, the parents felt that these warning indicators should have encouraged staff to repeat scans or tracings ($n = 3$ parents). There could then have been an opportunity to visit the NICU to see babies in similar circumstances ($n = 1$), to talk to other parents who had faced similar situations ($n = 1$), to discuss matters with a neonatologist ahead of the delivery ($n = 1$), or to have a paediatrician present at the birth to make an early assessment and take appropriate action ($n = 1$).

Two cases deserve special mention because differences in the couple's perceptions appeared to influence management and satisfaction with their care. One father worried when his wife was sent home after removal of a cervical stitch, believing that she should have had a Caesarean Section then and there and that this might perhaps have prevented the subsequent birth trauma. His wife, however, had been insistent that she should be allowed home. In the other case the mother believed that an early abnormal CTG was linked in some way to the defect with which the child was born, and that earlier intervention might have increased the options available to her. The father, on the other hand, said that he was not so sure that such a link could be made.

# Adequate information

Four sets of parents expressed a wish for a more detailed explanation of the risks and problems attached to the diagnosis. Such information as they had been given could have been usefully supplemented by leaflets. Inconsistency of messages was a problem for two families, and false reassurances were unacceptable to another.

# Seamless care

Fragmentation of care posed problems in five cases. One mother who had to undergo surgery while pregnant found herself being shunted from a surgical ward, where the staff seemed not to recognise that she was in labour, to an X-ray department where she found the staff unsympathetic about the pain of adopting strange positions while in labour, and then on to the labour ward where the staff appeared not to know how to attend to her surgical wound.

# Caring approach

The overall care was seen to be deficient in a number of other cases – it was generally poor ($n = 4$ parents), the ward or reception staff were impatient or unpleasant ($n = 4$), and the mother's basic needs were sometimes overlooked ($n = 1$). The approach of the medical staff was regarded as critical and where the consultant obstetrician was perceived as having undeveloped 'people skills' ($n = 5$), or anyone was intimidating or humiliating ($n = 2$), the parents were left feeling angry or distressed. Two parents from separate families said that they felt very disempowered: one was a young father who felt too scared to articulate his opinions; the other was a mature professional woman who overheard staff ridiculing the way in which her difficult antenatal period had been managed.

# Sensitivity of handling

During this anxious time before delivery the parents felt vulnerable. Two mothers were unhappy about being roomed in with mothers and babies when they were contemplating problems in their own birth experience. Two others felt under an unwelcome amount of pressure to terminate the pregnancy.

# THE LABOUR AND DELIVERY

The numbers of operative and normal deliveries have already been described in the previous chapter. It should be remembered that 14 women who had emergency Caesarean Sections and three who had planned sections had also laboured for some time prior to the operation.

# Complications during delivery

## Birth catastrophes

Parents who experienced unexpected catastrophes in labour described a sense of shock and unreality which remained with them. The pain of delivering a full-term baby and having something go tragically wrong at that point appeared to be devastating, and many wept as they recalled the event a year later, as well as soon after the event.

For some the shock was sudden – the fetal heart suddenly disappearing, the cord prolapsing, the uterus rupturing, a placental abruption occurring, the neonate stopping breathing when in his mother's arms. For others the tragedy unfolded more gradually. They described the dreadful feeling of hearing the fetal heart dropping, of seeing the evidence of fetal distress, of waiting endlessly for the baby to return from resuscitation, and of fear mounting. For yet others the delivery itself was a shock. One mother was recovering from an operation herself and the birth occurred so swiftly that the baby was delivered by the surgeon and anaesthetist. Another mother was fully dilated when she was transferred to the labour ward from the X-ray department.

> It was like being between the devil and the deep blue sea. In the labour suite they didn't know how to deal with the septicaemia and everything else. But then in [the surgical] ward they didn't know how to deal with labour. I can remember speaking to the girl the night before about how scared I was about going into labour. I just feel ... they knew over the weekend that they anticipated I would go into labour, so why didn't they say to me then?
>
> (P36: mother of preterm baby)

## Preterm delivery

Parents who experienced preterm labours talked of a different kind of pain. It was a shock to be labouring so much sooner than anticipated, but their expectations were not as high and they appeared to be more guarded in their hopes for the outcome. Some were encouraged to continue the pregnancy for as long as possible, often at some cost to the mother. In one case the mother lay with an opened cervix for two weeks. Another said that she was fully dilated for several days. These women described ambivalent feelings, wanting to fight for the child but fearful of what lay ahead for them. When delivery was delayed for some time they often experienced conflicting advice about the chances for the child and the relative risks and benefits of delivering at that point. With nothing to do but lie wondering, these comments could assume worrying proportions. Several mothers talked of taking strong action to try to fight for their babies. Some tried to deal with the pain of labour without recourse to analgesia because they felt that it might be detrimental to the health of the baby. One mother refused to see family members in case she got upset and that proved harmful to her babies.

Parents greatly appreciated a calm approach at these times:

> Even then [when I was transferred to the room where they would be born] they were relaxing us. They just kept making us laugh. Every time they tried to put in my epidural I was shaking with laughter. They

even went to the point of hiding all the travel incubators . . . they hid all the neonatal staff and all the equipment so when we went in we didn't see all these people which I think was [helpful] because if we'd walked in and [seen] 30–40 people we'd have thought [shock horror!].

(P35: parents of preterm triplets)

They all have this incredible sort of serious optimism – it's like being seriously cautiously optimistically pessimistic – all in a oner. There wasn't any hand-wringing or anything like that. It helped you stay very, very calm.

(P25: mother of preterm baby with asphyxia)

## Multiple births

For parents with multiple pregnancies there was a particular sorrow attached to the stillbirth of one baby when the others were living. In one case, neither parent ever saw the child who was stillborn. One mother refused to hear what had happened for several days. Another couple said that they felt very confused about seeing the stillborn infant when they were trying to relate to the living siblings, but were persuaded by the staff that it was the best thing to do. In another instance, the mother was not told of the death until all of the babies had been born.

## Necessity for transfer

Transfer to a specialised Unit far from home became necessary for some couples, with all the additional stresses that such a dislocation involved. In three cases subsequent additional transfers were required as complications developed which necessitated even more specialised care.

## Loss of control

Fathers graphically conveyed the bewilderment and shock of being caught up in a situation which was quite out of their control. Two of them were far away at the time, and one was uncontactable, but others were present in the labour ward and recounted the agony of watching helplessly as emergencies gathered a momentum of their own.

I'm just horrified when I think that [my husband] didn't have anybody [to show him where to sit and everything], he was just wandering the corridors.

(P46: mother of baby with brain damage)

One young father was shocked by the experience of being in the operating-theatre, not prepared for what he would see or experience, and feeling 'useless'. One recalled watching for half an hour as doctors battled to resuscitate his child, and another recalled waiting for five hours while staff struggled to stabilise his baby. The experience recounted by another father was of being 'grabbed to sign a form' while his partner was being anaesthetised, of being 'pushed about' and 'excluded' in the stampede that followed a sudden emergency. He fully recognised that the priority was to get the baby out, but nevertheless he felt sidelined and on the fringes of this drama in which he had such a vested interest. At one point he could see the two rooms where his partner and child were both being worked on, and he vividly recalled his fear that he might lose both of them.

# Contact with the baby

Ten mothers (17%) and 9 fathers (15%) had the opportunity to touch their baby briefly before transfer to the NICU. A further 12 mothers (20%) and 23 fathers (39%) merely saw the baby before transfer, although for most it was a fleeting look. Two of the mothers had wanted to see or hold their babies in the labour ward, but the fathers were happier to have them go straight to the NICU.

# Information givers

Although many parents had recalled no discussion of potential problems during labour, many more were given information at the onset of or during labour when things started to go wrong. Only two families recalled no information being given about possible problems during the entire period of pregnancy, labour and delivery. In one of these cases the baby had an undiagnosed cardiac defect and the other baby was born prematurely. One couple were unsure of the identity of the person who was telling them what had happened, but for the majority of the parents (33, 56%) it was the labour ward staff who provided information during labour and delivery. Sixteen couples (27%) were informed by staff from the Neonatal Unit, in 10 cases by a consultant neonatologist.

> I really appreciated the fact that he [the neonatologist] came to see me and that he spent as long as he did. What I liked about his approach was he didn't pull any punches and he would talk to you and he never gave you the feeling that he had to go anywhere else or do anything else. You had as much time with him as you wanted really.
>
> (P25: mother of preterm baby with asphyxia)

In a further three families, basic information was first given by the local labour ward staff, and then a consultant neonatologist filled them in on the detailed explanation. In just one instance it was the postnatal ward staff who took responsibility for imparting this information.

# Information conveyed soon after the birth

Six families (10%) had no recollection of being given any information about potential problems at this stage. On occasion parents had to wait a long time for further information – while babies were being resuscitated, stabilised or assessed – but 51 sets of parents (86%) reported that some information was imparted at this stage. Half of the couples (29, 49%) were given information together, and in three of these families the mother was given information on her own as well. Five mothers were alone when the news was given to them. However, in 17 cases (29%) the mother was not in any fit state either to be told or to take in what was being said, and it was the father who listened to what the staff were saying at this point, although the mother was physically present at that discussion in five instances.

At this stage, when parents were given early information it was often before a definite diagnosis had been made, and five families recalled being advised that the next 12, 24 or 48 hours were critical, and that everyone would need to wait to see how the baby responded during that time. But in some cases the problems the baby faced were very evident from the outset. Fifteen sets of parents (25%) were given gloomy prognoses at this early stage, with doctors holding out little hope of recovery. In 11 of these 15 cases the babies were preterm infants at the edge of viability. Three infants (one of them a preterm baby among the 11 cases just mentioned) had obvious severe congenital anomalies. Three had suffered severe asphyxia, and in each case the time to resuscitate had raised serious doubts about the future outcome. However, 13 couples (22%) recalled being given false reassurances at this point, which they subsequently felt had been counter-productive.

# Improvements

In total, 38 sets of parents (64%) felt that this part of the proceedings – during pregnancy, labour, delivery and the period immediately following the birth – could have been handled better. Again it must be remembered that the outcome was an unhappy one, and this might well have coloured their perceptions. It must also be borne in mind that 11 women (19%) delivered in local hospitals and were referred to the study Units later, so their criticisms relate to hospitals other than those directly involved in the study.

## Earlier transfer

A number of the parents whose babies were transferred to the study Units wished that they had been referred in sooner. They felt that potential problems might have been detected sooner, and a better quality of expert care might have materially affected the outcome.

## Better preparation

Having things go catastrophically wrong was a shocking experience, and a few families wished they had been better prepared for what was coming. Some pointed out that, in general, new parents-to-be know little of the hazards of childbearing, and perhaps more should be done to raise awareness of the difficulties which might be encountered, and the implications of antenatal screening tests, perhaps in schools or in early pregnancy. A small number felt that more monitoring in pregnancy might detect problems earlier and give parents more options to abort the pregnancy or go for earlier treatments.

A few parents who had had preterm babies pointed out that in their case preparation could have been given. A visit to the NICU prior to delivery might have prepared them better for the shock of seeing tiny babies in such an alien environment. The consequences of early delivery could have been explained to them beforehand.

> I think now that at that stage [early in pregnancy when you know your babies are likely to be born prematurely] you should be taken up to the Neonatal Unit ... if you see a 24-week baby and you see all the machines and maybe even talk to some (of the mums) ... it helps you to understand, Wow, this is what it's like ... To make a better informed choice I think it would have been good to go up and see the reality of it and speak to the neonatologist and paediatricians up there.
>
> (P12: mother of preterm triplets)

In cases of multiple pregnancy where preterm birth was expected, parents suggested, opportunity should also have been given to book into antenatal classes earlier.

## Earlier intervention

The management of the labour and delivery was one of the main sources of concern. Eleven families (19%) felt that earlier intervention might have averted the catastrophe, and five (8%) felt that a specialist should have been called in sooner. Three couples felt that monitoring had been inadequate. Sometimes parents had tried to tell staff that intervention was required, but eight families (14%) felt staff were not really listening to what they felt to be wrong. In six of these eight cases the parents held the staff partly to blame for the outcome because they had not paid attention to the parents' concerns.

> Before it all got out of control in the delivery room, I said to the mid-wife – my husband was there at the time – I said to her, 'You know I've always had this fear of my original scar bursting.' And she just laughed and she goes, 'Oh well, that never happens. Don't worry about that.' But I'd even brought it up, so it should have been in their minds. You'd think somebody would have stood back and said, 'Wait a minute, there's some-thing not right here.'
>
> (P 5: mother of baby with asphyxia, whose uterus ruptured)

## Greater sensitivity to fathers' feelings

Fathers felt that they were sometimes not accorded the right amount of involvement. Three reported being excluded from the scene of activity against their wishes. One said he was not called from home soon enough when things started to go wrong. However, one was given too prominent a position – he was placed on a high stool from which he could see every detail of a surgical operation – which he found was not to his liking.

## More staff

Parents were seriously concerned about the shortage of staff, which meant that mothers were left unattended or students were given too much responsibility. Some of the 7 parents (12%) who identified this as an issue felt that, if trained staff had been vigilant in attendance, important warn-ing signs might have been detected soon enough that something could have been done about them and the tragedy that occurred could have pos-sibly been averted.

## Substandard care

The actual standard of care was deemed to be poor by 9 sets of parents (15%), who cited factors such as unhygienic techniques, deficient equip-ment, being left with legs in stirrups for 100 minutes whilst waiting to be stitched, and not getting pain relief because the keys to the drugs cupboard had been mislaid. Care was too fragmented for 7 families (12%), and one mother drew attention to the difficulty of repeating a history to several different people while coping with the pain of labour.

> *Mother*: Her head was actually crowned and the midwife went away out. I found that scary. She went out the room. I didn't know what to do . . . I hadn't been to any classes to do any of my breathing or [anything]. The only reason I knew [anything] was through watching it on the telly . . . but when she went away when the baby's head was crowned I didn't know how to breathe . . . I know it was only 2 to 5 minutes, but anything could happen in that time . . .
>
> *Father*: I was quite worried about that as well . . . I was quite annoyed at that, I think because you're the only other person there and obviously you're trying to be helpful to [the Mum] and she doesn't know what's going on. It feels as though it puts a lot of pressure on me as well, to be able to know what to do. All I wanted to do was press the button to get her to come back in. I just felt they were away far too long. I really did . . . I know they see it all the time but *you* don't. You've never been through it before.
>
> (P 58: parents of preterm baby)

Doctors, midwives and clerical staff all came in for criticism of their attitudes and behaviours. In some instances doctors were perceived to be insensitive ($n = 8$ parents), incompetent ($n = 4$) or disrespectful ($n = 2$). Parents who were struggling to deal with the shock of an emergency Caesarean Section found it offensive to have the surgeons laughing or discussing shopping centres during the operation. A father was incensed by the comment of a junior paediatrician that his baby 'might not be a genius.' Shortly after giving birth to a child with problems, mothers found it insensitive of doctors to discuss the next pregnancy or say they should consider being sterilised. Certain midwives were perceived as dismissive ($n = 2$), rude ($n = 2$), too casual ($n = 2$), complacent ($n = 1$) or negligent ($n = 1$). Reception staff were considered by one couple to be unhelpful when the mother arrived in very premature labour.

Many parents spoke of the need to see the baby soon after transfer.

> I was [in the NICU] within hours of waking up, which was wonderful. They didn't say, 'Oh no, no, you should stay in bed,' or something. They realised that that was my need therefore they did what they could to get me into that wheelchair and up . . . The postnatal girls who looked after me were wonderful. They just said, 'You're going to be very busy and you're going to be on your feet a lot and you're going to be sore,' and they said, 'We're going to offer you lots and lots of painkillers and you just take whatever we throw at you.' And I thought, 'That's what I

need. I need to be on my feet.' None of this, 'You're going to be sore, therefore you must rest' . . . and I think I have made an incredibly quick recovery because of that.

(P46: mother of baby with brain damage)

But many parents experienced long waits. One mother felt particularly sad that her visit was delayed when she had specifically requested an epidural anaesthetic so that she could be mobile and visit her baby early on.

# Inadequate information

The extent and level of information conveyed created problems for a number of parents. Twelve sets of parents (20%) had experienced unacceptable delays in being told what was happening. They realised in many instances that all staff resources were drafted into working with the baby, but they wished that someone had just popped out to keep them in the picture. A further six sets of parents (10%) felt that the explanations they were given should have been more understandable and detailed. However, for three couples the information given was wrong – they had been falsely reassured that all was well. In all of these instances this reassurance had come from midwives – one of them a student midwife – and the parents commented that unless the midwives had the full facts it was not in their province to offer such platitudes.

Parents were sometimes left in limbo after the infant had been transferred to the NICU. One mother had an elective Caesarean Section, after which the parents were told that the baby had a chest infection but was not deteriorating. The father went home, but telephoned several times through the night and was told the baby was doing well. The mother, who was still in hospital, was told nothing, and no one offered to take her to see the baby:

> She was born at two minutes to one and I got to go to the ward [from Recovery Room] I think it was nearer seven o'clock and I got to go and see her then. The nurse took me up before she took me to the ward, so I got to look at her then. And I never got to see her again until the [next] morning. I didn't know I could go and see her. Nobody actually came to say to me, 'If you want to go and see her we'll take you in the wheelchair.' I worried the whole night. Nobody came to say, 'We've phoned and she's doing very well,' or anything. You know what it's like when you're in hospital, you don't like to push the nurses, and we didn't think there was an awful lot wrong. Obviously I was worried all night.

(P7: mother of baby with cardiac anomaly)

## Broken promises

Three sets of parents (5%) objected to promises being made but not kept. In one case this was a promise to a father that he would see his baby in half an hour, but it was actually three and a half hours before he was admitted to the nursery. One mother was promised that she would have her membranes ruptured (ARM) by a certain stage of labour, but the procedure was delayed by a long time. She felt that the severe fetal distress might have been detected sooner if they had done the ARM when she wanted it, much earlier on.

# Discussion

It is evident that parents perceive shortcomings in the service provided ante- and intranatally. As we have pointed out, attention must be drawn to the possibility of bias in that the outcome was tragic for all of these families, and things which irritated or angered them might not have done so had they left with a healthy live baby. But, in the perception of some of these parents, factors such as shortages of staff and substandard care were associated with a sense that the disaster might have been avoided if the service had been optimal. Although we made no effort to establish cause and effect, the fact that these vulnerable parents felt this was so is sobering, and adds weight to the call for more resources.

Being heard is an important part of being in control. The parents in this study lamented the fact that staff just did not listen to them when they felt that something was wrong. In all of these families something *was* seriously wrong, so it is understandable that most felt that this had also contributed to the outcome. The majority of them reported serious complications arising antenatally or during delivery. From the evidence of the outcomes, their concerns would seem to be borne out by the data. For example, only one of the mothers who went into preterm labour was in false labour, but many of them were not believed and were sent home. Few of the women who delivered preterm remembered being told of the risks of prematurity. However, these were the families in which things did go wrong. Many women present in early labour, and in many cases their fears are unfounded. Frequently judgements have to be made on the basis of little evidence, and we have no objective way of knowing whether appropriate assessments were made for these particular families. But their concerns must be heard and taken seriously. Whether or not crises might have been averted, parents were left dissatisfied, and opportunities to discuss the consequences of preterm delivery were lost because staff did not seem to believe them.

Information is also empowering. A considerable number of these parents felt they were not always appropriately informed. It is understandable that warning of impending problems was not often given during pregnancy. If everything is going according to plan, there is no necessity for discussing difficulties. When problems do present, sometimes circumstances influence who is told what and when – individuals may be unavailable geographically, mentally or emotionally. At the time of a delivery crisis, attention is often focused exclusively on the baby – these parents remind us that they may be left unsupported with no knowledge of what has happened or what is being done. Their urgent needs and concerns must not be forgotten.

Around the time of the delivery, only half of these couples were given information together. Many of them regretted not having the support of their partner at this time. One-third of the women felt that they were in no state to hear serious news, because of the effects of anaesthesia/analgesia or exhaustion. A few fathers were unavailable. News of this nature is hard for a parent to hear alone. Clinicians need to bear such criticisms and regrets in mind under such circumstances.

Another difficulty identified by these parents is that of fragmented care. Only about a quarter of these families recalled being given information at delivery by paediatric staff of any grade, still less by a consultant neonatologist. Many couples who were known to be likely to have preterm babies reported that they were neither seen by a paediatrician nor had an opportunity to visit the NICU. When the child is later transferred into the care of the paediatric team, not only is everything very unfamiliar and frightening, but also the doctors and nurses are strangers. They may well tell parents a different story. Confidence is shaken.

What is said is also of crucial importance, and it may impinge on future confidence as well as present understanding. A worrying number of parents reported being given false reassurances. Obviously at this early stage all of the facts of the case are not always known. Furthermore, many parents express anxieties during delivery, and midwives and obstetricians reassure them to good effect. However, some of these parents knew they were at risk. One-fifth of them had a history of infertility; it is known that such women are at increased risk of having a perinatal death.[101,102] As we have seen, the mother whose previous Caesarean Section scar was rupturing felt patronised and falsely comforted. A midwife reassured another couple that their child was crying lustily on the resuscitaire, but they subsequently found out from post-mortem findings that he had never cried. The experiences of these parents remind clinicians of the dangers of rushing to offer platitudes without foundation. Not only may parents be left feeling that staff were negligent, but also trust in future care may be undermined.

# Conclusion

- It is important to listen sympathetically to pregnant women who are concerned that things are not as they should be.
- When things do go wrong, these women need to be kept informed of developments and not offered false reassurances.
- Involving the paediatric team at an early stage helps to foster confidence and reduce the dangers of fragmentation of care.

# CHAPTER 6

# When things went wrong

The possibility exists that the point at which staff detect problems might not coincide with parental awareness of trouble. Our respondents were asked about the time when they were first alerted to the possibility that things were not going well and that the child's life might be in question.

 A few parents drew attention to a difference in the time at which staff started to alert them to possible problems and the point at which they personally assimilated the news. For example, one family was told soon after delivery that something was wrong, but they did not really accept that it was serious enough to threaten the child's life until 5 weeks later. Another family would not let themselves take in the truth until just hours before the baby died. Both points have been taken into account but, unless specified otherwise, it is the time when parents accepted the reality to which we refer in this section.

It must be borne in mind that at the time they were asked this question they all knew that the baby had subsequently died. It is likely that if the outcome had been good, some of the warning signs they cited would not have been interpreted so pessimistically, either at the time or subsequently.

## When parents realised things were going wrong

For one couple, realisation of trouble came antenatally with the diagnosis of a severe congenital anomaly. Two other couples who were told of possible serious malformations during pregnancy did not cite the antenatal period as the time when they first believed the outlook was poor. The onset of preterm labour alerted 9 couples (15%). For a further 8 families (14%) things started to go wrong during labour.

However, for the majority the sense that things were going wrong only came after delivery. For 18 sets of parents (31%), this realisation came within hours of the birth. For 5 families (8%) it was not until day 2. Nine families (15%) were alerted between day 3 and day 7, and a further 7 families (12%) were not alerted until about 2 weeks after birth. For two families (3%) their hopes were initially high, and the reality of a poor outcome did not impinge until 8 or 11 weeks later.

> [We built up our hopes] to begin with, yes. The doctors kept trying to knock us back but we didn't listen. He was doing so well. They *told* us he was doing so well. We could *see* he was doing well. And our hopes just rose with him. And even when he came through the operation ... and he was still doing OK, at that point our hopes were definitely high. So it was quite a shock [when he deteriorated].
> (P3: parents of preterm baby with congenital anomaly)

> [The neonatologist] said these hiccups had been seizures and that it was a very common sign in a child that was being deprived of oxygen, or had been. A seizure or a fit doesn't necessarily have to be a whole spasm, it can just be a slight twitch to the hiccups that he had been having. But then when they stopped, we thought, 'This is great!'. So obviously we were starting to build our little tower of bricks. But every time we got a couple of our bricks built, we were always getting another slap in the face. It was an emotional rollercoaster ... When the fits stopped, and he's breathing on his own, and the body starts to move when you touch [him], we had great optimism ... But then we always went on to find out these things were grossly abnormal. When the fits stopped that was the way of saying the brain was dead.
> (P20: mother of baby with asphyxia)

It was only the sight of a written report of what had been said during their meeting with the consultant that convinced one mother. The description was exactly the same as what she had heard verbally, but seeing it written down, and realising that the staff did not expect her baby to live, reinforced the reality.

# Factors which alerted parents to the possibility of a poor outcome

Given the difficulty many parents had in taking on board the enormity of what was happening, it is important to establish what it was that alerted them to the fact that things were seriously wrong. Some families demonstrated a degree of optimism at the time which they themselves later found surprising.

> *Father:* They highlighted a few things which, to the layman – well, they weren't apparent. For example, he had a big head, he had a short neck, he had slightly strange ears, he had a heart problem. There were a few items they mentioned. Looking at him . . . the big head: [our daughter]'s got a big head, I've got a big head. So it's a family trait. He did seem to have a bigger than average head. Fine. Again his ears: they seemed to think they were slightly low – whatever, and they had these funny lobes which I think I've got, too. So we were minimising things. And the short neck: again you saw him lying there and I couldn't really say he had a short neck. So they flagged up a few things which probably objectively [were odd] . . . OK, they've got to do that obviously, but it seemed a more darker picture than you'd think as a layman . . . I'm sure they were right to point these things out, but we were looking through rose-tinted glasses and you do tend to dismiss them.
>
> *Mother:* They always say these things trying to cover themselves. They always manage it on BBC every week, on Children's Hospital! That's it, whatever his problems you think, he's in the best place . . . whatever happens, almost certainly they'll manage to sort it out.
>
> (P6: parents of baby with congenital anomalies)

Others described a growing realisation. For example, one couple was told at 2 weeks that their preterm baby had a swollen abdomen and must return to Intensive Care. She developed severe necrotising enterocolitis (NEC), but they remained optimistic. It was not until a month later when she deteriorated following major surgery that they entertained doubts about her survival, but it took a direct statement from the consultant to make them realise that they might lose her.

In one case it was the development of a problem antenatally which sounded alarm bells for a father. He had been pessimistic since the onset of hydramnios in pregnancy, his experience with animals having influenced his expectations. His wife, on the other hand, had been more optimistic that any problem would be correctable.

In 13 cases (22%) it was a sudden dramatic event which first alerted the parents – a cord prolapse, the fetal heartbeat dropping suddenly or stopping, a pulmonary haemorrhage, a pneumothorax, a dusky episode, or a sudden deterioration in the baby's condition. When the staff avoided their eyes during the event or failed to reassure them, the parents knew things were serious.

An extremely preterm birth alerted 8 sets of parents (14%) to the potential for a bad outcome. Once the baby was born, whether prematurely or at term, there were a number of warning signs which parents perceived as significant indicators of trouble: poor colour ($n = 7$), limp, lifeless condition ($n = 2$), sleepiness ($n = 1$), the baby being whisked away and not coming back for a long time ($n = 4$), there being no news of his progress for a long time ($n = 1$), or the parents not being taken to see him ($n = 1$). But sometimes initial concern was allayed and it took future developments to alert them to the possibility of grave problems.

For 24 sets of parents (41%) it was the onset of a clinical problem which made them seriously concerned about the outcome. These included problems with the lungs ($n = 10$), bowels ($n = 4$), brain ($n = 5$), intubation and ventilator ($n = 3$), gangrene ($n = 1$), patent ductus ($n = 1$), consciousness levels ($n = 1$), fits ($n = 1$) and temperature control ($n = 1$). The general appearance of the child alerted a further 7 sets of parents (12%) to serious problems. One mother said that as soon as she saw the 'vacant eyes and clenched fists', she knew. For others the signs were less obvious, but the child just looked ill.

It took direct information about a poor outlook or deteriorating condition to ring the first alarm bells for 17 sets of parents (29%). When the staff told them there was nothing more that could be done, or that they held out little hope for the baby, the message was clear – the situation was grave. However, one father came by such information by chance; he overheard staff referring to his baby as 'that poor wee boy', and he knew then that the situation was bleak, although nothing had been officially said.

The whole demeanour of the staff conveyed to 12 parents (20%) that things were critical – serious expressions, a worried exchange of glances, a hand held to a forehead, staff avoiding eye contact, a cessation of rigorous handwashing and other precautions, and evasion rather than reassurance. These behaviours spoke to the parents before any words were uttered.

> They took about 5, 10 minutes to bring [the first twin] back to me and when they didn't bring [the second one] back to me and the midwife was [patting my arm] and saying, 'It'll be all right. It's going to be OK. He's OK. He's OK,' I knew. I knew then that there was something wrong. It was like they were comforting me . . . and the way she looked at me . . . I felt there was something wrong.
>
> (P40: mother of baby with asphyxia)

It was all very calm but you could tell there was something wrong . . . how could I tell? Oh, by their faces. There was no heartbeat – well, they couldn't detect it. I was saying, 'Should I be panicking here, girls?' And they were [saying], 'No, no, no. Everything's all right.' And then it was into a cubicle and it was: 'On to your side quickly, please, quickly. Leave your handbag.' Then it was, 'Could you get the registrar through.'

> Then I said 'Should I be panicking *now*, girls?' 'No, no no, you'll be fine.'
> You could just tell by the look on their faces ... then it was, 'Could
> you sit into this wheelchair, please, and breathe some of this oxygen.'
> And now I was well panicking. Next minute I was upstairs.
>
> (P21: mother of baby with cardiac anomaly)

When the parents had difficulty reaching the baby because of the number
of staff around his incubator ($n = 3$) they became seriously concerned for
his welfare. Sometimes it was the events which preceded any discussion
that gave real cause for concern before anything was said. These included
a 'summons' to see the consultant ($n = 3$), or the medical staff coming to
the ward to see the parents ($n = 4$), or being woken in the night ($n = 1$), or
a telephone call from the hospital ($n = 4$), or the appearance of a specialist
in a suit ($n = 1$), or the arrival of the police at their door ($n = 1$). Such
experiences were out of the ordinary and indicated unexpected troubling
developments.

> It was someone that we didn't know [the nurse looking after our baby on
> this occasion] ... she was chatting away [telling us about the baby being
> settled and doing well] and, 'You're seeing [the consultant] in a wee
> while. He needs to talk to you about a couple of things with [the baby].'
> And as soon as she said that I knew. Suddenly it changed from *we've
> asked to see the consultant* and suddenly now it's *the consultant wants to
> see us*. And I knew that there was going to be bad news.
>
> (P20: mother of baby with asphyxia)

> The suits came in – the men in suits! That's when we knew something
> was wrong ... Well, four people came in; one man in a suit – it felt like
> more! ... Something's wrong. Why are four people coming to tell me my
> baby's got wet lung? Something's seriously wrong. And then he took a
> seat and that was it. Our world fell apart at that point.
>
> (P21: mother of baby with cardiac anomaly)

It came as a shock to one mother to see her husband so upset. She had
known him for more than ten years and had never seen him in tears
before. It was that more than anything which conveyed to her the seriousness of the situation.

# How information was imparted

## To whom

Although the majority of couples (37, 63%) were given bad news together,
for a variety of reasons it was sometimes conveyed to one parent alone
initially. The mother on her own was given the bad news at this point in

the case of 13 families (22%). Given that the mothers were usually in the hospital much more than the fathers, this was unsurprising. However, in one instance the information was given over the telephone; in another case, the mother was told on the ward but the father was telephoned at home and given the news, too. Two of the women rang home to tell their partners themselves. Seven of these 13 mothers shortly afterwards had further discussions with the doctors with their partners present. One mother reported that the news was given first to her own parents, who later explained to her what the doctors had said.

In 7 cases (12%) it was the father who was given the information first. In three of these families the father chose to tell his partner himself what had happened, but the other couples had discussions together later with the doctors. (Data are missing on this point for one set of parents.)

## By whom

The 56 sets of parents who talked about this part of their experience recalled being given the information about the problems by a variety of people. Thirty-six families (64%) heard via a member of the paediatric staff. Of these, 15 were told by their baby's named consultant neonatologist, 8 were told by a paediatrician other than the named consultant, one by different junior members of staff, with the senior registrar imparting the most serious news, and 12 families were told by a combination of different neonatologists and paediatricians, or in one case an advanced nurse practitioner.

As many as 20 sets of parents (36%) reported a series of different information givers. Ten sets of parents were first given information by obstetric or labour ward staff and then by the paediatric team. In three of these cases a third layer of information givers was added when they were seen by a specialist. Local paediatricians in smaller Units imparted initial information to three sets of parents before the study Unit paediatric staff took over the role. For a further six families the information that was initially given by the neonatologists was added to by specialists who were called in to give an expert opinion. In the last case, policemen gave the first indication of a serious problem when they called to find the mother whom the hospital had been unable to contact. The neonatologist filled in the medical detail when the mother arrived at the Unit.

## Others present

Parents reported that there was almost always someone else present when this initial information was given. Most although not all consultant neonatologists were accompanied by a neonatal nurse. Only four parents said that they were entirely alone when they were first given news of serious problems – two mothers and two fathers. One mother reported being visited in her single room by the consultant neonatologist accompanied by the consultant paediatrician from the smaller Unit where the baby had been born. She felt that they were conspiring to tell a story which absolved anyone at the delivery from blame, and she was distressed that they had done so when she was alone and vulnerable. Other family members were present in only three cases – the maternal grandmother on each occasion.

## What was said

For some the news was of a hopeless situation from an early stage. An undeveloped trachea, a grossly abnormal heart, lethal combinations of anomalies, or catastrophic asphyxia beyond treatment were all conditions which left no room for hope of improvement. As many as 20 sets of parents (34%) reported being told unequivocally that there was nothing more that could be done.

At this stage, 14 sets of parents (24%) remembered being given a clear diagnosis enabling them to label the problem – a syndrome ($n = 4$), a specific heart abnormality ($n = 5$), a congenital anomaly ($n = 4$) or a known bowel problem, NEC ($n = 1$). However, for others the actual diagnosis was rather more elusive. The underlying factor – for example, prematurity – did not of itself necessarily lead to death, but it rendered the child vulnerable to other problems which could be life-threatening or damaging. The complications arising from events such as birth trauma or preterm delivery created their own problems, but were indicative of the greater insult. When asked what they had been told, parents could only enumerate the various complications and sequelae which followed the initial precipitating event. A picture of a bleak outlook could take some time to emerge fully as test results accumulated and the baby's condition worsened. Parents told of information about brain damage ($n = 28$) or lung damage ($n = 23$) or of other complicating factors, and how they gathered all of these threads together to form a composite picture of problems which together gave cause for serious concern and led to their worrying about the futility or wisdom of continuing treatment.

Other parents had no overarching diagnosis, but rather described a series of discussions which started off with a rather vague sense that all was not as it should be, and gradually built up to a picture of deterioration or seriousness. For example, one couple reported being told initially that the baby was ill but the doctors did not know why. Drugs were commenced to control her convulsions and to 'protect her brain.' The doctors next queried whether she was reacting adversely to her mother's milk. After three weeks the parents were told that the baby had a syndrome related to enzyme function, but that it was so rare that the doctors had to seek confirmation of the diagnosis overseas. It was not until five weeks later that the parents were finally told with certainty that the condition was incompatible with life.

In another case, an early diagnosis of a hole in the heart was followed at two months of age by more serious news of three holes. Major surgery was discussed, but a chest infection developed. At four weeks doctors discussed various abnormal characteristics which troubled them, but confirmed that tests had revealed no chromosomal disorder. The baby's temperature began to fluctuate dramatically and her condition gave further cause for concern. Although early scans had shown a normal brain, careful checks now showed that her brain had stopped growing. The parents were told that she had only days to live, and they prepared themselves for her death. In reality she lived for several months.

Five families (8%) were given false reassurances early on which were later seen to be erroneous. Diagnosis was sometimes impossible at the outset, but by sharing their 'hunches' doctors sometimes rendered themselves vulnerable.

> I didn't want a Down Syndrome baby; I wanted a baby who was perfect. But I was told that it was a Down Syndrome baby. It took me how many days [to come to terms with that fact]. I was upset, but the one thing we had worked out in our own minds was, we've got a Down Syndrome baby, we've got to make him the best Down Syndrome baby. We've got to give him 100%. Why did [the consultant] tell me that he was Down Syndrome when he wasn't Down Syndrome? ... They should have been 100% certain, not just telling us he was a Down Syndrome, making us go through five days of hell ... I said to that [consultant], 'You may be wrong.' And he told me for definite he wasn't wrong ... I said 'If you're wrong, you'd better come and tell me; you'd better be the man to tell me.' ... But he didn't, it was [another consultant] that came and told me. As far as I'm concerned that's out of order because he should have come back and said it, because he was the one who told me my laddie had Down Syndrome.
>
> (P 38: father of baby with congenital anomaly)

More than one family was advised that their baby had features characteristic of Down Syndrome – in no case was this the reality. The parents' reactions varied. In one family the father was angry that 'wrong' information had been given, and he doubted the ability of the neonatologist. In another case the mother was more sympathetic to the medical quandary: it had taken a week of increasingly worrying developments for the specialists to diagnose the actual condition, and she appreciated the dilemma of dealing with anxious parents while waiting for a differential diagnosis.

Nevertheless, in general parents preferred to be kept in touch with medical thinking, even if this meant saying 'We think there is something wrong but we don't yet know what it is.' Being told the baby was 'a bit wheezy' or had 'a simple chest infection' or was 'a wee bit cold,' and subsequently discovering that the child actually had a life-threatening condition, undermined confidence. One island couple described their experience graphically. The mother had travelled to the mainland for delivery – in itself a disturbing transition. When her baby was born, the midwife tucked the child in beside the mother because she felt cold. She was seen by a junior paediatrician who also reassured the mother that the baby was fine. It was shocking for these parents to have the consultant neonatologist subsequently tell them that she actually had one of two serious heart conditions and would need to be referred to a specialist centre even further away from their island home. The heart specialist diagnosed a lethal anomaly, and the child died shortly afterwards in this very distant Unit.

# Satisfaction with this part of the proceedings

Two sets of parents were unable to assess the adequacy of the staff's management at the time of informing them of serious problems, and information was unavailable from one other mother. A number of respondents commented that the news is so far from what parents want to hear that this must colour their perceptions to some extent.

> It's only because she died that we're super-sensitive. [That insensitive comment from the midwife] probably would not even have been noticed. Because you retrace every single thing when something's gone wrong and you remember everything. But then if everything had gone all right we'd probably have forgotten [what she said] or maybe not even have remembered.
>
> (P21: mother of baby with cardiac anomaly)

Other parents commiserated with the neonatologists, recognising that they had an unenviable task. They wondered how anyone could cope with repeated exposure to this kind of stress.

Nevertheless, even given the unpleasant nature of the task, 21 sets of parents (36%) were satisfied that this part of the proceedings had been handled as well as it could have been. One couple could only appreciate this in retrospect. In the absence of tangible evidence of a problem, they became convinced that the only thing that was wrong with their baby was due to the drugs being given to stop her convulsing. As neither of them had seen any fits, they disbelieved the staff's observations. After a period of great tension, they reached a point when they insisted that they were going to take the child home. The neonatologist refused to allow them to do so, but withdrew some medication. As a result, the fits returned and the mother, seeing them for herself, was persuaded that something was indeed wrong. It took many months to obtain conclusive evidence of a serious disorder, during which time, by their own admission, they continued to show hostility and suspicion. It was only much later when proof of a lethal condition was available that they could look back with regret at their behaviour and express their admiration for the skill and tact of the doctor.

Twenty-six sets of parents (44%) felt that this part of the experience was generally handled well but there was some room for improvement, and a further 9 families (15%) felt that it had been handled badly. In three cases the parents were unhappy with the care they had received in their local hospital, but were entirely satisfied with the service provided in the study NICU.

# Areas for suggested improvements

Although 35 sets of parents overall commented that they were not entirely satisfied with this part of the experience, an additional 10 families had some suggestions for improvement, even though they described themselves as satisfied overall. Thus 45 sets of parents (75%) contributed a total of 171 comments that were critical of the way in which this part of the process had been handled. No attempt had been made to prioritise these elements, since the distress of one person cannot be compared with that of another. Numbers in parentheses (*n*) indicate the number of families making this point. It is important to bear in mind that these were factors remembered some months after the event, and that they must therefore have impinged on the parents with some force and clarity. When the parents were struggling with such a traumatic experience, these additional irritations and grievances were therefore significant, so a detailed catalogue of events is provided. Many of them are idiosyncratic, but together they provide a picture of what constitutes good practice.

Suggested areas for improvement related to communication, the approach of staff, the quality of care, facilities and problems associated with transfer to another hospital.

# Communication

Communication problems were by far the commonest cause of dissatisfaction. Exploration of the nature of the difficulties revealed many sources.

*Inadequate explanation* (n = 12)

Ten of these families all referred to insufficient or incomprehensible information, but in addition there were parents who, whilst they did not cite this as an area for improvement, nevertheless registered regrets in other forms. A number of them reported overhearing facts about their babies before they were told officially.

> When the shift changed out I didn't leave. I wanted to know what was going on. I stayed there so they had to do their shift change while I was there. I found out this was the best way to find out what was going on. Also I wanted to find out what all the monitors were doing – [they only told me] if I asked. I found that if you asked they were willing to tell you. But they'd only tell you so much, then you'd to ask a little bit more and then they'd tell you a little bit more until you got the full picture. I got on really well with the midwives after a few days. I've no qualms about them at all. It was just the doctors weren't very forthcoming with information and I still didn't know there was this massive haemorrhage.
>
> (P9: father of baby with cardiac anomaly)

Others lamented the fact that they were not made aware of the seriousness of the baby's condition, and had therefore not rushed to the cotside to spend every moment with the child while they could. They later regretted this missed opportunity.

Conflicting information was a source of distress for one set of parents. A lack of concrete evidence was cited by another family; they simply did not believe the doctors because they could not substantiate their hunch that there was something very wrong with the baby.

*Long silences* (n = 9)

When no information was conveyed for long periods, concern mounted and parents became upset. As one mother put it, 'It was torture. It was the uncertainty. That was horrible. It was terrible. That's what will stay with us.'

> I think what might have been useful is if when we arrived or maybe an hour or so later somebody maybe came and explained to us why we couldn't go [to the NICU].
>
> (P1: mother of baby with asphyxia)

It was very distressing for parents to face long waits for information.

> [Five days after she was born] they came – still to this day yet I think it
> was the most terrible thing – about 5 o'clock teatime, [to say] one of the
> consultants wanted to see us regarding the condition of [the baby] at
> 8 o'clock. We just sat there and we went numb. That was the longest
> three hours of our lives . . . Three hours we had to sit and we were ima-
> gining everything. We were saying, 'Oh they're going to tell us to switch
> off – they want the ventilator switched off,' something like that . . . the
> time scale was diabolical . . . as soon as they know they should let [the
> parents] know. Why should the rest of the place know and you don't?
>
> (P 36: parents of preterm baby)

Furthermore, such perceived disrespect seemed to make the doctor of so
much more importance than the parents.

### Lack of support for the mother when bad news was given (n = 6)

It was traumatic to be given very bad news without someone present to
offer support. One mother actually had her sister in the room when doctors
came with bad news, but the sister was asked to leave and the mother was
entirely alone while she was being given devastating information.

### False reassurance (n = 6)

False reassurance undermined confidence in the staff.

> Maybe the midwife went a wee bit over the top with her assurances.
> I remember at one stage she hugged [my wife] and she said to us, 'I pro-
> mise you nothing is wrong,' and even though I was quite hopeful that
> nothing was wrong I remember thinking, 'You shouldn't do that. That's
> maybe going a bit too far.'
>
> (P 27: father of baby with cardiac anomaly)

### Ambivalent messages (n = 5)

Where bad news was given it was confusing to have staff later back-
tracking, toning down the message and leaving the parents unsure about
exactly what was being conveyed.

> Don't gutter round about. Just hit me with it. No matter how hard it is at
> the time at least I know where I'm going. I would want it like that. In all
> honesty I don't see you're being nice to somebody by not telling them the
> whole truth because it's got to come out some way. You're just delaying
> what's going to happen and I felt the hospital did that with us. In a way
> I'm actually glad [the junior paediatrician] thought we knew everything
> because she came out with it and just said everything in a way we
> understood it. She said, 'Your daughter's got chronic brain damage,

she's got hydrocephalus, she's blind. You're never ever going to get her home. She's never going to cross your front doorstep. You'll never be able to cuddle her. You'll have to put her into hospital. You can't touch her. Every time you try and touch her she'll scream. The only bit of comfort she'll get is if you put the music on.' How hard that was at the time [but] when we look back now that was a relief because at long last somebody'd said to us what was [*really* happening rather than trying to describe the] worse case scenario... If you think things are going to be bad, tell it, don't hide it because at the end of the day your 'kindness' isn't going to work [in our interests].

(P36: parents of preterm baby)

When [the neonatologist] in the referral unit came in to see us, he sat us round the table and he said, 'She's going to die.' We were absolutely distraught there and then. We thought she was going to die that night. And then he came back to us and we were told something different again. What was hard was you saw one doctor, they told you one thing; you saw somebody else, they told you another, and you just didn't know where you were half the time. I think what they really needed to do was to consult together before coming to us to clarify between themselves which pieces of information they would give us and then give us it all at once, not in bits and pieces... Even that time when [the neonatologist] spoke to us, my Dad was present as well and we all believed, from the way he put it across, we all picked up the same thing, all four of us and the next day he said something different.

(P9: parents of baby with cardiac anomaly)

The effect of these mixed messages was compounded when the news was passed on. As one father said: 'You go and tell everybody and then you go back and tell them [it's not good news after all]. It does take its toll.'

If nurses evaded answering questions, parents thought that they knew more but were concealing the truth. If they used language among themselves which the parents could not understand, it excluded them further.

### *Too many or inappropriate information givers* (n = 3)

Some funnelling of information through one key individual was recommended. Information from different sources could be confusing. However, the identity of the primary information giver was important. On one occasion a junior paediatrician blurted out new facts that had not yet been imparted by the consultant.

I had seen him having hiccups and I had said to the nurse, 'Is that [the baby] got the hiccups?' But she didn't actually bother too much. She just said, 'Oh is it? Just time them and see how long he has them for.' But this was obviously her way of not letting us get too alert and aware and worked up and worried. They're very good, the nurses. They're very dedicated. So he was lying there and his little chest was jumping out and in. And it went on for about half an hour, 40 minutes. It was late at night – about 11 o'clock. . . . There was this young doctor . . . she swung round in her chair – and this would be the only time I would say I ever had any problem in all the care he had – and she just said, 'About these fits . . . .' I just did not know what she was talking about. And another nurse who was caring for [the baby] as well, they all just looked. They obviously thought that we knew what they were talking about and I didn't have a clue. And it was 'Oh, I think we'd better go to the quiet room.' And while we were in the quiet room, it was then that she went on to tell us she would have to go and call in somebody from outside because she didn't know very much about them and couldn't actually finish telling us. She'd probably have been better saying nothing until we'd seen [the consultant neonatologist] . . . she just blurted this; she didn't have a very good manner the way she just came out with it.

> (P20: parents of baby with asphyxia)

### Erroneous or incomplete information (n = 4)

Although few parents actually identified factual inaccuracies as an area for improvement, implicit in others' stories was a recommendation for accuracy. Names and details should be correct. Prognoses should be confident. Two sets of parents felt that they should have been given statistics to enable them to assess the risks for themselves.

### Inappropriate approaches to communication (n = 8)

Two sets of parents wished that the neonatologist had been proactive in imparting information. One of these couples had been introduced to the consultants on the ward in passing, but had not spoken to them properly before being told that things were going wrong.

They were always very good at saying, 'Now if you want to see any of the doctors, just ask.' But of course we never ever did. I always felt, the nurses are there, they're giving us the information . . . We'd always be informed if they were going to plan anything. And when [the consultant] asked to see us, the nurse had said it's just for a routine chat to keep you up to date, I thought, 'Well, that's great, it's the first one that we've really had.'

> (P6: mother of baby with congenital anomalies)

The parents concluded that it had been 'very much our fault' because they were told they could do so but they suggested that it might be better for there always to be some discussion with the consultant, even when things were going fairly smoothly. One other couple commented that 'When you know nothing, you don't know what to ask for.'

One father was seriously disturbed by the experience of being at the centre of many pairs of eyes when bad news was imparted. His anger and hurt were still evident more than a year later.

> A [specialist] had come from the [Children's Hospital] and I was there just myself. And he wanted to speak to me but it was going in one ear and out the other. And the nurse said to me 'I don't think you heard half the things he said to you there.' I said, 'I didn't.' All I could see was all the nurses looking for a reaction from me. That's how I felt when the guy was speaking to me. Everybody was all around and he was going on about this and that. I couldn't even tell you half the things he said to me . . . I was in a daze because I felt that embarrassed. He was standing there talking to me like I was a wee laddie and I was on trial. The thing that was going through my head was 'Are they wanting me to [cry] or are they wanting me to do something [else]?' He really embarrassed me.
>
> (P 30: father of baby with asphyxia)

A highly intelligent couple were resentful of the staff's underestimate of their capacity to understand what was happening. Another set of parents disliked the 'amateur psychology' which prompted staff to show them pictures of surviving babies when they were being told that in their case the baby's condition was very serious.

In two cases families disliked the 'softly-softly' approach. One mother had requested that she should be given the full facts from the outset so that she knew what she was 'up against.' Instead, she reported, bad news was given to her in drips. She came to dread the next session as each piece of news was worse than the last, and she was always fearing that there was more she would have to adjust to in the future. The other family reinforced the view that bad news is better delivered 'straight', believing that in their case staff had been 'too kind' and should have been 'more harsh.' Their baby presented with vague symptoms which were controlled by drugs, but the parents felt that the drugs themselves were responsible for her problems. They made a series of demands for medication to be withdrawn, and declared their intention simply to take the child home. Eventually, after many complex tests, the child was found to have a serious but rare disorder, and reflecting back over the experience they accepted the wisdom of the medical management. This father used the illustration of a dog – if there is something wrong with its tail you can try cutting it off little by little but that is not as kind as chopping it all off in one go. They concluded that it would have been better if they had been told unequivocally that the child was seriously ill, she had to remain on drugs, and there was no question of the parents taking her home.

Although the suggested improvement here was to give frank information, no matter how bad, one set of parents appealed for positive messages to counterbalance the negative ones. Something gentler might have helped to break the unremitting gloom of constant bad news, these parents felt, and would have given them something to cling on to. It is noteworthy in this context that several parents commented that the consultant became synonymous with bad news, and two parents said that they were 'terrified' of him as a result. Parents in general valued a gentle and sensitive approach alongside frankness and direct truth-telling.

Any talk of future pregnancies when the baby was dying could be interpreted as insensitive, but in the case of one father the remarks seemed doubly hurtful, as he had had a vasectomy.

# Approach of the staff

The expressions used to describe behaviour are either those used by the parents or those which best convey their perceptions of the attitudes of staff.

### The consultant obstetrician

One mother with a bad obstetric history was incensed by the consultant not taking the trouble to come in when he was telephoned to be told she had presented in labour. She believed that, had he been present, he would have ordered a Caesarean Section and prevented the subsequent severe asphyxia of the baby.

### The consultant neonatologist

A small number of parents felt that the consultant failed to appreciate their vulnerability and tried to overwhelm them with his knowledge and opinions. Young couples seemed to be particularly vulnerable. When the parents personally felt very insecure, a confident approach was sometimes perceived as patronising or disrespectful ($n = 2$), unsympathetic and arrogant, 'thinking he knows it all,' ($n = 2$), abrasive and upsetting ($n = 2$) or prejudiced ($n = 1$).

> I always felt that they weren't giving us the full picture because, as well as being partners rather than [married], we were also classed as kids. We weren't given any respect for the fact that we were the parents just like anybody ten years older... it was a life or death decision on the spot ... once again it was like we were the kids; 'If you can't come to a decision then we'll make the decision for you,' [that's what he said]. We were getting pushed into the decision and if we didn't come to a decision then the decision would be made for us. All of this was in the same

30 minutes that we had gone up [to the Neonatal Unit for the first time]. I was still an emotional wreck; I didn't know one thing from another. We were still sitting beside [the baby] and we were getting all this information thrown at us and we were having to decide ... I just felt like I was back at school – headteacher, naughty schoolkid.

(P28: parents of preterm baby with asphyxia)

In two cases parents were troubled by the consultant's apparent indecisiveness. When one baby deteriorated, the consultant on duty said that he could not decide to withdraw treatment because the baby was his colleague's case. The parents had to wait many hours until morning for the named neonatologist to come in to make a decision.

Two consultants made promises which they did not then keep. The parents felt that they became less trustworthy as a consequence of this.

Several sets of parents who were doctors or nurses themselves, or who came from medical families, said that the doctors treated them differently. In most cases this was not thought to be a helpful thing to do, as in this situation they were first and foremost vulnerable parents. One non-medical father had problems with the neonatologist speaking to his wife on a level which he could not understand. He did not like to see her in 'professional mode' when it was their child under discussion – the 'human side' of care was missing. He also objected to her translating the information for him. The tension resolved when the mother adopted 'mother mode' and the consultant picked up on the altered cues, treating them both just as parents.

As has already been mentioned briefly, one mother was greatly disturbed by the apparent underhandedness of the consultants. The neonatologist came with the consultant paediatrician from her local hospital to see her when she was entirely alone, and tried to explain away the events at delivery. The mother said that throughout the encounter she was 'totally out of control.' She felt that she was 'being ganged up upon by them both. I was defenceless ... it was like they knew I was the weak one, I was the soft one, I was the pushover one.' When they had gone and she had time to analyse the situation, she put a different complexion on their visit. She reflected that one of the doctors had seemed very ill at ease. By using the phrase 'If a lawyer was to look at this,' he had introduced the idea of negligence which had not previously occurred to the parents.

### The specialist

Two families considered a certain specialist who had been brought in to provide an expert opinion entirely unequal to the task. His interpersonal skills and communication were judged to be poor.

He never once looked me in the eye ... every time I asked him a question he answered [my partner] and it wasn't her who was speaking ... he

looked at his feet quite a lot! If you look somebody in the eye as you tell
them, then you know they're telling the truth.

>                                (P38: parents of baby with congenital anomaly)

Furthermore, his explanations were inadequate.

> [He] was there because he was a specialist . . . He's diagnosed [this rare
> syndrome] . . . but we never saw him again. Well, if he knew so much
> then he should have come and told us more . . . He's the one that diag-
> nosed it. He's the one that stopped the treatment, if you ask me . . . That's
> what hurts me: somebody has made the decision that that's what he had
> but nobody has explained to me why they came to that conclusion . . .
> when is he going to come and explain it to us? Because until he explains
> there's a lot of unanswered questions in my head.
>
>                                (P38: father of baby with congenital anomaly)

## The junior doctors

Insensitive approaches were cited by three sets of parents. One doctor
made a crude joke about the baby in the parents' hearing. Another used
an expression which the father found cruel.

> [The baby] was in his incubator and I had asked them about what the
> prospects were and at that point [shortly after a premature delivery].
> I was wanting to get some information about the prospects in relation to
> brain damage – survival wasn't really what concerned me. I was told by
> this young guy who was on duty that day, 'Well, we'll do some scans later
> on in the week' – these being ultrasound scans of the brain – 'and we
> won't know until then, but your son might not be a genius.' I didn't say
> anything about that at the time; I just wore that comment but it cer-
> tainly struck me as being a completely ignorant thing to say to anyone
> in that circumstance who's obviously very concerned and anxious about
> what's going to happen to their son . . . I'm expecting to get bad news, but
> I don't expect to get it in that form.
>
>                                              (P18: father of preterm baby)

In the third case, a doctor was sharp with a mother who needed to be
checked out prior to transfer to the study Unit, and yawned in her face.
Strong accents were thought to be problematic at a time when parents
were struggling to assimilate unpalatable information, and were mentioned by one couple as a source of dissatisfaction at this time.

## The nurses

Inflexibility troubled three sets of parents. They were confused when certain nurses insisted that policies be adhered to when others had been more

flexible and sympathetic to their special circumstances. A set of grandparents who had been involved and supportive were suddenly denied entry to the nursery. One mother was told she could not hold her baby because it was after 7.30 p.m.

> She wasn't very nice. Out of all the nurses [our baby] had, I didn't like her ... [she wouldn't let us have him out of the incubator after 7.30 p.m. but] the [named neonatologist] had told us we could hold him any time. But luckily she went off and we had lovely nurses after that. It didn't matter what time we sat there till, or how long, or even how many were round his bed – it was, 'Do you want [to hold him]? We'll move all the [paraphernalia around him]'. That nurse wouldn't let anybody else hold him. At that point they knew [the baby] was going to die and his grandparents were always there and I think she could have. If they know the baby's going to die they should let the grannies and granddads hold them. It might be a bit much for the baby, but for five minutes? You've not got a lot of time.
>
> (P 38: mother of baby with congenital anomaly)

> The first time – because grandparents were allowed in the [study] Unit, – [my husband's] folks came in and I said, 'Oh, you'll need to wash your hands, and take your watch off and jewellery'. And they came up and said, 'Oh, what are you doing?' I said, 'Well, they're just washing their hands', 'Oh they can't touch the baby'. And I said, 'What do you mean, they can't touch her?'. And by this stage we knew that she wasn't going to live. They said, 'Oh, it's hospital policy – no contact ... and that was really hard for me, because they'd never held her. By that time I'd been building up and building up – I lost it. I said 'You don't know what it's like for me.' I said, '[My baby] might never come out of here alive. You just haven't got a clue.' Sometimes you got the impression from them it was just another baby on a conveyer belt – just another number. But to us it's our child and they take away your right as a parent and I think that was what was really hard because you've got no control ... The thing is *my* mum had been up and she had got to hold her. You see it depended on who was on. But I think they should be a bit more understanding towards parents ... Now they didn't feel like grandparents because they hadn't been able to hold her.
>
> (P 9: mother of baby with cardiac anomaly)

A perceived lack of sympathy was a source of concern for some couples. Two fathers reported seeking reassurance only to be curtly told to accept the reality of the situation.

> I was sitting talking to [my baby] and I was saying, 'Come on, wee man, get your head together. You're going to be all right.' And one of the

nurses said to me, 'Be realistic. Have you not listened to what the doctor's told you?'... That really did hurt me. I must admit that hurt me.

(P 38: father of baby with congenital anomaly)

Many months after the event one mother was still distressed by the off-hand way in which she felt one nurse had treated her baby, and by her loud and insensitive manner overall. Another mother was horrified when a nurse said to her that if the baby stopped breathing she should just give her a pat. The casual way in which the nurse seemed to treat apnoeic episodes was very far from the terror the mother experienced at being put in a position of responsibility for taking appropriate action. A father was hurt by the nurses' dismissal of his ideas. After closely watching his daughter's responses he had a hunch that adding fortifier to her feeds was causing her to vomit. He suggested this to the staff but found that they would not listen. Subsequent events appeared to confirm his intuition, leaving him frustrated that they had not responded appropriately to his observation.

Inconsistency was cited by two families. One mother was asked to say whether she wanted a Caesarean Section. She said that she did, and she was then told she could not have one. She was left feeling insulted and disempowered. Having just been told that his child could die at any minute, one father was bewildered when he was advised by someone else that it was late and he must leave the hospital now. Although they did not cite inconsistency as a problem, another family captured the effect of a mismatch between verbal and non-verbal messages:

The very first time when the nurse came in smiling, I had this vision straightaway everything was going to be OK ... but then I suppose if she'd come in all sullen-faced I'd have known straightaway everything was bad ... I think it was more the reassuring nursey-type smile. I mean nurses smile, don't they? You don't often see them walking round with long faces ... but I did remember afterwards thinking it was a strange mix of emotions – the smiling and the terrible news.

(P2: father of baby with cardiac anomaly)

Indiscretion was an area in need of attention for one family. The father overheard the nurses discussing their case as he passed an open door, and he learned some unpalatable truths about the prognosis which troubled him greatly.

# Quality of care in the NICU

Anything which kept the parents from the baby was potentially a source of distress for them. They cited long delays before seeing the baby ($n = 6$) or being able to hold him ($n = 1$). There were so many staff clustered around one baby when she was being transferred to a transport incubator that the parents could not get near her. Not only did they feel excluded, but the mother had no opportunity to kiss her daughter before she was taken away to the referral Unit. Since her condition was grave, this was a source of acute distress.

Having too many people involved was a second source of dissatisfaction ($n = 3$). Too many different faces meant that parents had to work repeatedly to establish new relationships, which was not an easy task when they were so vulnerable. One couple believed that the constant change of nursing staff resulted in them overlooking problems with the baby's circulation. It was only when gangrene set in that they were alerted, and the condition was then too advanced for treatment. The parents felt that the same person observing the baby regularly would have detected the problem early on, and they might have been able to take preventative action.

Perceived poor standards of care were troubling. Two families cited unhygienic practices. They noticed lapses of standards such as dropped needles being re-used or blood being spilt and not wiped up. However, it seemed rare for them to pass comment to the staff. One couple feared that delays in intervening had increased the dangers for their child.

When it came to the management of families at this time of things starting to go wrong, parents suggested a variety of factors might be improved. It seemed to them incongruous that distressing procedures should be undertaken on the baby when everyone knew he would not survive ($n = 2$). Monitoring or testing seemed to be superfluous and insensitive. The focus of the staff came in for criticism by three further families. One mother felt that staff spent too much time filling in charts and writing notes, rather than watching the babies. Another couple was troubled when an especially kind nurse visited them at one point, even though she was now assigned to another area, only to be reprimanded by a senior nurse. They felt that such sensitivity and caring should be encouraged, not crushed. The third couple found it incongruous that when parents were grappling with the prospect of losing their baby, staff laughed, joked and behaved as if nothing untoward was happening.

Two families commented on certain practices which they had found frightening. Moving the baby's incubator to another space without warning the parents caused great distress. One family found it distressing when alarms kept ringing although nothing was wrong. They felt that they were made to worry constantly and unnecessarily, but they also feared that this form of 'crying wolf' might obscure real emergency situations.

Other practices were annoying ($n = 2$). One couple really disliked being screened off in the nursery. It was claustrophobic for them and, they felt, troubling for other parents. The other couple resented being asked to wear 'silly aprons.'

# The quality of care in the labour ward or postnatal ward

Medical care was perceived as deficient by a few parents. Great faith was placed in senior consultants' expertise, and if junior doctors were slow to call them, parents could be left feeling that the delays contributed to the tragic outcome ($n = 2$). One further family wished afterwards that they had insisted on a Caesarean Section, as they felt that intervention had been too slow.

The support parents would have liked, but which they did not receive, was cited by a number of families in this context. In one case the midwives in the labour ward were too upset themselves to be supportive of the parents. Four families felt that the postnatal ward staff tended to isolate mothers in their situation. They were left alone in single rooms or quiet areas when they were feeling isolated and depressed. Some parents interpreted this as staff being scared to enter their rooms. One mother felt that the midwives failed to appreciate that she was simultaneously grappling with other major domestic problems. They had pigeon-holed her in the context of this baby and this tragedy alone, and they did not really listen to her other troubles. Three families found it disconcerting when the staff did not know what was happening to their baby in the NICU and behaved inappropriately. Fragmentation of care was troubling, and parents found it difficult to have to get to know so many staff at a time when they were pre-occupied with more important issues. Also, when the mother was some-times on the ward and sometimes in the NICU, her basic care, such as postnatal checks and pain relief, tended to be overlooked.

Three families had found the staff insensitive at this time. One mother was distressed to hear staff making inappropriate comments about her baby's ambiguous genitalia. Another couple was stunned by a midwife's bright and cheerful banter when they were overwhelmed by sadness. She seemed impervious to their cues, and they 'hadn't the heart' to point out the iniquity of her behaviour lest they hurt her feelings. Another mother did not identify this factor as a criticism, but independently recommended that mothers' notes should be marked in some way so that staff were alerted to the special sensitivities of those with very sick babies. In the third case, a mother was distressed by a midwife 'laying into' her about her smoking. Although she herself wanted to give up the habit, she felt it was wrong for anyone to try to deny her a crutch at such a time, and to do so with such harshness.

# Facilities

Five families found the ambience poor for conveying bad news. The association of bad news with features in the decor was strong. Parents shuddered as they remembered colours, decor and pictures in the room or area where they were told that their child might die. A Moses basket left in the room, and mothers wheeling in prams, were too distressing for couples who had just found out that their baby would never leave the hospital.

Poor basic amenities were cited by five sets of parents as areas in need of improvement. Having no accessible or sufficiently private telephone line was distressing when relatives had to be contacted. Malfunctioning lifts, or lack of toilet paper in the lavatories, could feel like neglect to parents who were already vulnerable and feeling a sense of injustice. One father had to go out to buy sandwiches because the food was so inedible. Being unable to park near the hospital added to the distress of another father, who was conscious of the waste of precious time which should have been spent with his baby and partner. When the child's life was destined to be so short, every minute was important.

The place where parents were housed was an important element in their care. Three felt that their own situation had been less than ideal. After receiving devastating news it was traumatic to return to a postnatal ward, to be surrounded by happy mothers with healthy babies, or to be under pressure to vacate a single room.

> I think it's hard [being in the postnatal ward] for me with other babies about . . . I had a private room anyway, but you still walk through a ward and you hear babies crying . . . All along I knew that he was probably going to die and I had to sit up amongst people that had perfect babies. And sometimes you'd hear them complaining because they hadn't got to sleep that night, the baby's kept them up and [I thought] you don't know how lucky you are.
>
> (P4: mother of preterm baby)

> It was horrific. Because, the phone was right outside the door and it was just people all day on the phone, 'I've had a baby girl. I've had a baby boy.' It was just awful.
>
> (P5: mother of baby with asphyxia)

> I was taken into the big delivery room which is for multiple births, and it's right next door to the resuscitation room and that was really, really difficult. I'm obviously delighted for all the other Mums having healthy babies . . . you can hear them crying. I was right next door to that and I thought, 'I might never ever hear mine cry. You're stabbing me in the heart here.'
>
> (P12: mother of preterm triplets)

The place where the parents were given the bad news was also important, and two families regretted the lack of privacy at this time. One couple
was told in the postnatal ward where they were very conscious of other
'normal' parents in the background. It was not easy for others to listen
to such a discussion, they felt, but nor was it right for the grieving family.
The very presence of happy new parents highlighted the injustice of what
was happening to them.

Parents clung to the first photographs they were given of their baby, but
in one case they found the quality of the photograph so poor that the child
looked much worse than in reality.

# Problems of transfer

Having been told that their child needed more expert care, two sets of parents felt keenly that delays in transferring him were detrimental to his welfare. Another couple was distressed when they were refused permission to
accompany the baby in the ambulance. Every moment with him was precious anyway, but more than that they were very conscious that the child
might die in the ambulance and that they should be with him. Attention
was drawn to the lack of official transport for the parents when the baby
was transferred to a different centre. Two fathers and one mother from
three different families experienced distressing problems when trying to
find the referral hospital. In one case a mother had to travel soon after
having a Caesarean Section:

> I got there on the Sunday night at quarter to nine because we got lost
> trying to find the hospital. I had to travel by car but I injured myself in
> the car because I asked [my husband's] sister, I said, 'How do you adjust
> the seat?' because I was getting really uncomfortable and I was in pain.
> And she said, 'Oh, there's a lever at the side.' Well, I pulled it and the
> whole seat just [shot back] . . . it was getting to about eight o'clock at
> night and I was getting myself so worked up because we couldn't find
> the hospital . . . and in the end we got into the town and we had to hire
> a taxi to follow the taxi to get to the hospital.
>
> (P9: mother of baby with cardiac anomaly)

> We were left to our own devices. It was 'She's going to [referral hospital for
> surgery]. Make your own way there.'. . . I had been working all day; it was
> a 2-hour journey back. I'd sat up all that time till 12 [at night]. And your
> emotions are high anyway, and then it was, 'OK, can you get to [this surgi-
> cal hospital]?' And I'm thinking 'Where the hell's [this hospital]?'
> I'd never been there before . . . and you're driving at that time of night and

thinking, 'Where am I going to get parked? Where am I going to go?' . . .
Should there not be a driver or a taxi?

(P58: father of preterm baby)

Once the parents were at the referral hospital other issues arose. Simply
being transferred hundreds of miles away from family and support networks at such a time was isolating for one couple. A breakdown in communication between the two hospitals and inadequate relaying of information
was upsetting for another couple. Finding very different practices obtaining in the referral Unit compared to those in the previous hospital bewildered another family. The things they had been able to do were now
forbidden, and the staff seemed to be censorious of their behaviour.

# Parental factors

For four other families there were problems other than those in the province of the staff. In two cases the father was far away at the time. In the
other two families the mother was heavily sedated and not able to enter
fully into the events which were unfolding at this time. The parents
regretted her unavailability at such a crucial point.

# Sources of support at this time

Only two mothers reported feeling totally unsupported at this stage in the
experience, and in neither case was there an opportunity to check the perceptions of their partners. In both instances the mothers underwent
operations and problems developed precipitately. In one case the uterus
ruptured and the fetal heart suddenly stopped. In the other case the baby
was born unexpectedly following an operation for another problem.

All except five sets of parents (i.e. 54 families, 92%) gave information
on the people who had been supportive towards them at this time when
problems were developing, and on the nature of that support. Their
responses have been analysed using the framework of Lazarus and Folkman, sources of support being categorised as emotional, informational,
providing appraisal/esteem, and practical.[103] Exact numbers are of little
value in this context, since it is the contribution of each group which is of
real interest, rather than how many individuals identified a given action as
supportive. However, there was a remarkable concordance in the stories
parents recounted in relation to the type of support different groups had
provided.

# Professional support

## *Doctors*

The support that parents looked for from the medical staff was both infor-mational and emotional. All of the parents were dependent on the doctors for information about their baby. They wanted this to be clear, frank and direct, without false reassurances or confusing circumlocutions.

> He handled it remarkably well. I think that's a tribute to the man more than anything else. There was no flannel. He knew what our concerns were going to be, I think, before he started talking to us, even though he'd never met us before. He put it to us very, very straight, which meant that by the time we came back to see him [two days later] we were in a position to discuss what he wanted to discuss and I felt that he dealt with that very, very well. I found the honesty of [the neonatolo-gist] very helpful as well. I don't want anybody trying to beat around the bush or to be giving me any half-hearted waffle. He just came straight to the point really, but nicely. . . tell us what we really want to hear then fill in the rest later. It was almost in the first sentence, 'I'm very sorry but . . .' It was appreciated that it was quick, because if he'd said about five sen-tences and then [the bad news] it's almost like delaying the pain.
>
> (P18: parents of preterm baby)

The manner of the delivery of news was crucially important, and parents spoke warmly of the sympathy, kindness and genuine caring which many consultants demonstrated.

> [The neonatologist] had the knack of saying all the right things in the right way. He was reassuring without being over-reassuring. He was being factual without being cold. He had the knack just right. He left you with the impression that whether he saved [our baby] or not, no one else would have done a better job.
>
> (P27: father of baby with congenital anomaly)

> [The doctor who came with the transfer team] said, 'We've had a lot of problems' – when they were preparing [the baby] for transfer to [the study Unit]. He said, 'We lost him and had to bring him back. He haemor-rhaged. He's got blood in his lungs.' When they tried to transfer him [to the portable incubator] he took [this bleed]. Then he said, 'Oh, but he's not dead!' [I just gasped]. 'But,' he said, 'he is gravely ill, we only give him a 20% chance of survival. Would you like to get him christened?' I went, 'From a boy that was born 5 hours ago and I was told that was going to have a 98% chance of survival, you're just hitting me [with *this?*]' He just went on and on . . . [By contrast] in the [study Unit] every person you turned to was a really caring person. They spoke away to you. They

told you what things were. *He* just told you [the facts] and basically it all went over my head. He was using words [I just didn't understand]. You've got that much coming at you. It was just the way he put it.

(P56: father of preterm baby with congenital anomalies)

Compassion was expressed in many ways – showing emotion when imparting bad news, being available when the family needed him, making the parents feel that they were valued and equal members of the team, explaining patiently but not patronisingly over and over again what had happened (using diagrams, different illustrations or analogies, or concrete demonstrations of serious problems), reassuring the parents that everything possible had been done, gently guiding them (sometimes saying what he would do if it were his baby), and making the parents feel that both they and the baby were special. Individuals also identified specific extras. One consultant asked the mother each day how she thought her little girl was doing. Another doctor set daily goals for the parents to help them to cope at this difficult time. One set of parents were overwhelmed by the experience and welcomed the consultant 'drip-feeding' the information in instalments so that they took in the enormity gradually but correctly. One consultant warned the parents that they might blame themselves but that they should not to be frightened by this – it was a common reaction and the doctors would talk to them about it at the right time. The parents also appreciated consistency, with one or at most two key individuals keeping them informed.

## Nurses/midwives

The support of the neonatal nurses was enormously valued by all of the parents without exception.

It's just like a wee family [the staff in the Unit]. We had a wee bit of withdrawal symptoms, I feel, when we came home with Twin 1. I missed them terribly. [You're going through something very powerful with them] and it's something only they know what you're going through. ...We actually had some great laughs up there – some fun times and some hard times ... but it had to be like that. You need that [humour].

(P10: father of preterm twins)

[The staff] they were so nice ... In a day and a half you felt you had known them for years.

(P13: father of baby with cardiac anomaly)

A number of parents also spoke of the support offered by midwives in the labour ward and the postnatal wards. Some of them specified individuals staying on beyond their shift to offer ongoing comfort and care, freeing them from the necessity to start again and get to know new staff at a difficult time. For a number of parents their support was encapsulated in simple overarching expressions such as 'they were brilliant', 'they're all so kind'. However, others unravelled the experience and gave insights into what it was that constituted support. It was predominantly emotional and informational, but in addition it was practical and appraising.

**Emotional support** was highly valued. Nurses/midwives outside the NICU could show that they were understanding of the parents' trauma in many ways. Labour ward midwives demonstrated their sympathy by seeking information about the baby on their behalf early on, or by visiting the parents and/or the baby subsequently. Postnatal ward staff showed their support by helping the mother to mobilise quickly so that she could be with her baby, or by personally taking her to the NICU at the first opportunity. A referral hospital nurse could show her understanding by transferring the baby of a multiple birth back to the place where the siblings were, as soon as was practically possible, so that the parents were not divided in their loyalties.

In the NICU, the strongest sense which was conveyed was that the help provided by nurses centred on comfort and sensitive emotional support. This might be demonstrated in many ways – by hugging, encouraging the parents to talk about their mixed emotions, openly showing their own distress when things went wrong for the baby, and telephoning staff elsewhere to advise them that the mother would need extra support because of recent developments. During this difficult time relationships were built up which parents treasured. Many of them had been impressed that the staff cared for them as well as for the baby, being sympathetic to their needs and wishes as well as to the interests of the child. When the nurses called in to see the parents, even when they had moved on themselves, the parents were touched and felt that such behaviour underlined their genuine interest in the family. When they troubled to remember each family member's name and details, or found an opportunity to slip into the postnatal ward to talk to a father who was struggling with his emotions in a sideroom, or helped to keep the baby going one more day to avoid his death coinciding with another family event, this demonstrated a sensitive awareness of the effect on this particular person or family of living through this trauma. Parents were greatly helped by the respect and love which nurses showed for the babies in their care. Mothers greatly valued the empathy which prompted nurses to reassure them that they would take great care of the child in the parents' absence, or to accord the baby little dignities beyond the standard management of a sick neonate. Having relatively few staff to relate to was helpful.

When the nurses took a personal interest in grandparents and other relatives and how they were participating or coping, this gave the parents the sense that they as a family were special, respected and held in affection. Some parents described the kindness of nurses towards their other children, sending letters from the baby or encouraging them to become involved.

Nursing staff also provided **informational support**. The parents valued the 'interpreting' or 'mediating' service they could offer when the medical information was dense or complex. It helped to have the facts repeated in more understandable language, or simply reinforced by repetition. If the neonatal nurse was present when bad news was given, the parents could consult her for clarification of what had been said or meant. They appreciated a frankly honest approach to information giving from the nurses – a direct question deserved a direct answer. Evasion undermined confidence and trust. If any facts were being withheld, it made the parents wonder what else was being hidden from them. Continuity of people and consistency of information were valued.

**Practical support** by the nurses was also valued. This took different forms. Parents appreciated the providing of accommodation for themselves and sometimes other family members, easy telephone access, and the facilitation of privacy.

The fourth form of support was **appraising**. The parents' sense of self-esteem was enhanced if the nurses encouraged them to be involved with the baby, pointing out the uniqueness of parental love and touch and smell. Being accorded status as a parent helped to counter their feeling of overall helplessness.

### Chaplains
Two families included the chaplain in their list of supportive people. In one case he gave parents the strength to take control and play things their way. In the other he managed to be with the parents but not 'moralise', and they found his presence immensely comforting and reassuring.

One of the best folk was probably the minister. We're by no means church people. We're unreligious. We don't bother about it. My whole family's like that . . . he was a cracking guy, really, really nice. Basically he was probably like [my wife's] friend. He wasn't like family, too close. He wasn't a doctor that knew all about [the baby]. He just knew basically what was happening to us. So we could talk away to him about this, that and the next thing, about how we felt. It was better that he didn't understand what was happening to [the baby] either so you felt on a level with him. He said to us, 'I'm not going to get you praying or anything. I'm just here to talk to you if you want.' He was really nice. And he was somebody coming to see us who wasn't bringing bad news!

(P 56: father of preterm baby with congenital anomalies)

# Lay support

Although it was clear that the parents looked principally to the staff in the Units for support at this time, as problems developed and they started to face the possibility of a bleak outlook, some parents obtained additional support from lay people. This took the form of emotional or practical support.

## Family

Twelve sets of parents cited the baby's grandparents as being supportive at this stage. They were there for the parents, loving them and caring for them. Six sets of parents mentioned other family members who telephoned, visited or were just there for them. Sometimes, however, parents felt overwhelmed by the family, and the need to support them could add to their own burdens.

All the family were trying to comfort us both. It got a bit much having all the family there – it was too much trying to look after them and trying to deal with our own [the baby's] problems. My mother wanted to stay with me all the time – I just wanted everybody out the way. Trying to arrange accommodation and . . . it was all left to us. And our family were saying to us, 'Well, what do you want us to do? Do you want us to stay? Do you want us to go?' And we didn't need that pressure of having to make a decision for them. We had enough to cope with ourselves. So I told them all to go. I didn't want to but I had to, for our peace of mind and our sanity.

(P 9: parents of baby with cardiac anomaly)

## Friends

Friends supported a further 7 sets of parents. Their help included praying, sharing a common experience, taking a father out for a drink at the pub to give him relief from the hospital stay, and reassuring a father that even if his child was abnormal he would still be loved and valued.

### Colleagues and acquaintances

Work colleagues popped in and out for short visits to support one mother, and because they were healthcare professionals, she believed that they had been instrumental in getting her VIP treatment. One mother observed that during this difficult time neighbours rallied round to offer a variety of forms of support, and by their sensitivity and practical help converted themselves from neighbours into friends. Staff from the nursery which one sibling attended took the child whenever it could be helpful to the parents while they were grappling with the problems presented by the new baby.

# Discussion

Given the sad outcome for these families, it is tempting to try to address all areas of complaint in an effort to eliminate sources of dissatisfaction. However, such an attempt would prove futile. First, some things are just not possible. For example, diagnoses cannot always be made instantly – some emerge gradually, while others rely on tests which take time. Delays in communicating facts are sometimes inevitable if the results of tests are unavailable, specialists are being consulted, or the neonatologists are engaged with other pressing and equally legitimate work. Secondly, fixed practices cannot be applied when there is such an infinite variety of parental needs. One mother may want bad news in small doses, to give her space to accept the reality slowly, whereas another may prefer one sledgehammer blow to avoid the fear of worse to come. Judgements must be made which rely on subjective assessment and a degree of intuition. Not only will the perceptions of the parents and doctors be widely different and their personalities sometimes clash, but each individual is fallible and errors will sometimes occur. It is more profitable to extract general messages which provide a framework within which clinicians can strive for increased sensitivity.

The key factors which emerge from our study relate to communication and compassion.

# Communication

These parents are being told things which they do not want to hear. Is it possible to deliver such information in a way which parents will find satisfactory? Both the literature[40,104,105] and our findings suggest that it is.

The *process* can be distinguished from the *content* of the message. However, it must be remembered that the way in which the news is imparted is critical in the memories of parents.[40,53,106] It represents a sort of watershed, and is remembered vividly.

Many attempts have been made to provide insights and guidance into what constitutes good practice when bad news is being broken.[36,83,105–108] Certain elements are seen as fundamental:

- to be told as a matter of urgency after the diagnosis, preferably by a senior doctor who is fully informed about the case
- to be told in privacy, if possible with their partner or another person of their choice
- to hold the discussion without interruptions and with sufficient time available for an unhurried conversation
- to be given honest and direct information, in straightforward language, by someone who conveys understanding
- to have control over the amount of information given
- to have the opportunity in subsequent conversations to ask questions and have information repeated, and to discuss the future
- to have information about services and support available to them.

It might seem pointless to reiterate these points. However, the fact that there were still parents in the late 1990s who did not experience these circumstances indicates that these messages are not always remembered. For example, time and again the point has been reinforced that parents should be told together wherever possible. But practice has been slow to pick up on this need,[104] and in our own study it is sobering to find that many parents were alone when they were first given news of serious problems. In some circumstances, (e.g. when a mother is unconscious or a father is abroad), such a practice may be unavoidable, but a number of these parents perceived no reason for not waiting until the partner was present. The catalogue of suggested improvements outlined in this chapter provides clinicians with a salutary reminder that parents will probably always remember the way in which they were told, and their memories will be coloured by whether or not staff observed the 'rules' of good practice. The small numbers who registered dissatisfaction with specific practices serve to underline not only the idiosyncratic nature of each couple's experience, but also the need for individually tailored care. For example, the majority of parents seem to favour early imparting of information. However, a few feel that they only worry unnecessarily if they are party to all of the suspicions the doctors may have and all of the possible explanations for the problems. This reality has been identified elsewhere,[104] but the finding that it was applicable in this Scottish population emphasises the fact that these differences span cultures and policies.

# Compassion

When it comes to communicating with parents at such a time, it is important to bear in mind that not only is the news unwelcome, but the parents are often in a fragile emotional state themselves. They use different coping mechanisms to try to stay sane in a situation which seems to be spinning out of control. Some parents categorically deny the seriousness of the situation, some maintain an inappropriate level of hope, some become aggressive, and others withdraw and become difficult to reach. All of them require sensitive handling.

In a number of studies of bereaved parents communication has been found to be deficient,[45,109] and there is clearly still scope for improvement. The keys to success seem to hinge on empathic awareness. Being sensitive to parents' informational and emotional needs,[106,110] and a combination of humanity, accessibility and approachability with professional skill,[36,104] coupled, where possible, with a degree of intimacy,[36] are crucial elements in negotiating the necessary balance. The parents in our study repeatedly referred with appreciation and surprise to the kindness and compassion they had felt when the messages being delivered were so hard to hear. The overall context is one of excellence, they report. However, any impatient doctor or arrogant specialist, and any inflexible or indiscreet nurse, influences the experience of families and diminishes their perception of the service provided. A chain is only as strong as its weakest link.

Yet it must be remembered that much is being required of the medical teams at this point. The initial news often has to be broken at a time when the staff have only just met the parents or hardly know them. The doctor or nurse him- or herself may be disturbed by the events which have precipitated this crisis. Subjective assessments are required of how much to tell and how to tell it. Many variables in the lives and experiences of the staff themselves may influence their capacity to communicate effectively and sympathetically.[12] In reporting only the parents' perceptions we have been able to make allowance for none of these additional elements. Nevertheless, they should be recognised. In order to be affectively aware, doctors must be insightful into their own emotions as well as sensitive to parents' feelings. It is paradoxical that in circumstances of a poor prognosis, the success of a person's ability to communicate effectively may be contingent on his ability to tolerate medicine's failures. Professionals vary in their capacity to tolerate situations where continuing treatment seems inappropriate, and this might conceivably have influenced communication practices for the parents in the present study. Particular cases affect individual staff at different levels, and some are harder to bear than others. On occasion mistakes must be admitted and the consequences lived with. Yet each of the couples in our study required empathy and compassion, irrespective of what was going on in the life of the person communicating bad news.

Moreover, individual professionals do not operate in isolation. Not only do they work with parents, but they must also interact with colleagues in the NICU, obstetric colleagues, other specialists, and staff in other Units who refer patients to the NICU. Sometimes differences of opinion and practice may strain relationships, and deciding just what to tell families may demand special skills and diplomacy if parental trust and confidence are to be preserved.

As a result of studying the experiences of these 59 families in depth, we can conclude that hearing that things have gone badly wrong is a profoundly traumatic experience, and the way in which the news is broken has long-term consequences. Individual staff can learn, through the insights provided by these couples, lessons which add detail and specificity to the overarching guidelines that are already available to steer them towards good practice.

# Conclusion

- Parents need frank, honest, direct information.
- They need to have the seriousness of the situation reinforced – to offer false reassurances or to soften the news is not a long-term kindness.
- The approach should be one of compassion, respect and caring.
- Healthcare professionals are the major source of support at this time.

# CHAPTER 7

# Decision making

There came a point in the lives of each of the babies in this study when serious doubts arose as to the wisdom of treating further. Deciding when to withhold treatment is one of the most troubling issues in our Neonatal Units today. Just when such a decision should be made and who should accept responsibility for making it has taxed the minds of clinicians, philosophers and lawyers for decades. As Gorovitz put it:

> The decision to forgo life-sustaining treatment must surely be as hard as any that arises in a hospital or within a family. Principles to guide such a decision are elusive, because whenever the question arises, some of our most cherished values are in conflict. We believe in the value of life, but it is not clear that all life has value no matter what. We believe that suffering should be reduced, but sometimes that means shortening life. We believe that patients' wishes should be respected, but that seems not always best for patients. We want doctors to be stalwart champions of life, but we fear their capacity to impose continued life. We want to be able to say, of a single case, 'enough is enough,' yet we do not want to undermine the general respect for life that protects us all.[111]

It is important to emphasise from the outset the gravity of the decision for the families concerned. All of our respondents were traumatised by this experience.

> [To stop treating] was the right decision for [the baby's] sake. Because she was suffering. But I wish things could have been better because I was suffering too. And no mother or father wants to see somebody so delicate and frail go through something unnecessary... It was one catastrophic thing after the other. It couldn't get any worse.
>
> (P9: parents of baby with cardiac anomaly)

> [Making that decision] – it does feel like you're pulling the plug on your own child.
>
> (P2: father of baby with cardiac anomaly)

Furthermore, the decision was being made at a time when the parents were tired and emotionally drained.

> At the time you're so tired and confused that it's difficult to know what *is* the right decision.
>
> (P43: father of baby with congenital anomalies)

Parts of the decision making sometimes had long-term as well as immediate consequences. A first decision for one young couple related to whether or not to have a Caesarean Section. This teenage mother went into premature labour, and the cord prolapsed. She was rushed to theatre, but when she had been prepared and was about to have epidural anaesthesia started, the consultant obstetrician advised that it should not go ahead because she had had three Caesarean Sections already and the outlook for this baby was poor. Her existing children were by men other than her present partner. This was her third pregnancy with him, but they had no live children. Having a Section this time round would have meant that he would have no children with her because she would have been unable to have more. The father observed that he could not see how anyone in such an acute crisis could make such a momentous decision.

Although most parents were devastated by the prospect of the possible loss, for some there was an additional real fear – that the child would *not* die. The consequences of continued survival were more unacceptable than death.

> My greatest fear was always that she would actually get through [the withdrawal] and live – maybe extremely handicapped, in a vegetative state. So that was always at the back of my mind. The longer it went on the greater the possibility.
>
> (P46: mother of baby with asphyxia)

Other parents, having steeled themselves to make hard choices, feared that their courage might fail them at the last moment, so overwhelmed with sadness were they at the prospect of the child's death.

> Getting guidance from the medical staff is actually [really helpful]. This standing back and letting you make the decision puts such a weight of responsibility on to you. But I can understand why they do it. . . . Once they've sussed out what your general opinion is, they can then help you to stick to that. Because it would have been very easy for us in the emotion of the moment to say, 'No, no, forget everything I said before, I want my baby to survive at any cost.' Because when you're actually up against it and you're looking at your baby, you'd do anything. But if you've already stated something prior to that, you need somebody to help you stick to that.
>
> (P25: mother of preterm baby with asphyxia)

Conscious of the dilemmas and complexities of deciding on behalf of neonates, and having established the opinions of doctors and nurses in NICUs around the country,[12] we aimed to find out the nature of the parents' experiences of and opinions about decision making.

# Who first mentioned treatment limitation?

It was the parents who first brought up the subject of treatment limitation in the case of 10 families (17%). In two cases the parents initially broached the question with junior staff before mentioning it to senior medical staff. For the majority, however, it was the doctors who first raised the issue.

The initial discussion was with the consultant neonatologist for most of the parents (41, 71%). A specialist colleague (cardiologist, geneticist or consultant obstetrician) accompanied him in three instances. It was the specialist (paediatric surgeon or cardiologist) alone who mentioned withdrawing to a further three families (5%). The remaining five sets of parents (8%) were unable to identify the person who performed this task beyond saying that he was a junior doctor or one of the labour ward staff.

Just one person took responsibility for the task of discussing treatment limitation with about half of the parents (28, 47%), whilst for the other half (31, 53%) more than one person was involved at different points. Almost all discussions of this serious nature were with senior medical staff. Only one family recalled anyone other than a doctor imparting this information, and that one case involved an advanced nurse practitioner. Around 90% of doctors cited were consultant neonatologists or specialists, and the remaining 10% were junior or unknown grades.

# Personnel involved

Both partners were present for discussions of treatment limitation in the case of 43 couples (73%). For a further 12 couples (20%), discussions sometimes involved both of them, but on occasion only one was present. Given that parents sometimes visited the nursery alone and fathers went back to work sooner than mothers, this was seen by the parents to be quite understandable, and was even on occasion invited. Only one couple had nothing but separate discussions with the medical staff on the subject. Three mothers (5%) had their own parents present during discussions on this subject with the medical staff.

The majority of doctors were reported to have taken a neonatal nurse with them or had medical and/or nursing colleagues in the vicinity when such a discussion took place. Parents spoke warmly of the comfort of having the nurse's continuing care, and of the benefit of being able to talk to her subsequently about what had been said. However, in one Unit it was more common for parents to have discussions with only the consultant present than for there to be anyone else present. Most of these parents made no adverse comments about the practice. However, two parents did make strong critical comments about the doctors who were unaccompanied by a nurse. In one case the father felt intimidated by the pressure he perceived that the neonatologist was exerting to make him decide. In the other case the mother mistrusted the consultant, whom she perceived as defensive. Her unease was reinforced by a midwife whom she reported as telling her never again to have discussions with the doctors without a member of staff or her husband being present.

Four sets of parents (7%) had the baby's grandparents present when the first discussion occurred. In three of these cases the mothers were single women who looked to their own parents for support at this time. In another family, the child in question was several months old when the idea of stopping treatment was first raised, and the neonatologist suggested that the baby herself should be there at the discussion. For subsequent discussions, six families (10%) had involved other family members at some point, and again three of them were single mothers. Some families welcomed the presence of other relations to ask questions or simply to listen to the poor prognosis and confirm the parents' understanding of the futility of treatment.

# Setting for discussions

Such serious discussions were usually conducted in quiet places such as a special room or area in the NICU, or the mother's private postnatal room, and for 46 of the 59 sets of parents (78%) this was the case exclusively. However, at least some of the discussions were held beside the baby's incubator for 7 families (12%), sometimes with screens to suggest privacy, and sometimes in the open nursery. Rarely, early discussions took place in the antenatal ward or clinic, or in the labour ward.

# Timing of first mention

All except one set of parents clearly recalled the time when the idea of treatment limitation was first introduced. The couple who did not do so initially said that the idea of stopping treatment was never discussed because they made it clear from the outset that they wanted everything possible done for their child. The consultant evidently thought such discussion had taken place, since the parents were referred as eligible for the study. Significantly, when asked specifically how many times there was discussion about whether to treat the baby, the parents responded with 'several times.' Gentle probing elicited a picture of the parents repeatedly imploring the doctors to do everything they could to save the child, and of the doctors trying to convey the seriousness of the situation to parents who would not let themselves believe what was happening. They described nurses periodically asking whether they would like to hold the baby out of the incubator, but themselves being unwilling to do anything which might be harmful to the baby. As a result, the baby actually died on the machinery, to the evident distress of the parents, who felt that the last part of the procedure was rushed and frightening as alarms rang and staff scrambled to get the child into their arms to die.

In one other case the two parents themselves perceived events slightly differently. The father felt that, from the way the consultant talked to them about what had happened at his first meeting with them, he was really asking them to consider treatment limitation. The mother, on the other hand, thought that it was not until later that he broached the subject. They discussed the matter of their different perceptions at length during that time, but could come to no agreement.

For only a minority of parents was there any discussion about treatment limitation before birth. Only three sets of parents (5%) had talked with the paediatric staff in this way antenatally. In two cases it was the threat of preterm labour which prompted questioning about whether the parents would wish treatment to be started. The fetus in the third case was known to be congenitally malformed, and the parents had many discussions with the neonatologist about how appropriate it would be to initiate treatment when the child's life expectancy was short. In two of the three cases the decision was made to offer some treatment initially and to see what happened. One of these couples had decided after careful thought that it was important for them that the child should be born alive and given the chance to survive on his own. If he could not, the parents would have done all in their power for him, and would not then be burdened by self-reproach. In the third family – one involving delivery at 25 weeks – the parents and neonatologist agreed not to resuscitate. However, when the child was delivered, the neonatologist himself was not present, and the junior staff who were *did* resuscitate. The child lived for many hours – time which the parents subsequently said they were very grateful to have had.

An additional three sets of parents (5%) first discussed the possibility of treatment initiation and limitation during labour, in all cases preterm labour. In only one instance was this with the consultant neonatologist. In the other two, the parents did not know the doctor concerned but thought he was a junior member of staff.

For 52 of the 59 families (88%), however, the idea of possibly stopping treatment was first introduced after delivery. Timing of the first mention ranged from soon after delivery to eight months after birth (*see* Figure 7.1). For the majority of families (37, 63%) this occurred in the first week of life.

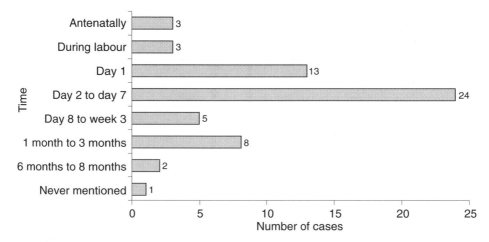

**Figure 7.1:**   Timing of first mention of treatment limitation ($n = 59$).

In the five cases (8%) where discussion was initiated soon after delivery, the gravity of the situation was clear to the parents as well as to the staff. Four of the babies were extremely preterm and in poor condition. The fifth child was severely asphyxiated, and the occupations and experience of this couple enabled them to understand the implications of what had happened during labour, when the cord had prolapsed and the monitor had shown prolonged severe fetal distress, and they both heard and understood the significance of information about absent reflexes and brain activity.

Three couples (5%) measured the time they first heard talk of possibly stopping treatment from the baby's death – 'just three days before he died' or 'not until the day he died.' In all cases these babies had lived for several months and the parents had become confident that they would live.

In two families (3%) where the first discussion took place at six months or later, the parents vividly described their sense of devastation. After so long it seemed incredible that suddenly they were hearing that there was no hope. Both babies were born very prematurely and both had numerous setbacks. But as they recovered from each problem and grew, the parents became increasingly convinced that they would live. One of the babies had a twin who also had problems but fought back each time, gradually growing stronger and surviving. The parents compared the progress of the two babies and felt sure that the second one would survive too.

# Times discussed

Twenty-one sets of parents (36%) could remember having just one discussion about treatment withdrawal. However, 10 of these families commented that following this discussion they were given daily updates which served to keep them in touch with the doctors' assessment of the baby's condition, with any changes and medical thoughts on the evolving situation. For 38 sets of parents (64%) there was more than one discussion about treatment limitation. Twenty-three sets of parents (39%) clearly recalled two discussions, and seven more (12%) remembered from three to five such sessions where the specific issue was brought up. The remaining eight sets of parents (14%) could not put a figure on the number of discussions, but remembered 'several' or 'lots.'

The time interval between the first and last discussions ranged from a few hours ($n = 16$) through a couple of days ($n = 11$) to a matter of weeks ($n = 11$), with one set of parents having repeated discussions over some 14 weeks.

# Initial information

The parents gave graphic accounts of what they were told when treatment withdrawal was first discussed. Clearly the encounters were etched on their memories, and it is important to remember that the messages were painful for them to hear.

> I actually took to hiding from them because I thought every time I speak to them they've got bad news. So I just took to avoiding them. If I saw them coming close I would just take off in the other direction because I didn't want to hear what they were going to say.
>
> (P 56, mother of preterm baby with congenital anomalies)

In most instances the parents recalled being given detailed descriptions of exactly what had happened to the baby. The accounts were sometimes backed up with diagrams or concrete evidence in the form of scans, X-rays or demonstrations of lack of reflex activity.

More than half of the sets of parents (32, 54%) recalled specifically being told that the baby would not live, or that there was nothing more that could be done to save the child's life. Where they could actually see visible deterioration, such as spreading gangrene or convulsions, it was easier for parents to appreciate the worsening situation. But where the decision related to the damage which they could not see, to brain or lungs or intestines, information had to be taken on trust. Parents were reliant on medical experts telling them about the probable outcome, often in terms of the quality of life to be expected. They were very aware that the facts given represented probabilities rather than certainties. Furthermore, some felt that, because they were clutching at hope, it was difficult for them to assimilate the information rationally.

A number of elements could be identified from the parents' descriptions of what was said. Sometimes they heard a definite recommendation from the doctor – that it would be best to let the child go, that surgery was too risky, or that the child should be given a chance meantime. More often the facts were explained, the futility of treatment was spelled out, and the parents were asked what they thought about possibly stopping. Some doctors used certain expressions to convey the bleakness of the outcome: 'We can't see a light at the end of the tunnel,' 'We must question the wisdom of continuing,' 'If this was my baby, I would let him go.' Many parents commented that those precise words, gentle but conveying a powerful and understandable message, would always remain with them.

Having the alternatives clearly spelled out provided something for parents to latch on to. Knowing that by going for option A they ran the risk of the baby dying without them in attendance in an ambulance *en route* to a distant hospital specialising in complex heart surgery, and that by taking option B they were going to put their baby through four operations, all of which carried a high risk of mortality or morbidity, and that the quality of his life in the interim would be poor, helped them to weigh up the relative merits of pursuing treatment or choosing option C – allowing a peaceful and pain-free death.

Inevitably the circumstances in which such decisions were discussed varied. Timing was one such factor. In a few cases parents reported that they themselves were requesting a rapid cessation of treatment but the doctor was seen to put brakes on the process. Two mothers reported anger at such a delay – why had the consultant mentioned stopping if he then recommended a wait-and-see policy? A few parents recounted several sessions where the consultant checked whether they were still of the same opinion. In other cases it was the parents who initiated delays; they requested one more day with the baby, or that the death was not arranged for a day with other family associations.

Sometimes the comments indicated that the parents should take their time to consider the decision and not feel pressured to commit themselves instantly. In other circumstances, however, time was not available for such a gentle approach to the final decision. Consultants had to reinforce the need to decide fairly quickly in case the baby died unexpectedly or when the parents were absent. A few parents described the irritation they felt at the time when pressure of this kind was exerted, even though with hindsight they could understand why it had happened. In about a quarter of the families the baby suddenly deteriorated, and either the staff or the parents seized the opportunity to say it was now time to stop treatment. In such cases parents were spared lengthy agonising before the death, but they sometimes questioned the decision subsequently.

Perceived rushed decisions could engender later doubts. The day after a surgical procedure one baby aged six and a half months deteriorated. The parents were requested to come into the Unit urgently, and were then told that it was only a question of time, but the child would die. They were offered two alternatives – either to withdraw treatment at once or to let the baby linger and die in an undignified manner. In all the months of progress and setbacks, they had never thought the baby might die. Faced with this stark choice, they decided that an unpleasant death was so abhorrent that they should agree to stopping treatment immediately. They subsequently regretted the decision profoundly. As the father explained, they could now never be sure that the prognosis was right. It would have been better to wait long enough for the parents themselves to see that the baby was slipping away. They would then have known that they had made the right decision.

> They should have given us more time. [We could have then have had a chance] just to see. It might have been a day – another day. He might have slipped away himself. We don't know. I'll never know. But they could have come back in another couple of days and said, 'Look, he is slipping away.' But we'd have seen it more ourselves. Then we'd have known.
>
> (P 34: father of preterm baby)

Where the idea of the baby possibly dying was new, having space to absorb the reality was important. It gave parents the opportunity to talk together in private, although not all couples found that specific discussion at this point was necessary, since they knew each other's views already.

Where the decision hinged on future quality of life rather than on the futility of further treatment, parents noted that other tactics were adopted. Being told that the medical team would watch and see what happened over the next hours or days reassured parents that a solid picture was being built up and no hasty decisions were being acted upon. Being given time to consider, but also concrete yardsticks by which to measure the gravity of the situation and the veracity of the doctors' diagnosis, was helpful. For example, knowing that there was just one more avenue to pursue, but if the baby did not respond then there was nothing else to try, or hearing that if the child did not rally in the next three hours the outlook was very grave. The vulnerability of and burden on the baby was underlined. It was similarly constructive when parents were given a sense of staged decisions: 'We'll continue to treat just now, but if the baby develops an infection we'll talk again about the wisdom of continuing.'

Practice varied when it came to prediction. It is clearly not a simple matter to estimate when a sick child will die. Some doctors made no such attempt. Parents were confused if assessments were given which subsequently proved to be wrong. To be told that their baby would not last the night put pressure on them to decide. If they delayed deciding, but the baby was still alive in the morning, their confidence in the medical foundation for stopping treatment was undermined. If the doctors were wrong on the question of how near to death the baby was, were they wrong in saying he just could not survive with such major impairments?

Rarely (in only two couples) the mother and father each perceived the messages that were given differently. The significance of this is best illustrated with reference to one of these couples, where the father believed that the doctor was asking them if he should help the child to die, whereas the mother thought he was telling them it was just a matter of time. This couple had strong views on what should happen. For the father, the worst scenario was that the baby should live with severe damage, and his greatest fear was that there might be no opportunity to allow the child to die. He deliberately distanced himself from becoming emotionally involved with the little boy until he knew death was inevitable. The mother, on the other hand, was involved and was comforted by doing 'mothering' tasks and expressing milk for him. Although she, too, intellectually believed that death was the best option for the baby, emotionally her instinct was to fight for his survival and she felt guilty for not wanting him to die. After the discussion they talked at length together about what had been said, but could reach no agreed understanding. Although they were a highly articulate couple, they were reluctant to ask the consultant for clarification of what he had actually meant in case they betrayed their 'anxiety to have him killed.'

# Subsequent information

As we have seen, 64% of the parents recalled more than one discussion about treatment limitation. In second and subsequent discussions about treatment withdrawal, the overwhelming emphasis was on the deterioration and damage incurred. Evidence of impending death, and the risk of the baby dying without the parents present, was pointed out. By this stage, parents were being encouraged to say when they were ready for treatment to be stopped, sometimes with a recommendation that that time had come.

# Conflicting messages

Clearly where more than one person is involved in imparting information there is a potential for conflicting messages. In considering sources of such conflict, it is necessary to bear in mind the fact that the parents themselves were often hoping against hope for a good outcome, or were sometimes in denial about what was happening.

> You kept on hoping. You'd go in and there'd be a dramatic change. And when you were in [with the baby] you kept on thinking, maybe he'll prove them all wrong. And because [just two months] before he'd been so well, you thought, 'Well, you never know' . . . I couldn't just have said, 'Let him go.' At the back of your mind you're thinking, 'He might just (pull round)' – a miracle or something. Because we'd seen him getting better. It's just something that you hoped would happen. That was the biggest thing – that he'd kept on going.
>
> (P19: parents of preterm twins)

> They'd always been giving us all the information and . . . they told you statistically the chances of survival, and as she was going through everything, we were warned that she would have problems with her breathing and that came about a week later than they said it would. OK, it was a fright but once you got over that, you wait for the next thing coming. And we just went on like that. So whenever I got called into the doctor's office, you always felt they were trying to put a downer on it almost. You were being so positive and upbeat about it – but you had to be, there was no other way that you could [deal with] it. Plus the fact that she fought everything anyway . . . you just thought, she's special she's going to go through it. Even just coming off the ventilator so quickly. So really it wasn't until after the operation he called us in and said, 'The next couple of hours are critical'. I was a bit worried at that point but I thought, 'No, she's going to get through it.' And then he called us in and said, 'We could lose her within the next hour' . . . at that point, that's when it was just a total shock. Both of us [realised there was no hope] at the same point, I think . . . but when we woke up in the morning, OK you're worried, but you just automatically thought, 'Yes it's OK, she's going to be fine. She'll get through it. It's just another of these things.' All we could think of was the scar [from the surgery] – what would the scar be like on her when she was older? . . . In your mind is that she's a wee fighter and you just expect that things are going to be OK.
>
> (P58: father of preterm baby)

> I didn't want to open the incubator because I was worried about infection. I still thought they were going to survive, you see. So I couldn't

touch them in the incubator because I thought all the heat is going to come out. I was worried, so I went home again . . . At the time I thought [I must protect them from cold and infection] but in retrospect I thought, well, if I knew that [Twin 1] would be switched off because of the cerebral haemorrhages [and] we'd made the decision and there was no going back on that, why was I worried about infection and letting the heat out of the incubator? And the only thing I can think of is that [I was in denial]: no, it's not going to happen. Or [perhaps I was] not even thinking about it. [So I was] still worrying about them, still caring about them and not wanting to touch them.

(P 33: mother of preterm twins)

Twenty-five sets of parents (42%) reported some tension in this area. For 14 families (24%) this was perceived as relatively minor. It arose in a variety of ways: an unclear picture in the early stages; a lack of knowledge in the local hospital which did not match the facts given by the experts in the study hospital backed up with sophisticated test results; or obstetric staff giving information which did not tie in with the paediatric picture.

However, for 11 families (19%) the perceived discrepancies were more serious, and some continued to feel great anger about the experience more than a year on. In recounting sources of conflict, a few parents commented that, to be fair, they must stress that with hindsight they were conscious that a level of confusion was understandable and possibly inevitable in their case. For example, where the condition of the baby was so rare, or the true picture emerged so gradually that no one could have been expected to diagnose it instantly, some confusion was unavoidable while tests were carried out or until time revealed the extent of the damage. Others volunteered that in their case it was probably their own lack of understanding, or their blocking of bad news, that caused the misunderstanding, rather than conflicting messages actually having been given by the staff.

The most commonly cited form of conflict arose from one person giving a better prognosis than another. Sometimes this spanned departments – for example, an ultrasonographer pronouncing an antenatal scan as normal, and a heart specialist saying that it showed an anomaly. Sometimes it crossed grades – a neonatal nurse giving false reassurances while the consultant gave a bleak prognosis, or a junior paediatrician telling parents a scan showed no deterioration when the consultant said it actually showed the reverse. On rare occasions genuine mistakes were made and individuals apologised – for example, one junior doctor misreading a test result and giving a good report when in reality the result showed a major problem. Where the conflict arose from differing messages from senior figures, parents seemed more upset than where juniors did not get things quite right – for example, a neonatologist saying a baby with necrotising enterocolitis (NEC) was doing well, and the paediatric surgeon telling the parents that the bowel was now irreparable.

In a small number of cases the conflict arose from the parents being given a wrong diagnosis – for example, a junior paediatrician diagnosing a simple treatable chest infection and the consultant neonatologist later saying it was a serious cardiac problem, or a consultant telling the parents that a baby had a relatively minor problem and a different consultant subsequently telling them that it was an untreatable and inevitably fatal syndrome. Similarly, an emerging diagnosis could engender a high level of confusion for parents as they assimilated each piece of information, only to have to revise their picture repeatedly.

False hope was another form of conflict which was universally perceived by parents as distressing. Although they might dread the approach of the neonatologist, they appreciated absolute honesty in the imparting of information. Unless he was totally frank with them they could not trust him. It troubled them when the consultants seemed to so sanitise their message that they were unaware of the enormity of the problem, or when nurses spoke of autopsy before the consultants had broached the subject of death. A similar level of honesty was required from all other grades, and parents found it upsetting when nurses tried to offer hope or reassurance when the family were struggling to take on board the clear messages from the neonatologist or specialist that the situation was very grave.

# The decision makers

The question of who, in the parents' perceptions, made the decision is such an important one that the results are presented in two ways. First we shall give the 'family' view and then the individual parents' opinions.

When the responses of all of the parents were combined, 25 of the 59 sets of parents (42%) believed that they were the ones who actually made the decision to stop treatment, with individual parents in four families (7%) adding that it was they alone and not their partner who had shouldered the responsibility. A number of parents spontaneously observed that it was part of parental responsibility to make decisions on behalf of one's child and, unpalatable though this one might be, it was still something they must do. It is important to emphasise, however, that no parent gave an impression of being abandoned or left to make this crucial decision alone. In all cases they perceived the medical professionals as giving them information to inform their choices, or guiding them, recommending on occasion, and sometimes confirming that they were making the right decision. One couple commented that it had been the doctors who gave them both permission and the opportunity to make this decision. More than one family felt that it would be easy for the parents to 'be selfish' and want to hang on to the live child, without fully taking into account the consequences for the baby: it required calm objective clinical decision-making to help them to guard against that. As it was, a small number of parents reflected with hindsight that they had perhaps added to the baby's suffering by not having the strength to make the decision sooner.

Six families (10%) believed that the decision was a joint one shared between themselves and the doctors. This has been differentiated from the earlier group, since the *actual decision* was seen to be shared rather than the *process* of decision-making. One family discussed with the interviewer the difficulties which might have arisen if they and the doctors had disagreed. They thought that they would have made strenuous efforts to 'hammer out an agreement' and, if that had failed, gone for outside independent arbitration. For them neither side had the casting vote.

In 18 cases (31%) the parents believed that the doctors had made the decision. Again this bald statement requires qualification. The majority of parents described a mutual give and take of information and cues, and some specifically added that the doctors were looking to them to give some indication of their own preferences and opinions. Many drew attention to the reality of the situation: it was the doctors who had the knowledge and experience, and the parents had little choice but to trust their ability to make a sound assessment. Two families added a rider that the medical staff had taken them, the parents, along with them as they came to this conclusion. A further two families said that the doctors had only been able to make the decision because they had established the parents' views beforehand. In four cases, although the doctors decided to stop treatment, it was the parents who decided when this should happen. One father would have preferred to make the decision himself, but since he was not in possession of enough facts and knowledge to do so, he felt that he had no choice but to leave it to those with the necessary experience and expertise. Time was against him in this, since rapid decisions were required in their case and he had insufficient time to search the Internet to obtain the facts he felt he needed.

Five sets of parents (8%) said that, although they had discussed withdrawal, it was the baby who actually decided because he had given up the fight. In cases where the baby deteriorated and death became imminent and inevitable, parents often interpreted this as the child telling them that he had had enough. Doctors sometimes used these terms to pave the way to stopping treatment earlier on, rather than continuing to wait and see. In one case, aggressive treatment was offered until the end as the parents wished.

The remaining four couples (7%) were divided in their understanding of who had made the decision. In each case the fathers thought that the parents had taken responsibility to some extent (in three cases jointly with the doctors), but the mothers all said that they had not. Three of the mothers felt that it had been the doctors who had decided, and the fourth mother thought that there had been no decision, but that the baby had resolved things by dying.

These figures represent 'family' responses. On this crucial matter, however – the question of who they thought had decided – each parent was specifically asked for their personal opinion. It appeared that in these circumstances consultants could sometimes manage to make both parents feel that there were different decision makers but both feel at ease with the situation. In one such family the mother was adamant that she could not make that decision, and even on the morning scheduled for treatment withdrawal she was still saying she could not go through with it. She believed that the doctor decided, whereas the father believed that the parents and doctor decided together. Both were satisfied. In another case, the father made a decision right away that it was not fair on the baby to resuscitate her repeatedly, and that she should be allowed to go. However, the mother was 'obsessed' with a need to cuddle her first. Once the baby was in her arms she then said not to reconnect the ventilator because she wanted to hold her as a normal baby. The child died within seconds. Both parents felt they had personally made the decision, but at different points.

At the first interview two fathers and one mother were not available to be asked who had decided. A further two mothers could not say who decided – one because she had been 'out of it' following surgery at the time, and the other because she was unsure who had decided. The remaining 103 parents gave an opinion, and Figure 7.2 shows the distribution of their responses. (Percentages are given as for all 108 parents.) Sixty parents (56%) believed that they had decided, 45 parents (42%) seeing this as their

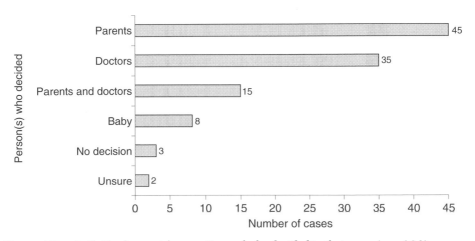

**Figure 7.2:**  Individual parents' perceptions of who decided in their case ($n = 103$).

decision alone and 15 parents (14%) seeing it as a joint decision between them and the doctors. For 35 parents (32%) the decision was seen to have been a medical one, and 8 parents (7%) believed that the baby had decided.

In each of the Units there was a mix of parents' opinions about who decided. However, when the parents were divided by Unit, noteworthy differences emerged (*see* Figure 7.3). Given the difference in numbers recruited from the three Units, comparative percentages rather than raw numbers give a better sense of the practices within the three Units. On a proportional basis, therefore, ten times the number of parents in Unit 1 felt that they had made the decision compared to parents in Unit 3. At least twice as many parents in Units 2 and 3 felt that the doctors took responsibility for the decision compared to parents in Unit 1. Far more parents in Unit 3 than in either of the other Units were left with a sense that it had been a joint decision.

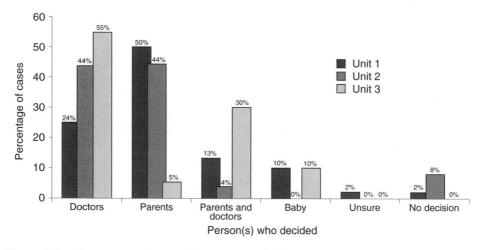

**Figure 7.3:**   Comparison of parents' perceptions of who decided in the three study Units.

When the practices of individual lead neonatologists were examined as they were perceived by the parents, it was interesting to note that some almost exclusively made the decision feel like a matter of parental responsibility, while others almost always kept it within the medical domain. In reality, however, the parents did not experience it in this polarised way, and others suspected that a degree of manipulation went on.

They make you feel like that is what they've done for you – [let you decide] – but it's not, it's done in a sort of roundabout way . . . It makes you *feel* like you've made the final choice but you haven't made the final choice.

(P42: mother of baby with brain damage)

Where the parents felt that they had personally decided, they saw the doctors as guiding, supporting and recommending appropriate courses of action for them to take. Where in their judgement the doctors made the final decision, they perceived them to be listening carefully to the family's views in balancing the factors and sometimes negotiating the decision with them.

# Did the right person make the decision?

Perhaps more important than the identity of the responsible agent was the question of whether parents were satisfied that the right person had made this decision. Parents of all persuasions could justify their opinions. For some it was indisputably a parental decision.

> I think it's our *right* [to decide]. Although having said that, the doctor's there to advise. But I think it should be [us] . . . Fair enough we never ever got her out of hospital, but she was *our* wee girl.
>
> (P10: father of preterm twins)

> We believe that the responsibility is ours. We made the [babies]. Therefore the responsibility for them starts that day.
>
> (P32: parents of preterm baby)

> I said, 'If it is this [rare condition] then I can't stand [the baby] going through any more pain and I want the machines turned off.' Because it was my decision. That was the only time I had ever got to make [a decision] about her future, and I knew that would be the right one because she had been through so much pain . . . it was my daughter, and it was my daughter's future. The hospital just did not seem to understand that at all. It was like that was their property, and whatever they said had to be done.
>
> (P31: mother of baby with congenital anomalies)

Nevertheless they welcomed confirmation that what they were choosing was an appropriate course of action.

> In a way you want them to make the decision for you, but now looking back on it I'm glad it was our decision. Then you've got nothing to blame anybody else for. But I do think you need some kind of positive guidance. [If there is no guidance one way or the other] I find that really difficult. I'm really intimidated. So the fact that we did get very positive guidance from [the neonatologist] I think is good. He gave us positive guidance and then left the decision in our hands, so it was a bit of both.
>
> (P25: mother of preterm baby with asphyxia)

He [the consultant] agreed. He thought I was making the right decision. I think he was glad that we had done that because ... he's the man in the know. He knows there's something not right there. I know I valued his expertise. They were his babies up there and he would do anything for them. And he knew deep down that there wasn't much hope.

(P10: mother of preterm twins)

Sometimes just a look or a shake of the head from the consultant was enough to confirm the parents in their decision. He did not always need to spell out his agreement.

Fathers in particular recognised the potential for allowing emotion to cloud their judgement. Some spoke of a need to remain detached until, as one put it, 'unpalatable decisions had been made.'

What actually went through my mind when [my wife was] still in the hospital and all this was going on, I'm thinking to myself, 'What would I do? Supposing he's dreadfully brain-damaged and just has a completely intolerable disability and they give us this wee boy home from the hospital, what would I do?' And I actually thought to myself, 'Would I have the guts to put a pillow over his face? Would I do that?' I couldn't answer it. But I mean, the fact that I even thought about that, that's how far I was thinking about all of this. What happened in the event was actually very easy compared to what I had contemplated. I'm one of nature's pessimists and from the word go I was worried he'd end up brain-damaged ... it was just something that entered my head. The fact that it entered my head I think is pretty extraordinary ... you need to be clear-headed about it to think what you're doing, but the trigger for doing it would be some emotional thing where you just got to the point where – if people do that to their relatives – they're actually at the end of their tether or they [can't deal any longer] watching the suffering of someone [close].

(P18: father of preterm baby)

For other parents it was a decision best left to the doctors. They recognised that parental interests might compete with the baby's interests.

If it was up to the parents, I'm sure most parents would feel like us that you would do everything and anything to keep your child alive. But that's because it's your child. And that's a very selfish point of view because that little baby – what are you going to put him through? [Our baby] could not have lived no matter what and we could have dragged that out for days. And I think that the paediatrician when he took a judgement there, not only spared [the baby] but he spared us as well.

(P50: mother of baby with congenital anomalies)

Doctors had the knowledge and experience to be able to decide for them.

> Leave it to the doctors. Take their advice, because at the end of the day you put that life in their hands, presuming that they know best, that they know everything. Which they do – of course they do.
>
> (P19: parents of preterm twins)

Even so, the task was not an easy one.

> When [the consultant] came to tell us about [the brain damage and the bleak outlook] I remember thinking, 'I wouldn't have your job for all the money they could give me. I hope they pay you a lot!' It must be so hard for them to admit failure.
>
> (P18: mother of preterm baby)

However, for a parent the burden could be heavy indeed.

> If you don't take the decision, you cannot take the wrong decision.
>
> (P17: mother of preterm baby)

> [We didn't want to make that decision] because that would be a decision we'd have to live with for the rest of our lives – thinking that we'd just given up on her.
>
> (P9: mother of baby with cardiac anomaly)

Still other parents felt that the baby was the best person to decide.

> I went over and I spoke to her. I wasn't bothering about anybody else. I just spoke to my girl. And she opened her eyes up, and [the nurse] said, 'She has not opened her eyes all night. The first time she's opened her eyes is to *you* this morning.' And I was chatting away to her and she was looking at me and it was like she was saying, 'Let me go. I've had enough.' I definitely felt she was pleading with me to let her go. But I couldn't. I couldn't do it – not there and then. I had to speak to her and that . . . I think she did make the decision. If her heart hadn't slowed down, the decision was to go on . . . because that would be her decision – I felt anyway. It was just something [the consultant] said to me and it always stuck up there [in my head] the day he said it with the first infection, he said, 'Her heart's still strong. As long as her heart's going as strong as that we'll keep fighting.' And that's what stuck in my mind to the day that she died. When her heart slowed, it wasn't functioning, and I thought, 'Right, I know it's not functioning right, that's her telling us' . . . it was her decision.
>
> (P10: mother of preterm twins)

Given all of these justifications, did parents feel that the right person had decided in their case? A breakdown by family revealed that, of the

59 families, 49 (83%) thought that the right person had decided, seven (12%) were unsure, and three (5%) thought that it was not the right person.

For the majority (83%) it had been the right person. A number of parents spontaneously commented on their confidence in the decision.

> I had no doubts. I wouldn't have done it [said to let him go] if I'd had any doubts. If the doctor had thought we were making the wrong decision, they would have given us more information to say, 'Well, maybe you are [making the wrong decision], but everyone was in total agreement with us. So I didn't doubt myself anyway, but nobody else did either. The people who knew the situation thought we were doing the right thing, too. So that made it easier.
>
> (P4: mother of preterm baby)

> I believe there was negligence there [at his birth] and I believe it was *that* that killed [our baby], so I have a clear conscience on [the decision to stop treatment later on].
>
> (P20: father of baby with asphyxia)

> I had asked [another paediatric consultant from the Unit] a few weeks ago, if he still believed in his heart that we had done the right thing, and he said yes, he had never doubted it. When you hear something like that, it does make me feel better knowing that people a lot more experienced than me can say we did do the right thing.
>
> (P20: mother of baby with asphyxia)

Two of the families who felt that it had been right that they – the parents – made the decision qualified their response. One of these families said that at the time they had very much wanted the doctors to decide, but now they felt that it had been right that they shouldered the responsibility themselves. The other couple added that they had only been in a position to make that decision because they had been given full information on which to base their assessment.

Seven families were unsure whether the right person had taken responsibility. In four of these families the parents felt that the decision had been theirs. In the other three cases all of the mothers and two of the three fathers thought that the baby had decided, while one father felt that it had been a joint decision between the parents and the doctors. Their uncertainty about the rightness of the decision stemmed from a variety of sources. For one couple it was a matter of general ambivalence; they could not say whether they had been the right people to make the decision to stop treatment, because the baby had just deteriorated and died anyway, and they could only hope that it had been right for them to state their preference. For two families the nature of the baby's death made them question things. In one case they said that if they had known the baby would definitely die they would have preferred the doctors to orchestrate a peaceful death, but the father knew that he could not himself have made the decision to stop treatment. Another set of parents believed theoretically that they were the only ones who had the right to say treatment should be stopped, but the father thought that it was much better if the doctors decided because the burden was too great for parents to carry. In one family where the parents had insisted on aggressive treatment until the end, the mother was left unsure of the wisdom of what happened. She felt that the baby had made the decision but it had been an unpleasant experience. Even so, she felt that it was probably best if the parents did not say that treatment should stop.

For only three families (5%) had it definitely been the wrong person making the decision. In one family the parents had taken that responsibility but they subsequently felt that it would have been better if the doctors had advised discontinuation of treatment, giving a list of reasons why they should stop. In a second instance the doctors had decided but the parents regretted the way in which things were protracted, and felt that if they had been in control themselves they would not have let the child linger for so long. The third family were simultaneously grappling with many other problems. Social workers were involved with them in relation to other children, and the father believed that these social workers were in league with the doctors and they had together decided to end the child's life. These parents were insistent that only the parents had the right to determine what happened to their children, whether it be where they lived or indeed *whether* they lived.

Of the 60 parents who felt that they had decided, only one father said that it had been too burdensome a responsibility, and even he believed that, despite his personal experience, it should be a parental decision. Only one mother said that she carried a heavy burden of guilt about the decision and she believed that the doctors had actually decided for her baby. Her partner did not share her guilt.

We put her in the wee Moses basket to go down to the mortuary and I just sat and looked at her. She looked like she was sleeping and I thought she'll be happy now. But that's when the guilt started. Because I looked at her in that Moses basket and I thought, 'I've put you there' ... We arranged her funeral. I darted about: I registered her dead and everything like that. I had to go up to the hospital to get the death certificate and I can remember walking into SCBU thinking, 'Oh no! They'll all be looking at me. I bet they're saying, "There she is, she killed her child."' And I can't get rid of that even yet.

(P36: mother of preterm baby)

# The extent of parental involvement

The parents were asked to expand on their perception of their involvement in the decision-making process. All except one couple could outline their roles to some degree. Two main activities emerged, namely participating in discussion about the decision (ranging from general participation in such discussion, through giving the doctors a sense of what they thought, to actually deciding what would be best for the baby) and determining the timing of the withdrawal of the treatment. All felt that they had been participants in the discussion, and 10 parents (17%) felt that they had decided the time of cessation of treatment.

> They had cornered us off, still in Intensive Care with screens round us. One of the two of them put her in my arms and they said that they were going to [reconnect] the ventilator and I said, 'No, I don't want to hold her with the ventilator.' And that's when *I* made the decision. They thought they were going to ventilate her to let my Mum see her, but I thought, 'No way, I'm not wanting that. I want her to die with dignity, I don't want her to die with a ventilator stuck down her throat'...When they took the ventilator away and [the consultant] looked at me and said, 'Are you sure? Are you sure this is what you want?' I said, 'I want her off the ventilator. I want to hold her. I want to kiss her without anything stuck down her throat.' And of course she could have slipped away on the ventilator and I didn't want that. I wanted her to open her eyes to me and she did . . . I just wanted her all to myself.
>
>                                                      (P10: mother of preterm twins)

However, a small number of parents (four sets) felt that their role had been limited by the circumstance of the baby deteriorating and dying before they could commit themselves, and in the case of a further two couples, although they *had* decided what to do, the baby deteriorated and this made their decision superfluous.

# Satisfaction with the limits of parental involvement

Decision making was a profoundly upsetting experience for parents. Analysis of their role in it prompted a small number of fathers to admit to being shocked to find that they did not want a child with severe disabilities. One mother said that she was appalled to find herself thinking it would be better that the child was dead. Others had hard questions to ask themselves. One father who had been brought up as a devout Catholic had a 'knee-jerk reaction' against the idea of stopping treatment. He admitted to being shocked at the suggestion that treatment might be withdrawn. But as the child's deterioration became more evident he concluded that careful withdrawal at that stage might be better than the alternatives.

> It was clear to me by that stage that he was going to die. I remember thinking, 'How would I prefer that he dies? Would I prefer that he dies in our arms or would I prefer to be woken up at 3 in the morning to be told that he's now died?' So I thought the former's preferable. The idea of switching off was almost abhorrent to me just instinctively, but then as I sat down and considered the alternatives, once I'd accepted that he was going to die – and I think [the neonatologist] had actually said that it was likely that he'd die within the next 12 hours ... and I remember thinking, 'So that will mean they'll probably be waking us up and telling us he has now died.' That's even worse – just leaving him and off we go and get some sleep and let him die – wake us up when it's all over, sort of thing. I thought that's even more abhorrent.
>
> (P27: father of baby with cardiac anomaly)

Three-quarters of the families (44, 75%) were satisfied that they had been sufficiently involved in the decision making, six (10%) were unsure and nine (15%) said that it had been unsatisfactory. Among the 44 families who had no complaints were both families who felt that they had made the decision themselves and those who believed that the doctors had taken responsibility. Some parents usefully qualified their responses. Five families found reassurance in the fact that everyone was in agreement and things worked out as planned. One couple was horrified at the very thought of being active in the decision-making process and only too glad to leave it to the doctors, whereas another couple believed that it was only by taking responsibility for the decision making that they were able to come to terms with what happened. Yet another couple observed that it was the parents who would have to bear the consequences in years to come, so it had to be their decision. For two families the degree of involvement had been right, because in the end the child had just died and they were spared the burden of deciding.

However, for the remaining 15 families who had reservations, things were not so clear-cut. Six families (10%) expressed uncertainty about their own involvement. Again there was a mix of parents who felt that they had made the decision themselves ($n = 2$), those who believed the doctors had done so ($n = 2$), one for whom it had been a joint decision ($n = 1$), and a family who believed the baby had decided ($n = 1$). The one family who felt that they would have welcomed greater involvement gave as their reasons for being unsure at the time that they had felt they had insufficient information upon which to base an informed choice, but they now felt that the decision was part of parental responsibility. One of the two families who wanted less responsibility believed they would have felt better about their involvement if they had had medical confirmation that they were doing the right thing. The other couple commented that, although they had not wanted to make the decision at the time, seeing it as a burdensome responsibility for parents, in retrospect they thought that it was right that they were asked to do so.

Three families did not indicate in which direction the burden of decision making should have gone. Their uncertainties reflected a sense that so much of the decision making was out of their hands and their experience was limited, so they really could not say with any conviction how much responsibility they would have wished to carry.

Nine sets of parents (15%) said that the balance of responsibility had definitely not been right for them. Of these, four families had made the decision themselves. Their reasons for not being entirely happy with their part in this were that they regretted not receiving reassurance from the doctors that they had made the right decision, they wanted to be able to blame the doctors, there was too little time to reflect, and they were insufficiently well informed to have taken such a momentous decision.

The doctors had taken the decision in four other cases. These parents believed that they should themselves have had more of a say, with two families wanting to shoulder the full responsibility. One of these two couples observed that the doctors tried to make parents *feel* that they had decided, but in reality it was the doctors who actually took responsibility. For one couple the decision came too soon, and although they realised that they were in no fit state to decide rationally at that point, they still regretted that the doctors had decided for them. One other family wished that they had personally taken responsibility because they felt the whole experience had been too protracted; they themselves would have stopped treatment much sooner.

In the ninth case where parents felt that the balance had been wrong, the decision was a joint one between the parents and the doctors. In this family the mother wished that she had been involved in the discussions much sooner.

# Consultation

The majority of the parents (44, 75%) did not feel the need to consult anyone else about the decision. Indeed, one couple did not even confer together, but they independently came to the same conclusion. A further three sets of parents (5%) had not sought other opinions, but they had discussed the matter with other people, and in two of these cases the parents clarified that they were looking for confirmation that they had made the right decision.

Nine sets of parents (15%) had consulted other people, specifically asking for their opinions. In almost all cases these others were family members, commonly the grandparents. Two fathers had relatives who were health-care professionals, and they both reported that it had been very valuable to discuss the salient issues with someone knowledgeable who could give them independent counsel. The fathers both emphasised that the consultation had been about the problems of prematurity and its consequences in general, and none of these relatives had attempted to enter into discussion about the specifics of this baby's condition and chances, leaving that to the neonatologists who were most intimately involved with the case. Some parents reported a degree of anxiety about what other family members might think of any consideration of stopping treatment, especially if they were known to have strong religious views about life. Indeed, this anxiety prompted some parents not to tell the grandparents that there had been a decision. However, a small number of those who feared recrimination felt that they should inform the grandparents even if it meant opposition. In all cases they reported being agreeably surprised at the level of tolerance and understanding that was shown.

Three couples had discussed the issues with close friends. Four had turned to other professionals – three to a minister of religion and one couple to their GP. In all cases these other professionals had highlighted the expertise and wisdom of the staff in the Neonatal Unit, and reassured the parents about the morality of what was done for babies whose future looked bleak.

Two other couples (3%) who were very young said that it had mainly been the grandparents rather than the parents who had discussed the situation with the consultants. They had then acted as go-betweens throughout the experience, as the parents had felt out of their depth and in need of the support of their parents in their bewilderment. In these instances it was less the case that the parents had consulted them than that they were full members of the decision-making team.

# Factors which helped parents to decide

The parents were asked what it was that had helped them to know whether or not to stop treatment. Of the 59 sets of parents, 56 families gave 145 responses. Only one couple talked of what had persuaded them to *continue* treatment initially – a hope that the child might possibly survive had encouraged them to give him a sporting chance. For this mother it was imperative to do everything she possibly she could to support him, and it was then up to God whether he lived or died.

> Me as the mother carrying [this baby] did everything that I could do for him so that at the end of the day it's up to God. If I do everything I can to give birth and then he doesn't live, then he doesn't live, but I've done what I can.
>
> (P50: mother of baby with congenital anomalies)

All of the other parents spoke exclusively of the reasons why they had felt it was right to let the baby go.

# The condition of the baby

By far the commonest factor was the condition of the baby. Visible signs of deterioration were a powerful motive ($n = 52$ citations). Convulsions, creeping gangrene, bradycardias, rising oxygen requirements, lack of responses, indications of heart failure, lack of growth, deteriorating electroencephalograms (EEGs) and increasing agitation due to brain haemorrhage all reinforced the truth of a bleak prognosis and helped them to realise that the damage was severe or that death was inevitable.

> [The neonatologist] quite often showed us. He'd lay her on the bed and take her by her hands and show us the effect of the brain damage. He'd hold her on her tummy across his hand and she was arched back – there would be no resistance there – and when he pulled her hands up and let go of her on to the bed, their arms were supposed to come up with the reflex and there were just no [reflexes] – she would just flop . . . he did that several times to see if there was any improvement.
>
> (P9: parents of baby with cardiac anomaly)

# The baby's suffering

The reality or prospect of the baby suffering was the next most often cited factor ($n = 23$).

> It's strange. I know there's people that don't understand because they've never been through it, but I loved him so much that I didn't want to lose him but I loved him too much to keep him suffering. I thought, 'You can't do that to him.' It was the hardest thing I've ever had to do in my life. God help anybody that has to go through it. . . . I mean you read about it. And I'd just sat there a few days before because one of the girls had lost her baby – she was 48 hours old – and I said,

'Oh, [name], how could you do that? Oh, I don't think *I* could do that.'
And there I was having to do it.

(P8: mother of preterm twins)

They used to put lines and everything into him. I feel sometimes we just
put him through too much . . . they were sticking lines into his arms and
legs. I feel guilty about that. I just sometimes feel we shouldn't have done
anything at all to try to keep him alive . . . but I'd probably do the same
again. He did so well to begin with though – he was strong and everything. You would always be saying, 'What if? What if?'. At least you
tried – but then I still feel guilty.

(P3: mother of preterm baby with congenital anomaly)

Parents spoke of the overwhelming sense of sorrow that the child's life was
filled with such unpleasantness, and of the paramount need to consider his
needs before their own wishes. Contemplating the alternatives to death
was 'too awful,' and helped them to accept the decision to allow the child
to die.

Definitely one of the factors that brought us to that decision [to with-
draw] was just wanting [the baby] to be left in peace – and watching
her deteriorate. Because they were taking blood tests every so often
and they say it's not painful and it doesn't hurt her. You're in the same
room and you hear other babies screaming the ceiling off because the
same thing's being done.

(P1: father of baby with asphyxia)

Nothing scared me [about] death. Nothing. Because at the end of the
day I kept thinking, 'If she dies she's out of her misery'. She's had
enough. She had been to hell and back. And she didn't scare me. I just
wanted her. I just wanted to cuddle her and kiss her and let her know I
was there.

(P10: mother of preterm twins)

Indeed, many parents were concerned about the whole experience that the
baby was going through, and for some ($n = 3$) it was a great need to have
the death itself dignified and gentle which made them opt for cessation
of treatment earlier on, rather than have the child die in his own time,
perhaps in the incubator and in distress. Death was inevitable, and they
preferred to have it take place in their arms with the child experiencing
the warmth and comfort of their love until the end.

What went through my mind was, 'How would I like this moment to be
remembered?'. And I wanted it to be remembered: the three of us
together, with him dying in our arms rather than with him dying on a
machine with us nowhere in sight. I did ask myself, in a year's time when

I look back on this day, which would be the nicest way to remember it? And I think that's what did it.

(P27: father of baby with cardiac anomaly)

# Medical information

Being given a very *bleak prognosis* ($n = 11$) specifically persuaded other parents to feel that death was a preferable option to continuing existence. However, as well as being given facts, parents were persuaded by the *arguments* that doctors offered. Interpreting what was happening and the importance of these physical indicators of trouble helped them to understand the gravity of the situation.

His approach was excellent. He was almost saying, 'Look, here are your three options – you tell us what you want for the best'. Because if you tried to work it out for yourself you'd probably think, 'Oh my God, there's 36 options here!' But instead you're concentrating all your efforts into the most important things; you're prioritising with his help.

(P50: father of baby with congenital anomalies)

However, some parents specified that it was the *clarity* of the information given to them which had helped them to see the wisdom of stopping aggressive treatment ($n = 22$). As one mother said, the neonatologist 'reiterated that the chances of him surviving were negligible and even that was generous', but, she explained, although the message was painful, the intention of the neonatologist was good.

The words were harsh, but they were real words; they reflected the reality. And he was very nice. I think he was just making sure that we were clear about what we were saying.

(P50: mother of baby with congenital anomalies)

Alongside the facts, the parents set the whole *tenor of the messages*; it was what they heard and saw in the staff's approach which helped them to trust in their expertise and judgements ($n = 13$) and to take on board the strength of the *neonatologist's comment that, if it was his child, he would withdraw treatment* ($n = 4$).

[*What helped you to decide?*] I think when that doctor came in on the Friday – because we had already been feeling it through the week that he was suffering, when that doctor turned round and said – his very words – 'If he was my baby, I'd say enough is enough.' And I'd already been saying that to myself. We just nodded when he said it.

(P8: mother of preterm twins)

# Realisation of the consequences of survival

Realising that the world was 'a cruel place which would be hostile' to a baby with such severe impairments was cited as a determining factor for one couple. The experience gained from seeing other babies dying around them helped one other couple to decide that continuing survival would be at too high a price.

# Support from the professional team

The ongoing support of the nurses and doctors was identified by seven families as a factor in their decision. It reinforced the wisdom of their choice. For one parent, *outside confirmation* from a perceived authoritative source helped at this point – a friend who was a GP who could detail the impact of such damage on the growing child, and confirm the horror of daily existence with such devastating impairments.

# Parental interests

Only one family said that it was their own needs which had helped them to decide it was time to stop. They could take no more.

> *Father*: To be quite honest, I put my hand on my heart – I just didn't want the boy home. As far as I was concerned, although he was my son, he wasn't part of my family. Because we've got a busy wee life in this house as it is, and there just isn't room for a handicapped child.
> *Mother*: It would have financially crucified us as well ... I felt the same. I didn't want [him here]. Basically he was a vegetable, that's all he was. To me I never had a baby.
>
> (P 39: parents of baby with brain damage)

However, one other couple initially secretly feared that they had made the decision for their own sakes. Privately each of them agonised over this thought. As the mother said, 'it was such a terrible thing' to think that she couldn't voice the fear aloud. They did eventually tentatively broach the subject to each other, finding relief in the open acknowledgement of their doubts and the conclusion that they could never have put their own needs above the baby's best interests.

> When we went into the [quiet] area I was thinking, 'Wouldn't it be terrible to be woken up to be told he'd passed away on that infernal machine?'. And the thought was going through my head, 'Am I doing this for me? Am I doing this because I just want to get home quicker and put this episode behind me once and for all? Or am I doing it for

[the baby]?'. You start to question your own motives. I didn't really know what my own motives were, I just knew I'd made up my mind that that's what I wanted to do [ – to withdraw the ventilator]. And even a couple of days afterwards that thought was going through my head: 'Did I do this because I was in a horrible situation and I just wanted to get out of it, or did I actually do it as an act of caring for [the baby]?'. [We eventually spoke to one another about it two days later.] I think we both concluded that if we'd thought that if there was even the remotest possibility of him living we would have stayed up until we collapsed with exhaustion. We both agreed that, yes, we would have done that, so we just put it behind us.

(P27: father of baby with cardiac anomaly)

# Was it the right decision?

## Mothers' opinions

By the time of the first interview, the majority of the mothers (51 of the 58 mothers who participated at this point, 88%) felt that the right decision had been made. A few of them harboured lingering doubts about the rightness of initial resuscitation ($n = 2$), the certainty of the prognosis ($n = 1$), or the cruelty of aggressive treatment ($n = 1$). Two families added that, although they were now confident that the right decision had been made because later information had confirmed it, they had earlier had misgivings.

Six mothers (10%) were unsure whether the right decision had been made. Two of them expressed a general feeling of unease about the accuracy of the prognosis, but the other four elaborated on their misgivings. In one case the mother was under the influence of powerful post-operative drugs and could not remember anything about the discussion or events, so she felt she was in no position to say whether it was right or wrong. Another was reluctant to voice her opinion because the death of the baby was so far from what she had wanted it was impossible for her to assess the morality of what had been decided. One mother could only hope that it was right because she could not bear the thought of the baby suffering. The anxiety of one mother related to the question of disability; she now thought that, even though the baby would have been impaired, there were plenty of people who would have been prepared to help her to care for the growing child, and he should perhaps have been given a chance.

Only one mother felt that it had been wrong. Deep down this woman had reservations about the prognosis, and felt that they should have kept treating in order to give the baby every chance of survival. This mother was dissatisfied with many aspects of her management, and felt that she had ample reason to mistrust doctors. She provided a detailed history of being given half-truths and wrong information, of being kept in the dark, and of errors in her own care. She herself had been gravely ill at the time of the delivery, and both she and her partner resented the fact that neither of them were informed at the time of the severity of her condition. Although by her own admission she had been very upset and 'hysterical' at times, she still felt that the neonatologists should have been more frank and direct in giving bad news. In her perceptions they had been too vague and too reassuring. The specialist who was brought in to confirm the diagnosis and prognosis had irritated and angered both of the parents. Five different consultants had shared the task of giving bad news, but the couple did not feel that they knew or had built up trust in any of them.

> For all the meetings we had we saw a different consultant every time, which I think is bad because then you're not getting to trust anybody. We had [the baby] for five and a half weeks, and in those five and a half weeks we must have seen every consultant in that place . . . five consultants, which I think is wrong because if you're dealing one to one with somebody you tend to build up your confidence in them . . . the day that they told us they were taking treatment away from [the baby] because the brain damage was so severe that was [Consultant 5] and that was the first time we'd met him, the first time we'd even *seen* the man. And I can always remember looking at him and thinking, 'I can't believe this. I've never seen you and you're telling me that you're taking away the treatment on my daughter because she's not going to live.'
>
> (P 36: parents of preterm baby)

As a result of all of these experiences, these parents could have no confidence that the bleak picture which was presented when treatment withdrawal was discussed was actually correct, and after the death the mother was left with many doubts and a sense of guilt which lingered for many months. Initially her husband accepted the situation and was strong for her. But he subsequently suffered a serious breakdown which they both agreed had been a late reaction to the grief and guilt associated with their traumatic experience of losing the baby.

# Fathers' opinions

Forty-seven fathers were able to say whether or not they felt that the right decision had been made. Of these, 42 fathers (89%) were confident that it was correct, although one commented that he had had some misgivings at the time.

Two fathers (4%) were uncertain whether or not the decision was right. They had no means of finding out, and could only hope that it was.

Three fathers (6%) believed that the wrong decision had been made. They felt that there was some small doubt about the prognosis, so the baby should have been given a chance, to see if he could survive. They believed that if they had seen for themselves evidence of the baby 'slipping away', they would have been more sure in their own minds that the prognosis was bleak and that withdrawal was the right option. Because there were no concrete signs that the doctor's predictions were correct, this father (who felt that the social workers and doctors were colluding to prevent them having children) was of the opinion, which he emphasised several times, that what happened amounted to murder.

In only one case did both partners express doubts about the decision.

## Parental opinion at 13 months

By 13 months only one mother and one father felt with hindsight that the decision had been the wrong one. The mother had watched her surviving preterm twin developing, and now believed that they should have kept treating the other twin. This feeling had been strengthened at follow-up when the consultant had admitted that he could not say categorically that the child would not have survived. The father, who believed a mistake had been made, now thought that his baby (who had hypoplastic left heart syndrome) would have had a chance of surviving if the defect had been detected earlier and the child transferred while she was still in good condition. Surgical treatment was available, but by the time the decision was made she was too ill for it to be possible to contemplate transferring her. Neither of these parents had expressed doubts at the earlier time of enquiry. Of the four parents who had felt that the decision was wrong initially, two were unavailable for a second interview, so it is not known whether they changed their minds. One was now unsure if the decision had been right, and the other was now satisfied that it had been right.

One year on, two mothers (4%) and three fathers (6%) were unsure whether they had made the right choice. Only one of these parents had expressed reservations at the earlier time. Then, as now, uncertainty related to an awareness that there was no cast-iron way of knowing what the outcome for these babies would have been, and the parents lacked the medical knowledge to be confident about this. But for one father reservations stemmed from its being a 'no-win situation' – for his severely congenitally abnormal child either choice was a tragic one.

Again, in only one family did both partners express reservations about the wisdom of the decision.

# Parents' own perceptions of why treatment was stopped

At both interviews parents were asked specifically why, in their opinion, treatment *had* been stopped. Although for a small number of families there had been no agreed decision to stop treatment, and the babies had died spontaneously, all of the families answered this question in some form. In the cases where death had intervened, the parents' responses related to the abandonment of all further attempts to keep the child alive. Parents often provided more than one comment. Numerical data are less important than the general feel of the parents' perceptions about this important issue.

## Perceptions at the time of first interview

Two main factors emerged, namely the baby's condition ($n = 93$), and judgements relating to future consequences ($n = 48$). At the time of the first interview, by far the largest category of reasons related to the baby's condition. Although all of these contained the idea that the child was very ill or damaged, it is interesting to see the ideas on which parents focused.

### *Medical condition*

|                                                        | Number of comments |
| ------------------------------------------------------ | :----------------: |
| Independent survival was not possible                  | 34                 |
| Nothing more could be done                             | 19                 |
| The damage was too severe                              | 19                 |
| Deterioration was already evident                      | 10                 |
| There were major structural problems                   | 6                  |
| The child was too ill for treatment to be effective    | 5                  |

In the case of two of these families, whereas the mothers believed that there were obvious signs of deterioration, the fathers suspected that it was an extra dosage of morphine which had actually killed their babies.

### *Judgements relating to future consequences*

|                                                        | Number of comments |
| ------------------------------------------------------ | :----------------: |
| Treatment was too burdensome for doubtful benefits     | 16                 |
| Future quality of life would have been too poor        | 16                 |

| | |
|---|---|
| The parents decided that it was best for the baby to stop treatment | 6 |
| The parents and doctors all thought that it was best for the baby to stop treatment | 4 |
| The baby had given up | 3 |
| The doctors said that it was best for the baby to stop treatment | 2 |
| The parents wanted a peaceful, dignified death in their arms | 2 |
| It was secondarily best for the parents that treatment be stopped | 2 |

The remaining comments stand alone, but provide useful indicators of those aspects which parents find persuasive. For one family, the strain of watching the child fighting was too great; the father decided that his partner could take no more, so he had advised that treatment should be stopped.

One father voiced a passing concern that a lack of resources had been behind the decision to forgo further expensive and prolonged treatment.

> When they first asked [about withdrawing ventilation] the question of NHS cash-starved resources – did they just want to clear him out and make room for someone else? – that thought did go through my head. I concluded in the end that [the neonatologist's] manner suggests integrity and confidence and all these sorts of things. And then [the chaplain] probably guessed that that was what I was getting at as well because he said, 'I can assure you that this idea of the sanctity of life is paramount to the people here [i.e. staff in the Neonatal Unit].' And I concluded that myself.
>
> (P27: father of baby with cardiac anomaly)

Subsequent events put these fears to rest. His baby son was born in a local hospital in poor condition and took a long time to resuscitate. Following transfer to the study Unit, a rare metabolic disorder was initially suspected. The baby's condition deteriorated rapidly, and ten hours later the parents were told that survival was impossible. Until that point the father had believed there was a chance for the little boy, and he was shocked at the suggestion made at this time that the treatment should be stopped. The mother, on the other hand, had been full of foreboding from the time when the baby had been whisked away from her following delivery and remained so long away. To her the ventilator and equipment did not represent life support, but they were just a temporary measure to allow the doctors to establish a diagnosis. It was only at the follow-up visit two months later that these parents discovered that the baby had a rare cardiac condition and had suffered cataclysmic damage which made his death inevitable.

An inadequate standard of care was the perceived reason why one baby had treatment withheld. This couple was told, two weeks after the onset of preterm labour, that there was a significant risk to the mother's health and future fertility if the pregnancy continued. On the basis of the available evidence they decided that it was right to deliver the baby, even though the chances of survival were slim. The child lived for only a matter of hours. The parents believed that an infection, introduced during a poorly conducted catheterisation and passed on *in utero*, was really the cause of the child's poor condition, and they cited this as the indirect reason why treatment was limited.

# Perceptions at second interview at 13 months

At the earlier point of enquiry all parents had offered a reason for the limitation of treatment. By 13 months after the death, the parents were considered to be robust enough to be asked separately what they thought, and 48 mothers and 38 fathers responded. One father and one mother said that they did not know why treatment had been stopped. The mother said that she just could not let herself think about it. Her child had been born prematurely at 28 weeks and had lived for over 100 days. The baby of the father who was unsure had been severely asphyxiated, and the mother in this case was certain that the child was deteriorating, damage was severe and there was no possibility of survival.

The reasons given by the two parents in each of the remaining families were essentially the same, but the way in which they explained them differed. As before, the reasons cited could be subdivided into factors relating to the baby's medical condition and judgements with regard to future consequences of surviving.

### Medical condition

| | Mothers: | Fathers: |
|---|---|---|
| Independent survival was not possible | 28 | 23 |
| Nothing more could be done | 9 | 6 |
| The damage was too severe | 9 | 8 |
| Deterioration was already evident | 9 | 10 |
| The child was too ill for treatment to be effective | 3 | 3 |
| Treatment was only prolonging the inevitable | 2 | 2 |

### Judgements relating to future consequences

| | Mothers: | Fathers: |
|---|---|---|
| Future quality of life would have been too poor | 14 | 11 |
| The baby had given up | 2 | 2 |

On a previous occasion, the parents reported, they had been told that the baby had been slow to revive after an apnoeic episode, and they were warned that it might not be possible to resuscitate him at some future point. But when the father asked at that point if they should decide about stopping, they had been told 'not yet.' There had been discussion of, but no agreement on, withdrawal of treatment. The mother just happened to be in the Unit when the baby deteriorated. She observed the difficulty that staff were having resuscitating him, and spontaneously asked them to discontinue efforts. As she pointed out, it had worked out smoothly because she was in the Unit and could instruct the staff to stop treatment, but it could easily have happened that the child died without them even being present, or during aggressive resuscitation attempts.

> *Mother*: We were very lucky that I was there [to say don't resuscitate when he deteriorated]. We wouldn't have liked to get a phone call in the middle of the night and that happen. We wouldn't have been involved so much. The fact that we were involved was because I was there and [my husband] got there very quickly so we were involved 100% because of the circumstances.
> *Father*: That's maybe a point worth picking up on. Because we were lucky. No one knew, I don't think, in that week. If suddenly he'd taken a turn for the worse two or three days earlier, no one from the hospital knew really what we felt about a decision . . . It was very quick downhill over three days or whatever . . . when's the right time for any hospital to come out and ask any parents, 'OK, maybe you might have to [decide whether we treat your baby or not]'?
>
> (P6: parents of baby with congenital anomalies)

However, not all of the mothers were satisfied. Some of the problems they perceived have been mentioned in earlier sections, but they are brought together here in a concise form to alert clinicians to matters of *process* which impinge on parental satisfaction. For 11 mothers (19%), the way in which the decision had been made was satisfactory for the most part, but they had small quibbles. A further nine mothers (16%) perceived their experience as unsatisfactory.

During decision making it was upsetting for mothers if the neonatologist himself was unavailable. Long delays (up to 9 hours) before seeing him whilst knowing that the news was very bad were traumatic for three mothers. It distressed another mother to have only irregular *ad hoc* meetings even though things were going very wrong.

Mothers were dissatisfied if communication was perceived to be inadequate. Three mothers felt that their discussions and decisions were too rushed. Three considered that they had been given insufficient information. Some cited a lack of continuity, with different people imparting information ($n = 3$), messages being indirect and ambiguous ($n = 2$), bad news being given to the mother alone, instead of waiting until she had support ($n = 2$), a consultant being a very poor communicator ($n = 1$), discussions being too public, with many witnesses of the parents' distress ($n = 1$), the parents being asked by nurses to go to the doctor instead of the doctor coming to see them ($n = 1$), and perceived arrogance among staff who seemed too sure that they knew what was right for the baby ($n = 1$). One mother felt that insufficient time was allowed for the reality to be absorbed before a decision had to be made. Two mothers were unhappy about the lack of continuity of nurses, which resulted in conflicting information or, in one case the mother believed, led to a failure to notice deterioration.

Some parents perceived staff to have a different agenda from their own at this time, and cited this as a source of dissatisfaction. One mother found staff too possessive of her baby, another felt that the doctors were keeping the baby alive to use as a guinea-pig, and a third believed that the overall service discriminated against the lower social classes. One mother expressed a strong belief that the doctors had colluded with social workers to kill her child. On the morning of the child's death, she had left the child 'wriggling and fine' and gone back to her own mother's house. During that day the child deteriorated. The hospital attempted many times over a period of five hours to contact her, but the mother and grandmother said that they did not hear the phone because they were in bed. Police eventually tracked her down, but further delays resulted from the family's reaction to their visit. By the time the mother finally arrived at the hospital, the tubes were still in position but had been disconnected from the ventilator. She was unable to reconcile the squirming pink child she had left with the dying baby she now saw, and she believed that the staff must have actively done something to bring about this deterioration.

# Paternal satisfaction with the *way* in which the decision was made

Of the 46 fathers who were able to comment on this issue, 29 (63%) were satisfied that the decision making had been managed as well as it could have been. One other father was satisfied at the time, but had since had doubts. At the time his overriding concern had been that they should be there cuddling the child as she died, and his greatest fear was that the death would be sudden and too clinical. After the event he was left wondering whether they should have waited longer to be quite sure there was no hope for the baby. Nine fathers (20%) expressed general satisfaction but had minor quibbles, and seven fathers (15%) reported dissatisfaction with the way in which the situation was handled.

Two fathers were dissatisfied with the long wait to see a consultant after bad news had been given – in one case 9 hours. Fragmentation of care with different people imparting information was a source of discontent for five fathers. One cited long delays in obtaining information, although he conceded that the doctors were themselves only very slowly building up a picture of a rare disorder. Messages were ambiguous in the perception of three fathers, and there was a lack of preparation for bad news for another. One father perceived a certain consultant as a very poor communicator.

The timing of events gave rise to some problems. Two fathers felt that the decision had been too hurried, leaving them with no time to absorb the reality. Another felt that fragmented care had resulted in a failure to notice deterioration.

In another case, the father's dissatisfaction stemmed from the unavailability of the mother to make a decision because of strong medication and great discomfort. Beliefs that the baby had been used as a guinea-pig while he was alive ($n = 1$), that the doctors had colluded with social workers to kill the child ($n = 1$), and that care was substandard for the lower social classes ($n = 1$), were expressed sources of dissatisfaction for the others.

The families who expressed dissatisfaction came from all Units and were cared for by a range of different consultants. No differences were found between families interviewed at three months after the death compared to those who were first interviewed later than this.

# Supportive people during this time of decision making

## Professional support

It was evident that parents looked principally to the professional team for support during decision making. Supportive people included neonatal nurses ($n = 31$ families), the neonatal consultant ($n = 28$), other doctors ($n = 16$), postnatal ward staff ($n = 6$) and a midwife ($n = 1$). Six families found a minister of religion helpful at this time ($n = 6$).

My need really was to speak to [our minister] . . . we didn't manage to get hold of [him] but we got hold of the new [minister] and I put the position to him and I said, 'Look, I just feel as though I'm being asked to kill my baby. How would God see it?'. And he said, 'No, no, of course it wouldn't be seen as murder because it's the machines that are keeping him alive at the moment. He couldn't sustain his own life at the moment'. . . . Once I'd heard that from [the minister], listened carefully to what he had to say and seen how [the baby] was overnight, we definitely arrived at the same conclusion. That was right from the beginning, but I just had to convince myself somehow.

(P2: mother of baby with cardiac anomaly)

Four families looked to GPs for support, two of whom were personal friends, and one mother found a health visitor supportive. One mother cited a counsellor in this context.

## Lay support

Some additional support came from the family in general ($n = 7$), the baby's maternal ($n = 6$) or paternal ($n = 1$) grandmother, aunts ($n = 2$), uncles ($n - 1$) or great-aunts ($n = 1$). Friends helped four families through this difficult time. The low numbers seem to suggest that lay people were of limited value at the time of decision making.

# Supportive actions during decision making

Support fell into the generally recognised components, namely emotional, informational, appraisal/esteem, and practical or instrumental support.[103,112] The exact numbers of parents who cited each given form of support are not relevant for two reasons. First, many cited several factors, all of which could be subsumed under one umbrella category, and secondly, many topics could be included in two or three categories. For example, encouraging a mother to be involved in caring for her baby constituted practical help, but it also provided emotional support and boosted her self-esteem.

## Emotional support

The overwhelming majority of comments from parents about the things which they had found helpful at this time related to emotional support. The compassionate approach of the neonatal staff was the one main factor which parents remembered with gratitude as supportive.

I could see that the man [the neonatologist] was really distressed himself. Then I felt, 'This is genuine.' He was actually in tears himself. 'Believe me,' he said, 'if there was anything anybody could do anywhere in the world,' he would have had them over to do it.

(P20: father of baby with asphyxia)

It was immensely confirming to know that their child's life and death had impinged on the lives of these professionals so profoundly. Their genuine caring, their obvious distress when things went wrong, their willingness to be with the parents through the whole trauma of decision making and withdrawal – beyond the call of duty or the boundaries of shifts – all spoke clearly of their commitment to each family. Several parents commented that the experience had been a revelation to them, and that they had no idea such a level of caring existed.

They were particularly appreciative of the sympathetic approach of the consultant. They used terms such as 'his lovely manner,' 'pitching it just right,' 'his caring and calm approach,' 'he was compassionate, not just clinical,' 'he inspired confidence,' and 'we felt he was on our side.' Although he had the unenviable task of giving them such bad news, nevertheless, where he did so with sympathy and gentleness, they valued his skill and personal involvement. They noted the consultants who were always around day and night, whenever things went wrong, the ones who never shirked duties or delegated the responsibility for giving bad news, and the ones who saw decisions through or who put their own cards on the table and gave the benefit of years of experience by offering their own recommendation. A number of parents spoke warmly of consultants who had made them feel like members of the whole team, and who had treated them as equals.

All of the parents without exception had found the majority of the neonatal nurses supportive, and many expressed wonder at the personal involvement with the baby which rendered the nurses themselves so vulnerable when the babies deteriorated and died. They pondered with concern the impact of an accumulation of pain for the staff who loved and lost so many babies. It was a source of surprise to many to find that the nurses cared for them, the parents, as well as for the babies, and many felt that they had become friends. Although only one couple (the parents who had had discussion with an advanced nurse practitioner) cited nurses as key people in *discussions* about treatment withdrawal, their continuing support through the *process* of decision making was highly valued.

> The nursing staff helped us come to all these decisions not through telling us anything, but by allowing us to ask questions and allowing us to talk to them for quite long spells sometimes.
>
> (P1: mother of baby with asphyxia)

The staff were still there doing everything they could [for the baby] – fighting. They were definitely fighting right till the end – right until the machinery was switched off. He was still getting his special feed drips – which costs lots of money. The National Health Service is so stretched for money, but even though they knew [the baby] had no chance, they kept on saying, 'Right, no expense spared here.' Until the final decision was made, everything was done for him. And that gave you a lot of comfort.

(P32: parents of preterm baby)

Several parents specifically mentioned the support of the chaplain at this point of decision making. Even where they had no religious beliefs themselves, they found it comforting to have him present. A number of parents noted their surprise that he had not tried to 'cram God or religion' into them, but rather had conveyed a sense that withdrawal of treatment was a legitimate part of the medical care of sick babies. A couple of parents added that they had specifically sought the chaplain's comments on the rightness of withdrawing. The fact that he was non-medical and not involved in the management of the case had strengthened the force of his reassurance about the morality of any decision to stop treatment.

> When the minister came up, he was offering us words of comfort and I asked him what his view on [stopping treatment] was. He said that of course it was our decision but, he said, 'The only thing I can tell you is that the sanctity of life is all-important to the doctors here and they would not under any circumstances have made that suggestion unless they felt there was nothing left for them to do. It's not a suggestion they would have made lightly.'

> (P27: father of baby with cardiac anomaly)

## Information

The second most commonly cited form of support was informational. Parents wanted frank and honest facts, although it must be noted that in two families the mothers said that they had disliked such blunt speaking, even though their partners had wanted it.

> *Mother*: I think sometimes [the neonatologist] could be a bit gentler the way he tells you. Because he's one of these people – he doesn't give you any false hope. He just gives you it as it is. I think that's why I called him Dr Doom! ... Every time he came to speak to me I got a lump in my throat ... You're under a lot of stress while you're in there, and I just wasn't emotionally stable for it.
> *Father*: But I liked that. I could identify with that and I prefer that. But not everybody can deal with ... Right from the moment she was born I wanted to know exactly what was happening straight away, and I didn't want anything hidden. I wanted to know up front what was happening, and I think I was like that all the way through. But I was frustrated and disappointed down in [the other hospital] because I wasn't getting that.

> (P9: parents of baby with cardiac anomaly)

Repeated explanations given without impatience, and apparently unlimited opportunities to ask questions of everyone, helped parents to assimilate the full picture of what had gone wrong and the bleakness of the future prospect.

> [This neonatologist] said, 'Look, if you have to ask me a hundred times, then ask me a hundred times; ask me *a hundred and one times* to be sure.'
>
> (P35: father of preterm triplets)

Invariably the parents looked to the consultant or specialists to give the serious information, but many appreciated reinforcement of the facts from other doctors and the nurses.

> I was terrified of [the consultant] and so was [my husband] . . . he was so nice in his explanation, I really can't fault him. He was lovely. [But] to have [the neonatal nurse] there as well made such a difference. It's someone who's . . . more near your kind of level . . . she could explain medical things in English terms . . . a mediator I suppose . . . and she'd ask you [if you understood]. Because in that sort of situation you're a bit scared, you're terrified, you don't know what to ask. You don't know what to ask, that's the problem and I think having somebody else there mediating between ourselves and [the consultant] and saying, 'Did you really understand what that meant? Well, that actually means . . .'. So that you do get things sinking in, which did help.
>
> (P12: mother of preterm triplets)

Facts which helped them to understand the futility of treatment, or the wisdom of stopping it, in turn reassured them that the right decision was being made and helped to confirm their trust in the consultant's professional guidance.

> It wasn't until we saw the brain scan that we actually understood exactly the extent of the problem. I was still convinced that no, no, they weren't right. You need your brain for this and you need your brain for that [things the baby was doing]. But the paediatrician that came to us on the Tuesday night and spoke to us and showed us the scans [the baby's brain and a perfect normal scan], he answered a few of our questions that we had. He explained . . . everything that we were seeing [the baby] doing was based on reflexes as opposed to actions from the brain. I suppose that helped us to understand why he was kicking his feet, and clenching our hands and things like that. That gave us a better insight into exactly what was going on. After we had seen the scans . . . then we made the decision that we were going to switch off the ventilator.
>
> (P23: mother of preterm baby with congenital anomalies)

For a very small number of parents, additional informational support during decision making had come from outside the team. People with experience of severely damaged babies were able to provide a stark picture which helped parents to take in the enormity of what might lie ahead. In two families where the parents were themselves experienced health-care professionals, one or both had looked to partners for lengthy discussion about the prognosis, and only required the essential facts from the consultant. The difficulty for both of these couples was in switching out of 'professional mode' into 'parent mode', and they were aware that their additional knowledge worked against them in some ways. Two other fathers came from medical families and found it helpful to discuss the situation with these informed relatives in general terms, leaving the specifics of the case to the neonatologist, although one father gave permission for the medically qualified grandfather to discuss the baby's condition at length with the neonatologist.

## Appraisal/esteem

Parents greatly appreciated acknowledgement of their special place as parents of this child with a unique attachment and role. Self-esteem was also increased when parents were praised for their way of dealing with this traumatic situation. One consultant personally complimented a family, and they reported verbatim what he had said. The effect was to increase their sense of mutual respect and to make the parents feel that they were an important part of the decision-making team.

## Practical support

This was the least commonly cited form of support at this stage. However, when the parents were burdened with pain and preoccupied with the outcome for this new baby, it was helpful not to have additional anxieties. Specific citations included having rooms, food and telephones made available to them, or passes to ensure ease of parking for themselves and grandparents. Family members and friends also provided practical support for a few parents at this stage, in the form of transport or help with other children.

## **Areas for improvement**

All of the parents were asked how they felt things could be improved at the time of decision making. In deference to the parents' wishes, it is important to remind ourselves of the context within which these comments were set. Discussing the death of a baby is a disturbing experience for parents. A small number of parents admitted to being 'shocked' or 'disgusted' at the very suggestion by the consultant that treatment should be stopped, or that a severely disabled child might represent an intolerable burden for their family.

> We had a meeting with [the consultant] again which I found almost shocking, and had I not been in a state of confusion and shock that he had come out with this nonsense, I'd have probably actually hit him, I'm sorry to say. We got taken into the room and he basically turned round and said that [the baby] is going to be brain-damaged, definitely handicapped and did we want to [stop treatment]? He made it as if he was thinking of *our* long term. And he said that there was a point we would be at where we couldn't say we wanted the ventilator turned off now because she's going to be handicapped. He said, 'Now, in the next couple of days, is going to be the time to say that.' And I always remember looking at him and thinking 'You're not turning my daughter's ventilator off because she's going to be handicapped. Whether she's handicapped or not she's our daughter and she'll come home.' . . . To be giving us that option was pretty much disgusting when our daughter was fighting for her life.
>
> (P35: father of preterm triplets)

Even when parents could see their baby deteriorating, it was still a shock to have someone say out loud that they were going to die. However, they recognised that when unpalatable information was being given, it was too easy to blame the messenger when the fault did not actually lie with him or her. Some mothers reported being hysterical or in denial at the time. Others were appalled at the prospect of making a decision of this magnitude. Some were fearful about the possibility of survival with severe impairment. And all of these different circumstances had to be accommodated by the consultants. In as many as 20 cases (34%) the first discussions about treatment withdrawal took place during the first couple of days of life, when there had been little time to get to know the family, and it seems all the more remarkable that so many parents felt that the information had been pitched appropriately for them.

Clearly, bad news *can* be conveyed and decision making handled well, and for most of these parents this was the case. Comments relating to less than optimal practice fell into five broad categories, namely communication, management, staff approaches, family responses and amenities. Some of the points duplicate those made in the previous chapter in relation to the time when things first went wrong. The fact that they resurfaced when parents reflected on the time of the actual decision making serves to emphasise their importance.

# Communication

## *Frankness*

The clear message parents gave was that they wanted full and honest facts. Anything less hindered their decision making.

> This is the most critical point in the whole [experience]. We didn't get any information about the risks. Because if you try to save a baby and it is heavily handicapped or blind or [whatever] then it's a very difficult decision to take for us. I would have liked some statistical data, like 20% are mildly handicapped and whatever. And we didn't get that – not at all. So we just knew there might be some handicaps ranging from almost normal to very heavily handicapped, but we didn't have any idea of the percentage. So not knowing this we cannot take the decision. How can we decide? If it was like say a 90% chance of having serious problems then we probably wouldn't have him treated . . . 'Do not treat' is the death sentence which we cannot, without knowing about the risks, we cannot take that decision.
>
> (P17: father of preterm baby)

Evasion worried them not just because they were unclear about the situation, but also because it left them fearful that other things were being concealed. Vague, ambivalent messages, soothing reassurances and even sanitised information which left them with false hope were unwelcome to all parents, although some did suggest that there was no need to be brutal in the telling either. Certain consultants were perceived as 'hovering' or 'shilly-shallying' – not coming to the point. It was not in the long term doing the parents any favours to be too protective.

Where parents felt that they were not being kept up to date with medical thinking they were not satisfied. One couple reported that for many weeks staff talked to them about what would happen when the baby went home, and suddenly they were told by a consultant that the child would never go home and indeed could not survive. Months later the father still conveyed his utter disbelief and bewilderment. It seemed astonishing to him that no one had given any inkling of the true situation. However, whilst most parents wanted full explanations and test results, two couples drew attention to the nervous energy expended when diagnosis proved elusive, numerous tests were carried out and they worried about the implications of each one, only to find each result was normal.

Criticisms of those consultants who failed to get the balance right for specific parents included reference to too casual an approach, a patronising tone, no eye contact, too negative an attitude and unintelligible jargon. Strong accents, even British ones, added an unwelcome extra barrier to good communication at a time of great stress.

## Consistency

Fragmentation or inconsistency could lead to conflicting messages, and it was sometimes very obvious. One couple was distressed by a nurse in the Unit telling them that the child was doing really well just before the consultant delivered news of a bleak outlook. At other times it was more subtle. One father regretted staying while the specialist examined his child, because he received a fragmented and impartial picture from answers to his limited questions. On reflection he felt that he would have been better off waiting until the neonatologist could have passed on the information in a broader and more understandable context, building on previous discussions.

A lack of internal consistency in the messages which were conveyed caused confusion. For example, if parents were told that the baby was dying and the dying trajectory was mapped out for them, it rocked their confidence if events did not occur as predicted. Furthermore, if what the parents were told did not match what they saw and understood it was worrying. Even at a fairly trivial level this could have implications, as was illustrated by the case of one father who was incensed when a consultant got the baby's gender wrong even though the notes stated that she was a girl, and she was lying naked in the incubator. As he said, it was 'kinda worrying if they can overlook the simplest of [details]' when the doctors are being entrusted with the most crucial decisions. If the incongruities related to serious medical facts, they were more frightening still. For example, one couple was told that their baby's brain had not developed, but they saw a baby who grasped their finger, who pushed them away if he wanted peace, and who cried if a painful procedure was performed on him. To them this represented a sentient, responsive child. For another couple, when the baby was transferred from one busy referral Unit to another, she left the first Unit with a diagnosis of respiratory problems. Initially they had seen a child struggling to breathe, but in the second Unit they found a child who was brain-damaged and obviously seriously ill. The parents were bewildered. The father repeatedly asked how his daughter could have gone in with one thing and come out with something very different wrong with her.

If the management of the baby belied what they were being told about his or her prognosis, parents could feel confused about the issues.

> By that time we hadn't given up on her, but at the same time they were giving her the massaging of the lungs and all the rest of it before they could take her off the ventilator assuming she was going to die. Now that was the assumption that everybody had made, so why give her the physiotherapy? I couldn't understand that. I just couldn't understand that. One minute the doctor's saying, 'I'm not going to do anything – we'll

try taking her off this ventilator.' Within an hour there's a physiotherapist in giving her physiotherapy! I mean, what the hell's going on?

(P9: father of baby with cardiac anomaly)

## Reassurance

Where parents received no reassurance that they were making the right choices they could feel insecure as a result.

At that time you want somebody to say, 'Yes, you're doing the right thing.' And nobody did. But I asked [the neonatal nurse when we had said switch off the ventilator], 'Do you think we're being cruel?'. And she said, 'No' . . . We wanted somebody to come and tell us there's no option here. Because we didn't have the guts to switch it off [at first]. We wanted somebody to say, 'It's just keeping her going for going's sake.' For this person to say, 'Look, you're not being cruel. You're doing the best thing.'

(P7: parents of baby with cardiac anomaly)

## Location

Parents did not like a lack of privacy, or large groups of extraneous staff hovering around them. One father described in vivid detail his sense of smallness and ignorance when a consultant brought a bevy of juniors who all stood over him as he sat on a low chair, not understanding the use of long medical terms and feeling greatly disadvantaged. He was still smarting from this humiliating experience, as he perceived it, more than a year after the event. On the other hand, the mother we have already mentioned, who was approached alone and unsupported in her own room, demonstrated the need for caution – privacy is not to be confused with secrecy.

## Support

A lack of support at this time could be burdensome. Mothers spoke of interminable waiting times until their partners arrived. Fathers recalled being telephoned at home or at work and not being able to remember driving back or being able to make simple decisions about what to pack. For other fathers there was a feeling of loneliness although they were not geographically distant from their partners. Several were facing the possibility of treatment withdrawal while their partners were still under the influence of anaesthesia or powerful drugs and therefore unavailable to them. Excluding family or friends could limit the potential avenues of help. Dismissing the parents' concerns or responding inappropriately was damaging.

*Father*: The chaplain . . . was pretty insensitive . . . he said it was his view or his opinion that it would be better with a termination because of the

cost involved with keeping these kind of [impaired] children alive.
Which we just thought was totally outrageous.

*Mother*: He said it to me. Because I did see the chaplain, because I was
really struggling with my conscience and knowing what was the right
thing to do, and so I did see him and I think he was trying to be helpful.
He didn't say it was his view, but he did say you could take the view
that it would be better to have an abortion because you have to remember that it's very expensive to keep babies alive in a Neonatal Unit, and
those resources are very expensive. Didn't really say anything because I
was just feeling very vulnerable.

*Father*: When she told me, I was wanting to go up and punch his head in,
although I'm not a violent person. I just thought it was ridiculous. Especially [for] a supposed man of the cloth to start thinking about resources
and cost – which we had done as well quite honestly, having spoken
with [the consultant obstetrician] who said that's not one of our concerns, the cost was really insignificant compared to what our views
were, no matter which way we went. Quite a different approach.

(P 50: parents of baby with congenital anomalies)

## Exclusion

Being excluded from discussions troubled some parents when the matters
under review were so crucial. It was disconcerting to overhear hitherto
unknown information about their baby on ward rounds or in passing, or
to have staff using incomprehensible language among themselves, or to
be excluded from team meetings about the child. A few young parents
resented the consultant speaking more to their own parents than to them.

## Timing

The timing of events was critically important to the parents' satisfaction
with their management. One couple felt that they were always one jump
ahead of the staff in asking questions, and wished that the doctors could
have introduced the topics ahead of them, and led their thinking. Another
mother reported being asked to consider stopping treatment, to which she
instantly responded in the affirmative, saying that it should be done now
rather than letting the baby suffer any longer. She was then taken aback
when the doctors advised the family to take their time, watch and wait 'a
few weeks.' On the other hand, one young couple felt that the doctors had
been too precipitate. In the father's judgement, each time they had tried to
wean the baby off the ventilator they had not left her long enough to establish whether or not she could manage unaided. As a result, the parents
were sceptical about their assessment that she was machine dependent
and could never survive alone.

I felt at times in the hospital that we were rushed into making a decision. I always felt there was so much emphasis placed on 'Get to know [the baby]. Take as much time as you want to know [him].' But at the same time you have to make your decision because if you don't make your decision he'll die on the ventilator. Every morning the doctors always came round and spoke to us and told us how [the baby] had got on during the night and things like that, but they used to emphasise that every morning to us: 'Take your time, get to know [the baby] *but* remember . . .'. OK, we were happy with that decision because we understood that [our baby] was going to die and there wasn't much point in sitting there day after day watching him, obviously breaking our heart over him, and knowing at the end of the day we were going to have nothing anyway. But I feel in some ways if we hadn't have been satisfied [it was the right decision] we would have been rushed into it.

(P23: mother of preterm baby with congenital anomalies)

Being required to wait hours, even through a whole night, before being able to discuss the decision was unacceptable to the parents.

## Management

On occasion the doctors or nurses introduced an element of incongruity. Limiting parental contact was one such practice. One couple was advised to put a dying baby back in the incubator, and another was advised not to stay all night. When the parents were considering a crucial decision about whether to allow the child to die, it seemed absurd to them to be hedged about by any such restriction. Their very vulnerability could render them less assertive than usual, and they rarely protested, but sometimes parents were left with lasting regrets. When they were going to have so little time ever with this child, it seemed right that they should make the most of every second.

Sometimes the overall situation seemed to present incongruity. For example, it seemed inexplicable to parents of large full-term babies for their child to be fighting for his life and losing the battle when other tiny immature babies were progressing well. Some found it really distressing to be exposed to this comparison and to encounter the other parents. The apparent injustices of life added to their sense of being out of control.

## Staff approaches

A mismatch between what was happening and the staff's manner was confusing for parents. It was disturbing to have nursing or midwifery staff being inappropriately jovial or cheerful. Chance comments could be wounding – being told that the baby was 'misbehaving,' or wondering aloud to a mother whether a first bottle of formula feed (which she had consented to) had triggered a reaction in the baby and started a serious problem. Delays in attending to the mother denied her precious time with the baby.

## Family responses

For a variety of reasons relatives seemed to be of little support at this time.

> Family was there for us, grannies and grandads were losing a grand-daughter, but it was us that were losing a child. And the only other people that knew what we were going through was the team. We were offered support from [our families] but we didn't want it ... I don't see that anybody else can know what we feel but – maybe it is slightly self-ish but – tough.
>
> (P35: parents of preterm triplets)

Informing relatives was painful.

> The hardest thing was the phone calls I had to make that day. Excited calls in the morning [when she was born], then phoning back about three or four hours later: 'We're going to [a referral Unit miles away],' then at night-time saying that she's not going to survive.
>
> (P13: father of baby with cardiac anomaly)

The reactions of family members sometimes added to the parents' burden. Relatives were hysterical, absorbed in their own grief, told the parents that they knew what they were going through, expressed false hopes, were silent, or went over and over the same ground.

## Amenities

As at the earlier stage when serious problems first presented, parents found the facilities to be inadequate at times. They cited a number of deficiencies. The position of private rooms came in for criticism if it meant that parents were constantly exposed to the sound of babies crying or to happy parents. If they were so secluded that mothers missed out on postnatal checks or they were forgotten or excluded at mealtimes, other problems arose. Conveying distressing news was made even harder if they were obliged to wait in a queue, to speak in a public place, or no telephone was made available to them.

While decisions were being made parents wanted adequate privacy from visitors to the Unit. They preferred a minimum number of staff to be involved. Some called for protection from the exhausting demands of too many relatives and friends.

They also reported having to waste time finding a parking space, or explaining their plight to gatekeepers, or feeding meters. These things were frustrating to parents whose only desire was to spend as much time as possible with their child while they decided on the best course of action.

## Additional pressures on parents

Some groups of parents cited special problems which they encountered as a result of their circumstances. Although they cannot be generalised to the wider population, they nevertheless merit a mention in order to alert clinicians to such potential difficulties.

Parents who were far from home and their support systems had additional problems. They sometimes had no one to bring them a change of clothes or money, nowhere to do washing, and no one to run errands for essentials. As one such family said, huge demands were being made on them to consider treatment choices for their baby, but they felt that the staff in the nursery isolated the management of those issues from their overall circumstances and undervalued the significance of their geographical displacement and sense of personal insecurity.

Special vulnerabilities were expressed by families with several babies where one or more died. When the survivors deteriorated the hurt increased, and discussions about treatment withdrawal and more deaths were acutely distressing.

# Discussion
## Deciding is difficult

Our study highlights the complexities of decision making for parents. It is well accepted that it is not easy for anyone, let alone a parent, to decide what someone else would choose when it comes to life-sustaining treatment,[113,114] especially when that someone is a neonate who has no history or expressed wishes to guide the choice.

> The prospect of choosing among evils in any context is not attractive. The forbidding character of such choices seems especially acute in those situations in which the evils faced bear directly on the life of a wanted infant, born to parents benevolently disposed to it.[115]

Competing interests may add to this difficulty. Unravelling the interests of the child from those of the parents is a complex matter, and the potential burden on the family must be considered if the value of their lives is not to be diminished.

In both the USA[116] and the UK,[12] most neonatologists have been seen to favour an 'individualised prognostic strategy,'[117] evaluating and re-evaluating each specific case as more and more information becomes available, the central tenet being that every baby is unique and his or her circumstances require consideration on their own merits. It is thought that the adoption of this strategy, rather than a 'wait until certainty' approach, helps to avoid two errors, namely the death of an infant who could have survived with a good quality of life, and the survival of a child with overwhelming disabilities.[116] Where a judgement is made that treatment is medically futile, it may be seen as a technical judgement. As such it raises no issue of values, and in theory requires no consultation with the family. 'Ethics is transformed into medicine.'[100] However, in practice, as we have seen, doctors do consult parents in these circumstances, and decisions are made about how long to prolong the life. Where treatment may not be futile but the consequences are burdensome, more troubling ethical questions arise and choices must be made. These relate not only to the question 'Should we treat?', but also to 'Who should decide?', 'How much influence should be exerted by others?' and 'Will they be burdened by this responsibility?'. And these were questions which our study addressed. We shall consider first the different options and then the implications of our findings.

# Doctors as decision makers

About one-third (31%) of the parents in our study believed that the doctors decided in their case, and most of these were happy to leave that decision in their hands. There are persuasive arguments for doing so.[12,36]

- Predicting and prognosticating, and assessing the burdens and benefits of medical treatment, are integral features of the decision-making process, and they are matters outwith the parents' domain.
- When doctors have initiated treatment they have an obligation to take responsibility for deciding when to stop it.
- Even many adult patients favour a passive role in decision making.

On the other hand, there are a number of hazards in leaving the choice to the medical team.[17,34,100,118–120]

- Both role and training may predispose them to be active in saving lives.
- Once they have started to treat, they may find it difficult to stop – the 'vicious cycle of commitment.'[121]

- It is questionable whether their decisions reflect those of their patients and their relatives.
- In presenting a case to the parents they may construct medical and ethical parameters which lead to certain conclusions which are so persuasive that the parents are left with few morally correct alternatives, and clinicians themselves have admitted that they are persuasive in the way in which they convey information to parents.
- The judgement of physicians in these matters is not simply technical. It is also 'shaped by their own interests and by adaptations to the stresses of medical practice, as well as by apparently high-minded concerns that are at best ambiguously patient-centred. Whether physicians report a patient as "terminal" or the possibility of recovery "realistic" does involve technical judgement, but technical judgement shaped by the distinctive values of their occupation.'[100]

# Parents as deciders

The majority of the parents whom we interviewed believed that they were instrumental, to some extent at least, in choosing for their babies. Powerful arguments have been proffered for parents to be the decision makers.[12,20–26]

- They are the ones who have to live with the consequences.
- They alone know their values, priorities and resources.
- Parental and family autonomy is the best defence for vulnerable children.
- Parents themselves *want* to be active in decision making on behalf of their children.
- '... the love which parents usually have for their children will be dominant in the decisions which they make in determining what is in the best interest of their children. It is to be expected that parents will act unselfishly, particularly where life itself is at stake.'[122]
- Parents respond better to a burden which they choose to carry.

However, there are also arguments against the parents being the people to decide.[8,27–29]

- Distress may cripple their thinking and understanding.
- They are often physically and emotionally exhausted.
- The responsibility may prove to be too onerous.
- Their own interests may conflict with those of the child.
- Their understanding of medical matters is limited.
- They have little preparation for such a crucial decision.

> The only decision I was given was the big one. Everything else – about any treatment right from the start – wasn't really asked. The only decision I had to make was the big one.
>
> (P15: father of preterm baby)

## Parents and doctors as joint deciders

Only a tenth of the parents in our study believed that the decision was a joint one. Clearly this involves a balance of the advantages and disadvantages of the two preceding choices. However, in joint approaches other influences are also at work. Zussman has suggested that families do have an effect on doctors and nurses, and that their relationship can influence decision making.[100] If families are attractive personalities, or are particularly demanding, or are very frequent visitors to the nursery, for example, a crack appears in the application of medical utility, and through this crack criteria of social worth, damage limitation or attempts to please may be introduced. In the reverse direction, it is inevitable that families will be influenced by the way in which information about the prognosis is conveyed by the staff,[123,124] and their perception of the compassion, sympathy and expectation of the professionals.

A joint decision is the one recommended by professional organisations. In this country, as in The Netherlands,[125] official guidance is that, not only are parents 'legally and morally entitled to give or withhold consent to treatment,' but 'the decisions of parents and doctors together should determine what course of action is to be followed.'[10] However, there are qualifications: 'the actual treatment decision will depend on the medical assessment of benefit' and 'parents cannot insist on enforcing decisions based solely on their own preferences where these conflict with good medical evidence.'[10] In essence the advice is that, whilst the decisions should be shared, doctors should take the lead in assessing clinical factors and parents should take the lead in determining best interests in a more general sense.

## The baby as decider

It is important not to overlook the small minority who believed that the baby decided. Instead of the adults consciously deciding that the baby is not for continuing treatment, a point may be reached where death occurs spontaneously or it is impossible to resuscitate the child. Where this happens the parents are relieved of the final responsibility. The question of choice then becomes a matter of technical judgement by the doctors, rather than one concerning the moral authority of the parents.[100]

Given these different approaches, does our study shed light on the best way to decide?

## Parents' own wishes

We have no way of knowing whether the doctors who dealt with these parents adopted an assent or consent approach,[17] or whether they agreed with the parents' understanding of who made the decision. We only know what the parents themselves thought. It is also important to remember that, with hindsight, the parents' own views might be different from those which they felt at the time, when emotions were turbulent and the end result and autopsy results were unknown.

That said, the parents gave a clear message that the majority want to be given the opportunity to decide, although the minority who found the very idea abhorrent must also be heard. This finding appears at first sight to be at odds with our earlier work,[12] where we found that only 3% of doctors and 6% of nurses thought that parents should be given this responsibility, although as many as 58% of doctors and 73% of nurses favoured a joint approach. Nevertheless, 30% of doctors and 14% of nurses believed that it should be a medical decision. These figures give pause for thought, in view of the finding of the present study that most parents believe they are capable of accepting this responsibility.

One of the principal reasons for protecting parents from this responsibility seems to be that professionals fear they will be overburdened with guilt.[12,17,27] Indeed, Rue has contended that guilt is one of the major components of such parents' suffering, because a decision to limit life is 'contrary to a powerful altruism that defends and nurtures the young and violates the deepest of parental instincts.'[27] (It should be noted, however, that Rue based this study on women seen in therapy, so it could be that he was speaking of pathological grief, rather than reflecting the emotions of parents involved in treatment decisions as a whole.) It is clear that in all such cases an element of regret may exist: 'One persists in wishing otherwise, even when one chooses one's course.'[126] These parents clearly wish that things had been other than they are. However, we found no evidence of such guilt.

The parents in our study did indeed express both regret and guilt in relation to a number of factors in their pregnancy, birth or postnatal period, but they did not express guilt about their decision to stop treatment, at least not within the first 13 months following the death. Indeed, one mother said that her guilt related to *not* wanting the baby to die when it was clearly best for him to go and another mother expressed guilt because she had *not* made the decision herself. We believe it to be especially significant that those families for whom the decision related to quality of life as distinct from the impossibility of survival did not feel guilt. All of this group of parents were certain not only that the right decision had been made, but also that they were the right people to make it. This finding has been supported by a small study in this area where researchers found that far from feeling guilt, parents were 'appalled' that such a decision could be made without their involvement.[62]

Although our research has revealed these different preferences, it is notable that whichever way the choices went, the majority of the parents were satisfied with both the decision and the decider. To summarise the relevant figures, as many as 83% believed that the right person had decided. By the time of the first interview, 88% were satisfied that the right decision had been made, and by 13 months this figure had risen to 97%. This suggests a service which is highly sensitive to parental preferences and cues.

# Parents' needs in decision making

If parents are to be involved in decision making of this magnitude, they need certain elements to enable a good process. An important finding of our investigation is that evidence to substantiate a poor prognosis is crucially important. Without it, doubts may always remain in the parents' mind about the wisdom of the decision to stop treatment. They need to *see for themselves* in an understandable form that the alternatives to withdrawal of treatment are worse than death.

Full and frank information is also a key component. Honesty is essential, and false reassurances are to be avoided:[127] 'Truth sometimes hurts, but deceit hurts more.'[128] The parents call for this information to be given by a single familiar knowledgeable person of senior standing, in a way which demonstrates empathy, equality and emotional availability, paced appropriately, given as soon as is practically possible, to both parents together or with another significant support person present, in a private quiet place, free from distractions. These preferences bear a striking similarity to those identified by a study of parents of children with developmental disabilities.[104] In this highly charged situation, however, it must always be borne in mind that what staff think they have said might not be what parents hear or understand has been said.[33] Moreover, parents may disguise their true responses in order to conform to what they perceive to be expected of them, as one professional, highly articulate and intelligent set of parents did when they went out into the car park to cry, rather than express emotion in the Unit. In their search for information we found that some parents ask the doctor what he would do if this were his child. As one mother wrote, 'I hated to impose demands of personal opinion on his already difficult role but was thankful, once again, for his honesty. If he would refuse treatment from his own informed opinion, our decision was clear.'[129] However, one paediatrician has advised colleagues to tread warily here – their task is to guide the parent towards a 'choice that is authentic and genuine for them,' and not to base a direction upon their own values and view of the world.[130]

The parents in our study support a system which ensures that they have regular meetings with a given consultant as a matter of course. It is frightening to be 'sent for' to see 'the top man' when things start to go wrong. It is also distressing to be seen by many different doctors and to meet unknown faces at times of crisis. Consistency and continuity help to engender trust and minimise conflict.[131] Part of this development of trust comes from admitting the parents into the thinking of the medical team – the transparency model.[132] This enables parents to take some part in the team's process of decision making even when it is based on largely technical issues, by sharing with them medical reasoning, paving the way for them to adopt a more significant role in subsequent decisions.[116] Part of it comes from the compassion and understanding which accompany the medical expertise, a fact which has been reinforced elsewhere.[100,133–135] When the message is hard to hear, a kind, sympathetic and understanding approach is highly valued. We found that special mention was frequently made of male consultants' caring and compassion. Not only was it particularly valued when it came from someone in such an exalted position, but comments seemed to reflect a sense that it exceeded what was expected of men. Male nurses were also singled out in this way. Nurturing seemed to be expected of females.[136]

It is clearly very difficult to pace events sensitively for all involved. Staff have expressed this concern[12] as well as the parents in the present study. In some circumstances, events dictate speed. On occasion, too, when death is inevitable and imminent, doctors must make unilateral decisions if an infant suddenly deteriorates and the parents are not available. However, if such emergency situations have not occurred, parents are dissatisfied if events are not paced in line with their wishes and needs. If the process is rushed they sometimes feel pressured to decide before they have properly assimilated the enormity of what is happening.[23] Reflections and doubts may occur later. If the process is too slow, they express distress at the protracted suffering they see. Some regret what they 'have put the baby through.' For others, serious doubts arise as to the wisdom of the decision: did the child really want to live? The timing of events is an important element in the overall management of decision making in these circumstances.

Our data draw attention to the key role of staff in providing support for parents at this time. Usual networks are of limited value in these circumstances, which are commonly outside the experience or understanding of friends and family. What the professional team do can make a real difference to the parents' ability to cope with the reality of the facts which are being given,[134,135] and it has been suggested that their compassionate concern, more than any other factor, will influence how parents respond to the loss of their child.[82]

The finding that certain groups encounter particular difficulties is a salutary reminder of the need for vigilance and individually tailored management. Very young parents, who may perceive authority and expert opinion negatively, require tactful handling if they are to feel that they have been respected as the parents of this child but not overburdened with responsibility. Too much may be expected of parents who are themselves healthcare professionals, and detailed knowledge of neonatal care should not be assumed. Parents who are transferred far from home can easily feel isolated and fearful, and their vulnerability should be recognised. The strain of waiting for an elusive diagnosis if rare conditions present sometimes induces powerful feelings of frustration or aggression, and sympathy is needed when dealing with parents whose emotions may be volatile.

These findings provide powerful insights into parents' experiences, and guidance as to the factors which help or hinder them at a crucial time in the process of decision making on behalf of their infant.

# Conclusion

- The majority of parents want to be actively involved in decision making on behalf of their baby.
- In order to do so, they need where possible concrete evidence of a poor prognosis.
- They require full, honest information which is consistent, preferably from one consultant and delivered in a compassionate way which is sensitive to their needs and wishes.
- Family and friends are of limited support at this time, and during the decision-making process parents need the empathic support of the professional team who are intimately involved in the care of their baby.

# CHAPTER 8

# Management of dying

The decision having been made to redirect care away from intensive therapy and towards compassionate care, priorities and needs change. Death is now the expected outcome, and efforts are focused on ensuring dignity and reducing distress to a minimum. As Isobel Allende put it when she finally accepted this change of direction for her daughter, 'we have passed the stage for efficiency and are entering the stage of love.'[137]

## Involvement in the dying process

Only three families in our study had no opportunity to be involved in the dying process, in all cases because the child had died before the parents arrived in the Unit. Although for most the opportunities included activities before withdrawal and death as well as afterwards, these parents were limited to doing things with the child only after death. One of these couples received a telephone call in the middle of the night telling them that the baby's condition had worsened. They were five minutes too late to see their son alive, and they expressed a sense of guilt that they had not been with him when he died.

Having the opportunity to participate did not necessarily mean that all parents did so. In one case the parents were not involved at all. A further five sets of parents elected to set limits to the level of their participation. For example, one couple who had a severely asphyxiated baby said that they just wanted to be called if he deteriorated, so that they were aware of developments, but they did not intend to go to the hospital because they could not face watching him die. Another couple from a minority culture left the Unit before their preterm twins died because they believed that the children were already dead in effect, even though they were still breathing. And in one instance, a couple remained convinced until the end that the baby would live. It was only during the last few minutes of her life that her mother would allow her to be taken out of the incubator to be cuddled.

In the majority of families both parents participated to some extent, but in one case only the father was involved and in three cases only the mother. One father initially persuaded his wife not to see the child at all, but after the death she insisted that she wanted to do so. She was subsequently glad that she had seen him, as it gave her an opportunity to appreciate his extreme immaturity.

Contact time varied. Some parents stayed for only minutes, others stayed for hours, whilst a few remained for several days and nights. It has to be borne in mind that while for some families this was their one chance to be with the child, in others it was the culmination of weeks of constant visiting.

> I hadn't missed a day at all in all those [13] weeks from the day they were born. I saw them every single day – for hours. I was going in at nine in the morning and it was five o'clock at night [before I left again] – a long day . . . [my husband] – the nurses – were saying, 'Have a day to yourself.' And I'm saying, 'No, I can't. It's my girls. I just wouldn't do that to them. They have to know I'm here.'
>
> (P10: mother of preterm twins)

# Parental differences

Differences were noted between mothers and fathers with regard to the extent of their involvement. What was right for one was not necessarily exactly right for the other. In almost all cases it was the mother who maintained the greater level of involvement. Thus where the mothers remained exclusively with the baby at this point, the fathers limited their time with the dying child, popping out periodically to attend to other commitments such as work or children, or as a break from the intense emotion. One father remained on the postnatal ward and just called into the Unit for short spells. Those who remained in the Unit with the baby sometimes stood back a little, taking 'second place,' to allow the mothers the bigger share of the handling and cuddling. This seemed to be a mutually agreed division of involvement. In most cases ($n = 7$) this stemmed from the mother's desire to be more closely involved than the father – she wanted to be the one to hold the baby, to collect the mementoes and to do the mothering tasks. The fathers expressed themselves as comfortable with this. As one father said, the woman's role was to mother the baby, and the man's role was to support and provide. Another mother observed that in their case it was more a question of her becoming extremely busy and going into 'autopilot,' while the father was 'lost in grief.'

A few fathers had been reluctant to stay for the actual dying, and had only done so because they were pressured by their partners. All of these men without exception volunteered that they were subsequently glad that they had been persuaded to stay.

A difference related to timing was seen in one family. Once the decision was made, the mother felt that they would know instinctively when it was right to take each next step. The father, on the other hand, was in a hurry to withdraw treatment, fearful that if they delayed the baby might die while he was still on the machinery, instead of in their arms.

> To be honest, once we'd agreed that we would [stop treatment when it was the right time for us] I was kind of in a hurry then to do it because my worry was he would die in that [incubator on the ventilator] before. I'd hate to be sitting there mulling over when the right time was and then to be told, 'Well, actually he's now passed away.' So I attached a slight sense of urgency to it. I wanted to hold him while he was alive.
>
> (P 27: father of baby with cardiac anomaly)

For a number of other fathers it was only once the decision had been made that they allowed themselves to start to attach to the baby. It had seemed imperative before that to remain sufficiently distanced to see the position clearly, and not to waiver from a difficult choice which was best for everyone concerned. Once they had given themselves permission to become emotionally engaged, that time with the dying baby then became extremely precious. These fathers were particularly keen to be actively involved in the later stages, having left things to their partners up until then.

Once the baby had died, differences were seen in a few families. Some fathers left and went home, leaving the mother with the baby. Two fathers fell asleep at that stage, exhausted from a hard day's work and lack of rest, but their partners spent the time savouring the child's existence and crying for all that they had lost.

For two couples there was a difference of conviction, one partner feeling great guilt or doubt and the other not. In one case it was the father who had grave reservations about withdrawing treatment when the baby had fought so hard to live, and he seriously considered asking for re-ventilation. In the other case, the mother was instantly racked with guilt when the baby died. The response of another couple differed inasmuch as they interpreted the baby's movements differently – to the father they spoke of pain, whereas to the mother they represented life.

# Warning of what might happen

Twelve sets of parents (20%) said that they had not been at all prepared for what would happen during the dying process as far as they could remember.

> I wasn't prepared for that birth and I wasn't prepared for his death either. I was completely out of control and I was petrified. I didn't want to be there, but I could not bear *not* to be. I didn't want [my husband] to have him. I didn't want anybody to touch him . . . nobody had prepared us for what was going to happen . . . They took the tube out and he lay there quietly in my arms and for a while I was able to look down at him. I still never moved from that position . . . and after a period of time I remember looking down and I looked at his hand and it was blue. It was from then on I was gone, basically. I could not bear to look at him after that. I was really, really frightened. I couldn't bear for anybody to come near me or take him from me because I didn't want to catch sight of his face, to see what was happening because I'd never ever dealt with that before . . . Two and a half hours later [the doctor] came in with the stethoscope [and certified him dead]. Now nobody had prepared me for that.
>
> (P20: mother of baby with asphyxia)

One couple felt that the staff were scared to predict anything. A further seven sets of parents (12%) said that they had simply been told that nothing was certain and nothing could be predicted.

However, the majority could cite specific information which they had received about what lay ahead. This information fell into the following six general categories.

# Procedures

Three sets of parents remembered the staff outlining the procedure for discontinuing treatment.

# Duration

Four sets of parents recalled being told that once the ventilator was discontinued the baby would die. Two others were advised that the heart might continue to beat for a time after disconnection. One father interpreted this as meaning for a few minutes, and was disconcerted when it kept beating for one and a half hours. Four other couples were warned that the child might gasp for a time, and again one of these parents was not prepared for gasping to continue for 20 minutes.

Parents were anxious about missing the death, and some described a sense of not being able to leave the room for fear of being absent at the critical time. Three families remembered being given a vague idea of when it might happen, from which they surmised how long that would be. One family was told that the death would not be sudden and unexpected. Two other families understood from what the staff said that the process would be swifter than it was – one baby took 20 minutes to die, and the other took two and a half hours.

A quarter of the families (14, 24%) were given some sense of how long it would take. Sometimes these parameters were vague:

- 'It will probably be quick' ($n = 6$ families). In five of these six cases the families did not think that the time it took was 'quick.' In one case they did not say how long it took, but commented that even the doctors were surprised at how long the baby lived. The other five babies took respectively 1.5, 7, 14 and 31 hours to die, certainly not a quick experience for their parents watching them dying
- 'It could be a few minutes, it could be hours' ($n = 2$)
- 'It could be a few minutes, it could be days' ($n = 4$)
- 'It could be days or weeks' ($n = 2$).

In only one case did parents report a longer prediction than reality. They were given an estimate of seven hours, but the baby died in just one hour.

> He only lasted the hour, and they expected 6 or 7 hours, so he wasn't as strong as they thought, so he couldn't have survived the operation [to repair damage and anomalies].
> (P 56: father of preterm baby with congenital anomalies)

# Physical changes

Two families remembered being advised that the child's colour would change as he deteriorated. Another couple was told that their baby would visibly deteriorate.

# Dignity and peace

Parents conveyed the impression that they had received general reassurance that the baby would be cared for in a compassionate way, his interests would be considered throughout, and the dying would be as dignified and pain-free as possible. Nine sets of parents were more specifically reassured that the death would be peaceful, with the baby just 'slipping away.'

# Relief of suffering and symptom control

A simple assurance that the baby would not suffer was the message that six families recalled. A further 15 sets of parents (25%) said that they were specifically told that the baby would be given morphine in sufficient doses to ensure that he did not suffer, or in one other case 'something to relax' him. One couple remembered hearing that the morphine would depress respiration and as a result could hasten death. In two other cases the adverse effects of morphine had been described to the parents, but the babies unexpectedly appeared to thrive on it. The parents of another baby who had had convulsions were assured that medication would control the fits during the dying process.

# Support for parents

The parents reported being aware that they could say if they wanted anything special at this time – it was for them to orchestrate matters in the way that best met their needs and wishes. Three families remembered specifically being told that the staff would do everything in their power to make the process as smooth as possible for them.

# The actual experience

The exact events at the time of dying were very varied, and whilst every death was significant and every account moving, each was unique, and for the purpose of analysis there would be little benefit in rehearsing all 59 experiences. However, some points merit expansion, although the numbers of parents reporting these matters are largely irrelevant.

# Length of time it took to die

Although many parents used the time they had with the baby effectively, the experience of a protracted death was harrowing for parents.

> There were some points at one or two in the morning where he decided to stop breathing and hold his breath for two or three minutes ...

and then he would start breathing so you'd been through [his death] 20 times and after 12 hours of that you can't keep on going – not at that level [of intensity] . . . if you've been holding your baby who's dying for the past few hours – and it is simply the worst experience you ever have – after a while, because you can't keep on hurting at that level, you start to come out of it a bit. You relax with it a bit more. The thing about it being as long as 15 hours is that after a while you're not crying any more and you can look at him and you can see his face and you can see the way his nose wrinkles. It becomes much more ordinary – you accept it more. And that contributed to why we wanted [his sibling] there. Because we don't want it to be this horrendous awful thing that nobody talks about that happened – this huge trauma. It was just a little baby who died. It's not scary; it's not frightening; it's just very sad.

(P25: parents of preterm baby with asphyxia)

It was evident that most parents expected the process to be quick.

They brought him [through to us after disconnection] in a nice little cradle. They said, 'Take your time.' Now he was still alive . . . He was gasping intermittently . . . I just thought when the tube comes out that's it, they're going to be dead. But it struck me [now] that no, they weren't. So I undressed him because I said, 'I want to look, I want to see, I want to remember, everything.'

(P33: mother of preterm twins)

What you tended to expect to happen is that he'd be brought and he'd be in your arms for 15 minutes, or half an hour and then he'd pass away. That would be nice and straightforward. But 15 *hours* later, the next morning, and he's still chugging away and you're looking at him and you're thinking, 'He's a fighter, he's surviving, he's keeping on going.' And there's nothing physically wrong with him apart from a couple of black eyes and the bruising. And that's when you go back and start questioning your original decision.

(P25: father of preterm baby with asphyxia)

When death did not ensue fairly soon after discontinuation, doubts sometimes crept in. Should they have resuscitated in the first place?

We felt like if they had just told us that [there was no hope before they resuscitated him after a week] we wouldn't have had to go through all this [agony for the next three weeks until he died]. I know people say it's nice to hold your baby and things, but you were just living on no hope because there wasn't any hope for him. He was really, really severely brain damaged and couldn't suck or anything, so he had no quality of life and it was no use pursuing that sort of thing. To be quite honest, it just prolonged the agony for so long. It felt like months to me ... it was the same routine day in day out for three weeks. If they had only just said to us what they told us the following day [that there was no hope] it might have just ended there [he wouldn't have been resuscitated on Day 6], and then we could have maybe got on a wee bit quicker, got back into a life again.

> (P 39: parents of baby with asphyxia)

Was the decision to stop treating right? If the baby was fighting so hard to live, should they not give him every chance? Was he trying to tell them that he wanted to live?

I didn't expect him to last for so long after they took the tube out. I felt because he was putting up such a strong fight, there was a couple of times I contemplated reversing [the decision and putting the tube back in]. It was really distressing. It felt like a lifetime.

> (P 20: father of baby with asphyxia)

The noises he was making – [my husband] said, 'Do you not think we've done the wrong thing? Do you not think the tube would be better to go back in?' And they were saying, 'No, no. This could go on for hours.' I even still then doubted we had done wrong – when he was not wanting to go. He was fighting to stay.

> (P 20: mother of baby with asphyxia)

More than a fifth of the parents (13/59, 22%) expressed reservations about the time it had taken. Four families reported that it had taken 3 to 6 hours from the time of withdrawal, two that it had been 7 to 9 hours, three that it had been 10 to 15 hours, two that it had been 18 to 21 hours, and in two cases it had taken 31 to 36 hours.

The experiences of three families are detailed in order to capture something of the variety of the circumstances and the trauma for parents.

## Case 1

It took one child with severe brain damage 36 hours to die. Even at the start of this long vigil the mother was already very tired after a Caesarean Section. The parents started off with the baby in bed with them saying their goodbyes. The baby continued to breathe, so they took turns to leave the room for a break. Eventually they themselves began to doze, so they put her into a cot beside them. The second night they put the baby to bed, said goodbye, and slept from sheer exhaustion. To their amazement, when they woke next morning she was still alive. Although intellectually they were very aware of the serious damage she had suffered, by this stage they started to question the wisdom of what was being done. By the third morning they felt that they could take no more. They were on the point of going home, leaving her in the hospital, when she deteriorated and died.

> We did take breaks, but we did feel that we had to be with her. That wasn't in question. But there's only so many times you can say goodbye . . . it does become harder the longer it is. Just being so tired you begin to get quite psychotic. I found those walls were beginning to close in on me and I really felt I had to get out . . . but I don't know how it could have been bettered. You can't escape it. You've got to go through it . . . But even if you knew that it was going to be 36 hours, what could you do apart from giving a whacking dose of morphine immediately she came off the ventilator?
> [*HMcH. You wouldn't have wanted that?*]
> I don't think so. It's this fine line I feel. It would have been kind of *convenient* to give it to her then but I don't think [it would be the right thing to do].

## Case 2

Another couple watched their baby with lethal anomalies dying slowly over a period of 6 weeks. They had dreaded the time when she would need morphine, seeing this as the beginning of the end. However, the child seemed to thrive on the drug, and they even took her home for a brief time, before a setback necessitated readmission. She remained on morphine for the rest of her life. Back in hospital, her condition deteriorated and she became totally unresponsive.

> [The consultant] came in and he then said, 'Well, I think what we need to do is put her on a much higher dose of the morphine, have her on the drip and really just see how she goes through the day.' And she was terrible that night. We had her in our arms and we thought, 'Any minute now she's going to go.' She was really [just lolling], really unresponsive. We just expected her to drift away.

Cheyne–Stokes breathing signalled the final phase. They prepared for her death.

> Then it got to the evening time, and I said, 'Right, I'm just going to change her nappy now, give her a sponge down.' We literally laid her on her cot, started to undress her and we couldn't believe it! She came to! 'Talking' to us, putting hands in our mouths, feeling our hair, gurgling away. I remember at that point we'd got her on the cot and I remember thinking, 'I don't believe this!' [A second consultant] came in . . . he saw the look on my face and I just said, 'I don't think we can go through this again' . . . . The thought that [the baby] could have come

back from that episode for maybe another week or so for us to have to go
through it all again . . . [was just appalling].

However, the baby died soon afterwards.

## Case 3

For a third couple the experience of preparing for death was repeated
several times. Their baby girl had a lethal congenital anomaly. On each occasion when treatment was withdrawn, they were advised to expect death.
She survived the first two attempts (being taken off the ventilator and
then having prostaglandins stopped), and they were eventually advised
that they could take her home if they so wished.

> We didn't know quite what was going to happen. [The named neonatol-
> ogist] said it could be over quickly or it could take a bit of time . . .
> he didn't want to commit himself to a definite answer. To start with he
> said she might go on for a few hours or a few days. And then after a
> few days, well, she might go on for a few weeks!

The baby remained at home for several weeks, returning frequently for
morphine injections. The parents recalled being told each time that these
might kill her, but she appeared to them to be getting better.

> She was becoming more aware. She'd started to move her limbs a bit
> more. Minor things but they were big things to us. They were noticeable.
> We were relaying this to [the neonatologist] but he thought we were just
> seeing them because we wanted to see them. But you have to remember
> the only time he saw [the baby] was when we took her back after she'd
> had a shot of morphine and she was out of it again. He thought we were
> just seeing things because we wanted to see them because we were her
> parents and we were grasping at straws . . . I was reacting with her –
> being a normal happy Mum. Because I think I'd forgotten – I'd put it
> out of my head – I kept thinking she was going to get better. I was
> seeing that many improvements I kept thinking, 'They're all wrong. The
> doctors are wrong. She's getting better.' [And she had after all defied
> their predictions before] so many times it was unbelievable.

When the baby was finally ill enough to be readmitted the parents did not
believe the prognosis of imminent death, having seen her defy expectations so often. As a result her death stunned them.

These three cases are illustrative of the experience of protracted dying.
For other families the process was much quicker and none of the parents expressed regret about this, although some did point out the discrepancy between what they believed they had been told and the reality.
More often they remarked that the speed with which the baby had died

indicated that the prognosis was right and the baby could not have survived. A swift death reinforced the wisdom of what they had decided was the best course of action.

# Unexpected happenings

Parents were sometimes caught unawares when things did not go as they had been advised or as they expected them to do. In some cases this came about because the child deteriorated rapidly. Events were then brought forward to allow them to be practically involved in the dying process. Sometimes unexpected developments shocked them – for example, continued breathing or unexpected colour changes after ventilation was stopped, the baby struggling or uttering 'screeches,' or breathing recommencing when they had thought that the child had died. This last experience was particularly upsetting, and parents described becoming hysterical or being rigid with terror during it.

> He was kind of choking; he was coughing, spluttering, gasping. The stethoscope was coming out but the minute she was coming over [to check his heart had stopped] he started again. I was just not looking. And then she would come again and he would start again ... I was just staring out into the ... corridor. My arm was numb. They were saying, 'Go and have a lie down, this could go on for hours.' But I couldn't even move. I was just so damn scared. I think it was more his noises that haunt me than the colour of his blue hand. It was going on for ever and ever and ever. Eventually I think [my husband] lent over to take him from me, but by the time he arrived in [my husband's] arms he was gone. It was two and a half hours later.
>
> (P20: mother of baby with asphyxia)

In one case the unexpectedness arose as a result of a decision being overturned. The couple had agreed with the consultant that their child would not be resuscitated. They were then taken aback to find that the junior staff had initiated treatment when the baby required resuscitation because they had either not known of or had not heeded the prior instruction. As a result the baby lived for 15 hours.

Sometimes plans had to be altered suddenly because of unexpected developments. On occasion the precise time of stopping treatment was changed because staff were not available. In one instance the delay was for four days because, the parents reported, they were told that a certain expert was required to do the post-mortem. Sometimes it was the parents who instigated delays, because they wanted family members to come in to say goodbye, or the mother was just not ready yet to let the baby go. Indeed one mother, who agreed in principle that it was the only right course of action, had such difficulty in letting go that she had to be helped by having repeated short-term deadlines and a form of countdown to enable her to accept that the endotracheal tube would be taken out at a specific time.

The enormity of what was happening during the withdrawal and dying, or the feeling of unreality associated with it, could make parents behave in ways which later surprised even them. Several fathers had slept during the dying process. One mother had spent the time before the death occurred in the nurses' office telephoning people to arrange the funeral.

# Fear

Many fears were expressed, some of which the parents said they realised were irrational but they were none the less real.

> *Mother*: Then I remember [the chaplain] telling me I must look at him. I must see him. But I didn't *want* to see him . . . [My husband] then came round and said I had to look at him – he was absolutely beautiful.
> *Father*: I took a photo of him and showed it to her.
> *Mother*: But it didn't register. And then they said, 'I'll bring him in.' But I said, 'Don't force him on me. Don't make me – don't make me look . . .' I felt I was lost in a world of my own. For as much as [my husband] was there and he was my anchor and he was supporting me, I was lost. And I was frightened like I've never been frightened before.
> [*In the end she allowed herself to look gradually*]
> *Mother*: He was absolutely beautiful. He was gorgeous. . . . It was the fear of the unknown I think.
>
> (P 20: parents of baby with asphyxia)

Several parents were afraid to bath, change or dress the baby in case they hurt him, even though they knew he was dying. One mother feared that the oxygen would run out and there would be a panic. Another feared leaving her dead baby alone, and could only go for a rest when the staff agreed to take the child's body into a room where they were. One mother was so fearful that the dead baby would change that she forced herself to stay awake watching. Another kept tucking a blanket around the dead child because he felt so cold.

For others the dread was of a different kind – a strong feeling of not wanting anyone else to touch the baby after death. They took the child's body home or took it to the mortuary or undertaker themselves to try to prevent this from happening. One mother described in graphic detail her despair when, after taking the baby's body home, she had to release it for autopsy. The pain of parting was devastating.

We brought him home on the night [of the day he died] then we took him back to the hospital for 9 o'clock the next morning. [The neonatal nurse who'd looked after him] came to meet us on the road outside the [hospital]. I was very distressed. Originally we'd just been going to give him to her in the car, but I didn't want to let him go. She took us into a room and left us for a bit so we had a bit more time with him . . . we had him back here after the post-mortem until the funeral . . . The thing is you're wide open, raw, emotionally and if I'd have had to hand [our baby] over to a nurse that hadn't looked after him I'd have found it impossible, I think – or to try and make some kind of connection with somebody at that time. So I think that was really important that it was [her] – but maybe it was just luck. But I think that is something they should really work to achieve . . . . We knew we were going to get him back but we didn't know for definite when . . . but also it felt that there was going to be a change in him – having had the post-mortem he was going to look different. He looked like he was sleeping that first day.

(P49: parents of baby with asphyxia)

# Taking the baby home before death

Three couples took their babies home knowing that they were going to die, although only one child actually did die at home. The other two couples had an arrangement that they would take the child back when deterioration or an emergency presented. They enjoyed having the baby at home with them:

I was over the moon! I thought finally we can use some of the things and put her in clothes and have her at home and try and be as normal as possible.

(P9: mother of baby with cardiac anomaly)

Nevertheless, they found the responsibility frightening initially.

It was terrifying. My doctor actually came in to see us and he said, 'Any time you need me, just ring me, night or day,' and he even gave us his home telephone number. But it still wasn't the same as having the security of having staff on hand.

(P9: mother of baby with cardiac anomaly)

These three couples took pleasure in showing their babies off to family, friends and colleagues. One couple specifically ensured that people who were in contact with their other child saw them out with the pram, so that when the sibling talked about the baby other people were in tune with her and could be supportive. A small number of other couples said that they were offered the opportunity to bring the baby home, but had declined because they felt that they would not have been able to stay in their homes if they had been associated with death in this way.

> I very definitely didn't want her to die at home. That was something we had discussed and thought no, because how would we feel about living here afterwards? Obviously it might have happened overnight while she was here and we wouldn't have had any say in it. If she'd lived here for a longer period and she'd had a *life* at home, we wouldn't have minded so much if she'd *died* at home, but because we don't think of her as being here, we think of her as being in the Neonatal Unit, so it's easier for us to handle if she died over there.
>
> (P51: parents of baby with congenital anomalies)

# Christening/blessing

Many families reported having the baby christened or blessed even if they were not church-goers. The ceremony served two main functions – performing the act in these circumstances underlined the seriousness of the situation and, with its special atmosphere and words, the ritual was comforting.

# Parental emotion

When asked how they felt during the time of the actual dying, parents recalled a sense of emotion so profound that they could not capture it in words: it was 'like a nightmare,' 'too dreadful for words,' 'the worst day of my life,' 'grief beyond belief.' Many parents wept as they recalled the actual moment of death, and it was very evident that this was one of the most painful memories to recall.

> We were obviously expecting him to die very quickly and he didn't, and he was chuntering away and chuntering away. At one point we got a bit concerned because he was whimpering and we were worried that he was in pain. And they said, 'With that kind of brain damage he won't be in any pain, but if it would make you feel better we'll give him some morphine.' You can know something up here [intellectually] but to hold a baby in that sort of state, who's whimpering and [grimacing] – it was just horrible. And also, we were very glad that we were having this opportunity to hold him in our arms, but it was just the most painful thing you could ever do in your life. And you just couldn't see yourself carrying on. Every minute I kept thinking I can't do this any longer. This

is just so painful. And I knew that if he was given morphine it would probably speed things up.

(P25: mother of preterm baby)

The trauma was indeed sometimes too great to feel at the time. Some parents described a sense of numbness – it was unreal being there waiting for their own child to die.

It was not painful [staying with our baby while she died]. It was at that time just a sort of depression. In some [situations] you can't feel any pain. It was very bad. [My wife] didn't cry. In such cases you can't feel anything [– you're numbed to the pain].

(P26: father of baby with congenital anomalies)

Others reported that at that stage they were distraught or hysterical. Even so, most parents did not wish to avoid this involvement. Rather the experience helped them to take on board the reality of what was happening in their lives. Witnessing the baby's inability to sustain life unaided, watching the deterioration for themselves, and holding the dead child in their arms; all these things reinforced the finality and in many cases the wisdom of what had taken place. Time spent with the baby in such circumstances was precious.

The reason that I've coped as well as I have is the fact that we spent that time [with the dead babies] and we shared and saw and lived death if you like, and dealt with it in our way. The time spent helped us to come to terms with it a lot quicker than perhaps we would have.

(P44: mother of preterm quads)

A few fathers expressed a feeling of anger at the injustice of what was happening. Some noted the incongruity of big babies dying while tiny preterm infants survived. Others, having listened to stories told by other parents, spoke of their own sense of injustice when the babies of women who abused their bodies survived, while theirs died. Some parents described a feeling of guilt because they had been unable to protect their child.

I knew he was going to die without oxygen. It was really, really hard for me. I felt [so alone]. Being a man I felt as though I should be able to fix this. I'm seeing [my partner] crying, I'm seeing [my wee girl] crying, I'm seeing my wee laddie dying. I didn't know what was going on. And I'm saying to [the nurse], 'I cannot watch this.' [But I did. I stayed and I'm glad I did now.] It was a long time to watch a baby die. I thought it would be over in an hour, an hour and a half. It just seemed to go on and on. He was still there and [my partner] was still treating him like a mother. That hurt because she was a mother and I was thinking, ['She won't be for long.']

(P38: father of baby with congenital anomalies)

Many parents noted a degree of ambivalence in their feelings. Alongside the horror of seeing the child slip away, or unpleasant changes taking place, was a sense of overwhelming love, peace and relief. Guilt mixed with the other emotions for some fathers when they realised how relieved they were that the baby was dead. The possibility of his or her continuing existence represented a worse dread for them.

> Wishing it would all finish ... not wanting him to die but wanting him to not suffer any more. It was tearing you apart seeing him suffer, but at the same time you still didn't believe it was happening. Very, very mixed emotions to say the least.
>
> (P2: father of baby with cardiac anomaly)

> Having been given your son in your arms [as he died], I was all over the place by then. It was tremendously important that I was able to do that rather than see my son die without feeling the way I should be feeling towards him. I was very grateful for the fact that I had that opportunity, very upsetting though it was, obviously. And when he did die it was like a tremendous sadness but a tremendous anxiety and an enormous weight had just lifted off my shoulders. That's the way I felt. Even at the time. I was glad that he was going to die. I felt it was better for him and it was better for all of us. But at the same time I felt really guilty about the way I was feeling. Being able to hold my son before he died was very important to me. Had I not had that opportunity I would have found it very difficult to live with myself having felt the way that I had. The overwhelming sense for me was the weight of anxiety had gone. Replaced with grief which I felt I could deal with. It was something which was incredibly burdensome and I found it very difficult to handle.
>
> (P18: father of preterm baby)

This last father highlighted the fact that although different emotions were competing, some were easier to live with than others. Sadness was natural and appropriate, and he would come through the grief process. The anxiety about a severely damaged child surviving, and the guilt of not wanting him to live, were much more burdensome.

Even the process itself created a sense of ambivalence. Each next breath reassured them that the child was still there, but each hour added to their fear that perhaps it had been wrong to withdraw treatment. They were simultaneously willing the baby to live and to die. The result was a time of concentrated anxiety and pain, but also of peace as they savoured each moment. It has to be remembered that a large number of these parents were already exhausted from labours, operations or sleepless nights, on top of the trauma of hearing a poor prognosis and knowing that the baby was so ill or damaged.

For one couple the ambivalence related to the fact that the baby's condition had affected their plans. Prior to his birth they had booked a foreign holiday, intending to take him, too. When he was found to have serious problems they decided to take the holiday anyway, although now he would not be with them. However, the baby did not die as swiftly as they had expected. His lingering death posed real problems. How could they accommodate going on holiday as arranged with leaving him behind still alive? They were increasingly ambivalent about going away, but felt that the break was what they needed. A relative offered to substitute for them and visit the baby, but in the end the child died before they were due to leave.

However, some parents reported positive feelings even though it was such a sad time. It was especially good for families who had had limited or previously no contact with the baby to be able to hold him close and do whatever they wanted with him. Even for parents who had already had contact with their child, it was a different experience once the tubes and machines had gone and they need no longer fear doing anything to jeopardise his chances of survival. For some parents there was a sense of relief, knowing that it would soon be over, the suffering of the baby would be at an end, and they need have no further anxiety about the consequences of a child with severe disability on the rest of the family.

A peaceful dying experience could bring its own comfort.

> We were so scared of 'the end' – all throughout the hospital [stay] from minute one – we were so scared of the end. But because it was so peaceful, and it was exactly how we wanted it, and it was quiet, compared to the [night before] which was horrible [with her struggling for breath and panting horribly]. She just lay and eventually just shut her eyes. But there was no gasping of breath and we were like, 'Oh, is that it?'. Because it was just so peaceful.
>
> (P21: mother of baby with cardiac anomaly)

As one mother said, the phrase 'dying with dignity' had meant little to her, but she felt that they now knew exactly what it meant. Parents expressed their enjoyment of the close contact, the privacy, and the realisation that suffering was at an end and things were now resolving in the best way for the baby. For several parents the closeness was so special that they were distressed if they had to be separated from the child for any reason at this time, or when events detracted from the peace of the dying – for example, painful procedures or evidence of distress in the baby. Some described themselves as 'lucky' that they had had this one last chance to pack a lifetime of loving into a matter of minutes or hours. A number of parents mentioned a sense of pride in their child even though his life had been so short. They sometimes realised that this pride was an essentially parental feeling which others might not share, and two mothers added that they did not want other family members to see the baby because they might mis-construe the changes taking place and perceive him as deformed.

# Place of death

Although a small number of parents also reported being offered the option, in only one case did the baby die at home. The majority (39, 66%) died in a quiet room away from the main nurseries. For parents who were present when the baby died in the nursery itself, a form of privacy was offered by screens (10, 17%), or the room was emptied of other babies and parents (2, 3%). In a small number of cases (4, 7%) the baby was taken to the room where the mother was being cared for. Parents were not present at the deaths of the other three cases (5%).

# Parents' involvement after the death

There was opportunity for the parents to remain with the child for as long as they wished, doing anything that they felt was right for them. Only one couple left before the actual death took place. Eight sets of parents (14%) stayed for just a few minutes, commenting that there was nothing more they could do now and they just wanted to get away from the scene of so much pain. However, nine sets of parents (15%) stayed with the dead baby for several days in a side room or special ward, wanting to be with their child while they still could. The rest varied in the time that they recalled spending with the baby immediately after he or she had died (*see* Figure 8.1).

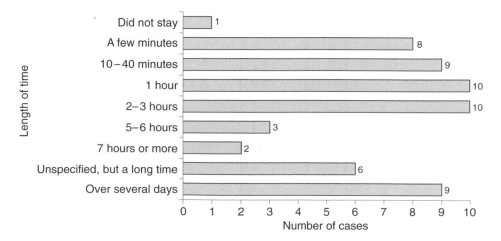

**Figure 8.1:**   Length of time parents stayed with the dead baby ($n = 58$).

The parents who were actively involved expressed their appreciation of the opportunity to do the things which parents normally do with their infants.

> It was really good because we were able to hold her [properly]. Before we were only allowed to hold her [low down flat in our arms], whereas I had always wanted to put her on my shoulder . . . we put her in between us [on the bed]; all the things you couldn't wait to do when you went home – we did all of them . . . I did most of my grieving that night . . . everything you could possibly think of that you know you're not going to be able to do I cried for that night – Christmas, birthdays, not being able to take the pram out . . . you're offered things and part of you is saying, 'What?'. But you're thinking, 'Well, if I don't do it, I'll regret it,' so you do everything, you take everything that they're offering you.
>
> (P 58: mother of preterm baby)

However, there was sometimes an initial reluctance to be overcome.

> At first I wasn't sure if I really wanted her [with us through the night after she'd died] . . . the first thing I thought of was rigor mortis, and change of colour and all these kinds of things, and I wanted to remember her as my daughter, being alive. But it seemed so natural when we actually did have her – just washing, actually holding her in our arms, no tubes or anything like that . . . to actually have her in bed between us was a good thing I think as well . . . so I think it was the best thing we could possibly have done.
>
> (P 58: father of preterm baby)

Some parents recognised at the time that it was now or never.

> [My partner] had fallen asleep . . . I couldn't lie in the dark with [the baby], I had to have some form of light, so I had put the bathroom light on. So I had brought [the baby] just to the bathroom door so I could see her but I didn't go right in because I didn't want her to come right into the light. And I read the SANDS* books . . . you want to do everything. No matter how hard it is, you want to do it so that in years to come, or in months, you won't think, 'Oh I wish I had done that.' But you had to make so many decisions right on the spot, whereas you're not used to doing that, you're used to saying, 'Well, give me a couple of days and I'll think about it.'
>
> (P 58: mother of preterm baby)

For the most part the parents set their own limits on what they chose to do, often guided by staff. However, some felt that suggestions indicated

---

* Stillbirth and Neonatal Death Society.

that the task was expected of them. They therefore 'conformed' but subsequently regretted doing so. Two parents cited bathing the dead baby in this context.

Other forms of involvement engendered mixed emotions.

> They asked me if I wanted to spend the night in the room with [the baby after she died] and I couldn't go through that. But there again as soon as, once they'd brought her [to me], they took her away for the last time, when I was leaving to go out of the hospital, I was [thinking], 'Oh God, I want to see her again.' It felt like I was leaving my baby in the hospital. But there again, I couldn't stand being there with all the other babies. It was dead weird.
>
> (P59: mother of preterm baby)

Having finally left the dead child, most parents were aware that they could return if they so wished. Thirteen families (22%) decided against going back to see the baby subsequently. For the remaining 46 couples (78%), returning was a mixed experience. Some did not specify the time they spent. Five couples (8%) brought the baby's body home either for the full time or for the night before the funeral. In one case the baby was at home in an open coffin, and it was only the smell which made the parents decide reluctantly that they must say their final goodbyes and have the coffin sealed. Six sets of parents (10%) spent many hours with the baby at a later stage on the day of death, in one case the couple then themselves taking the body to the undertaker. However, most parents limited their time to brief visits the following day ($n = 16$) or two days ($n = 1$), at the mortuary or funeral parlour ($n = 5$), or just before the funeral ($n = 5$).

> *Father*: It did actually help [spending time with him at the mortuary]. You didn't actually want to go away – you wanted to take him with you. That was the feeling you had . . .
> *Mother*: Although he was really cold and everything, it was just really comforting to hold him. To give him that last cuddle. To be very close.
>
> (P19: parents of preterm twins)

It was a very personal decision. One father went daily to see the baby, but his wife found the 'heavy, cold, lifeless' body too upsetting, so she declined to go again.

For some it was right to go back repeatedly to spend time with the child while they still could, while others welcomed the opportunity to take family members to say their goodbyes. But a number of parents regretted going back. Changes had taken place which haunted them, and they wished that they could have retained the earlier image of the freshly dead child who appeared to be simply sleeping.

I don't know. He didn't look anything like himself when I'd seen him [after he died]. [But] knowing he was lying there [in the funeral home], I couldn't *not* have gone.

(P53: mother of baby with congenital anomaly)

We went in to see her [in the mortuary next day] but it was pretty hor-rific because she looked nothing like she did. After she died she went very pale but then she came out a lovely rose colour – not *pink* pink but a lovely glow to her skin. And she looked so beautiful and peaceful. And when we went to see her in the mortuary the next day, I think what had maybe happened was they'd laid her with her head to the side after she died and with her having poor circulation, the blood had all come to the surface and she was very purple down one side and she had three white marks, you know like if you push your finger in [and it leaves an indentation] and it was like that. We were horrified when we saw her. It looked nothing like her. It wasn't the baby we remembered.

(P9: mother of baby with cardiac anomaly)

The experience was further marred for this last couple in that the mortu-ary was stark and appeared dishevelled.

It should be more sympathetic and more friendly. I know it sounds petty now, but the Moses basket she was in, the cover of it was dirty.

# Autopsy

All except one family were asked to give permission for a post-mortem examination. Broaching the subject was clearly a very delicate matter. Six parents reported being shocked and upset when it was raised, especially if the baby was still alive at the time.

I just hit the roof. I turned and I said, 'Don't you dare – don't you dare touch him again!' I apologised afterwards [to the neonatologist] . . . but I just didn't want anybody cutting him open . . . He was sleeping and he was in his wee outfit and in his wee shawl and that was the way I wanted him to stay.

(P9: mother of preterm twins)

[The consultant said, 'The baby's] going to die. We expect her to die by the weekend. She's not going to pull through. She's in a very, very bad way' . . . and right at the back of it, 'Now I think for medical research and for future pregnancies for yourself,' he said, 'you should think about getting a post-mortem done.' [My husband] just said, 'No way.' [The baby's] still alive! [News of her bad condition and the talk of a post-mortem] all came out in the one sentence. He said, 'Well, just think about it.' And I said, 'No, she's been through enough.'

(P 36: parents of preterm baby)

Some parents described the arguments and approaches of the consultant as being the persuasive factors.

He just said that although he was caring for [the baby], he had to think about me and my future pregnancies, any genetic things and [a PM] was what he suggested.

(P 52: mother of baby with congenital anomalies)

In one case it was another parent who persuaded the father.

Although it was explained to us very nicely and very well [by the doctors], I think it was really speaking to another parent about post-mortems that convinced us. Because it's not *their* baby at the end of the day that's getting cut up ... they would probably say *anything* to get us to say, 'Yes,' – you can't expect them to say, 'It's not nice.' This [other dad] knew and I think maybe he knew our fears so [when he reassured us that it was done very sensitively and that he had lovely photos of his son after post-mortem and you'd never know] ... that made us feel better.

(P 21: father of baby with cardiac anomaly)

Other families had their own strong views on the subject. In one such family the mother said that she was adamant from the outset that she did not want one, and she resented the way the doctors kept bringing the subject up. In her judgement they were only wanting an autopsy to reassure themselves that they had made the right diagnosis – they should have been certain of that *before* the child died. Others, whilst not overtly expressing such a sentiment, conveyed non-verbally a sense of distress about to the idea of cutting a baby.

Final decisions varied. Of the 58 sets of parents who were asked, 22 (38%) refused permission. One or both parents in a further 11 families (19%) were initially reluctant, but were persuaded that it was the right thing to do. For three of these it was reassurance that the procedure would be carried out delicately which persuaded them to agree. In total, 36 families (62%) consented to autopsy. In three families the parents themselves differed in their response to the request, and in only one of these was the procedure carried out, the mother going along with a very strong wish on the father's part to have an autopsy.

# Reasons why parents consented to autopsy

Those parents who consented to autopsy were asked to give their reasons for doing so. These are listed in Table 8.1, according to the parents' own definitions.

**Table 8.1:** Reasons why parents consented to autopsy ($n = 36$)

| Reason | Number of families |
| --- | --- |
| To obtain answers | 23 |
| To determine genetic factor | 13 |
| To help other families | 9 |
| To give doctors more information | 3 |
| To give meaning to the baby's existence | 2 |
| To confirm that the right decision was made | 2 |
| To confirm the diagnosis | 1 |
| To provide evidence for litigation proceedings | 1 |

Pooling the ideas which the parents cited, the principal reason was to obtain answers to their questions, the second commonest motivation was to help others, and the third commonest was to obtain information which might influence subsequent obstetric choices.

> You try to find some sense in doing it to her. Our heartbreak could be somebody else's gain.
>
> (P21: parents of baby with cardiac anomaly)

> I said to [the doctor], the best reason for getting the post-mortem done was so we knew in our own mind that we were right in making that decision – we knew what was wrong [with the baby]. And it turned out that there were far too many things wrong with her.
>
> (P10: father of preterm twins)

This man's wife, however, pointed out that the autopsy might *not* offer them this reassurance.

> It might have been there was nothing majorly wrong. And [the consultant] explained that to us. He said, 'Now you know if they do a post-mortem it might come back [with] a [result that it] was only an infection, which seems so cruel after what she's been through – to kill her in the end.'
>
> (P10: mother of preterm twins)

# Reasons why parents declined autopsy

The reasons why 22 families declined to give permission for autopsy are listed in Table 8.2. For them it was undesirable or unnecessary, but their stated reasons are differentiated.

**Table 8.2:**   Reasons why parents declined autopsy ($n = 22$)

| Reason | Number of families |
| --- | --- |
| Did not want the baby cut up | 9 |
| Already knew why the baby had died | 8 |
| Baby had been through enough | 6 |
| Too intrusive/shocking a question | 5 |
| Doctors should have obtained answers before they withdrew treatment | 2 |
| No more questions to be answered | 1 |
| Did not want anyone even to touch the baby after death | 1 |
| Could not cope with removal of the brain | 1 |
| Doctors were doing it for themselves to confirm their diagnosis | 1 |
| Did not want the baby to be a guinea-pig | 1 |

Viewed overall, then, the prevailing fear was a dread of the child being mutilated, coupled with a wish not to have anything else done to a baby who had already been through so much. The second commonest reason was that the parents had no unanswered questions.

# Comparison of families who agreed to autopsy with those who did not

These data from so few families are not robust enough to permit calculations of statistical significance, but some interesting differences emerged between the two groups who did or did not agree to autopsies. Notable differences related to diagnosis, the consultant concerned and the age of the child.

As Table 8.3 shows, the majority of babies with a diagnosis of asphyxia or brain damage or congenital anomalies other than heart defects did

**Table 8.3:**   Comparison by diagnosis of babies who did have an autopsy with those who did not

| Diagnosis | Autopsy | No autopsy |
| --- | --- | --- |
| Asphyxia or brain damage | 9 | 2 |
| Congenital anomalies (excluding cardiac) | 7 | 2 |
| Cardiac anomalies | 2 | 4 |
| Preterm | 18 | 15 |

have autopsies. However, twice as many babies with cardiac anomalies did not. Of the 33 families with preterm children, 18 sets of parents consented to autopsy (gestation 22–31 weeks, age range from less than 1 hour to nearly 9 months), whilst 15 couples did not (gestation 23–28 weeks, age range from less than 1 day to 6 months). There was no difference between the average gestation or ages in the two groups.

The second difference related to the approach of the doctor concerned. In the three study Units it was stated policy for the consultant in charge of the baby to seek consent for this procedure. One couple reported also being visited by a pathologist who on more than one occasion tried to encourage them to consent. The number of referrals to the study by different consultants varied, and although all except one family were asked if they would consent to an autopsy, the circumstances of each case varied and may well have influenced the extent to which persuasion was employed. It is not possible to compare individual practices in any meaningful way, but the data suggest that consultants' rates of obtaining consent vary. In one Unit where no one other than the neonatologist ever seeks consent, and taking comparable numbers of referrals to the study, one consultant obtained permission for 89% of his referrals, while a colleague had 80% declining autopsy, even though the babies concerned had the same spread of diagnoses.

The length of time for which babies live may be germane to consent. As many as 82% of the babies (9 out of 11) who lived for 1 day or less had autopsies, and 75% (3 out of 4) who lived for more than 3 months did so. By contrast, only 52% of the 44 babies who lived for between 2 and 92 days had autopsies.

# Mementoes

All parents retained mementoes of their baby's short life. Most shared them with the interviewer, and it was evident that they were greatly treasured. In one family the house had been burgled while the family was away on holiday, and the most distressing part of the experience, the mother recalled, was that the intruders had disturbed these treasured mementoes. However, although these items were sacred to the parents, the responses of other people were reported to be mixed. Such reminders were said to be 'morbid,' 'too distressing' or even 'shocking' for some.

All of the parents had photographs of the babies who had died. In almost all houses these were very evident. Indeed, several families had enlarged copies displayed in prominent places around the room. In some of these the babies were clearly dead. Most parents were eager to share their photographs with the interviewer, but one mother declined to show hers to anyone (even family members), saying that they were too private for public scrutiny. Footprints, handprints, hair, namebands, incubator cards, certificates, clothing and toys were all stored in the memory boxes or albums of most parents. Many also had videos, but at the time of the first interview the majority said that they had not yet watched them because the pain was still too raw. A few parents had put the cassette into their machines by mistake and reported being extremely upset by once again seeing the events so close to the death. Nevertheless, they were comforted to know that such a record was available for the future. Less frequently cited but still treasured were other tokens, including a computer diary ($n = 5$ families), nail clippings ($n = 2$), cordclamp ($n = 1$), splint ($n = 1$) and tubing ($n = 1$).

# Involvement of other people

Forty sets of parents (68%) reported that other people were involved around the time of dying, although very few had anyone else present at the actual death. The identity of these additional people varied: the parents' own parents ($n = 40$ families), the baby's uncles and aunts ($n = 18$), the baby's siblings ($n = 4$), unspecified relations or more distant relatives ($n = 6$) and a close friend ($n = 1$). In one instance a work colleague popped in, not knowing that the baby had died, and became involved to a minor degree.

These other people were involved inasmuch as they came in to say goodbye, or were there for the parents before or after the event. For many it was a brief encounter, the parents preferring to be alone with the baby at this time.

> We were told on the Wednesday evening and it was like shock. Then having to try to phone everybody to tell them not to come through – we didn't want anybody there – that things weren't as we wanted them to be and we wanted to be on our own, no visitors. And there was very little time for us because all through the Wednesday evening after we were told, we knew that every minute counted and we wanted to make every minute precious and have something to savour and hold on to. And that was going to be *our* time.
>
> (P20: mother of baby with asphyxia)

# Support during the dying process

It was very evident that parents looked principally to the consultant and the nurses for support at this time. Many expressed their gratitude for the depth of caring and genuine compassion which they experienced.

Everything was perfect in an un-perfect situation ... They weren't detached from them and although they were that busy with the kids there was always somebody there and coming to the door to see if you wanted anything and to see you were OK. They were really, really professional. But it isn't just a job to them, they really do care. Even [the named neonatologist], he really cared as well. A doctor, he sees that many cases and obviously it's his job, he's trained to speak to people, but it was coming from the heart – you could see it was coming from the heart.

(P4: father of preterm baby)

Other family members were rarely mentioned, and the impression was given that this was an essentially private experience which the parents had to live through themselves. On the other hand, the staff with their intimate involvement in the baby's life and their experience of similar events were in a position to steer them through these uncharted waters and offer such comfort as could be realistically provided during this extremely painful stage of the process. The satisfactory and unsatisfactory elements of their experiences are described in the following sections.

# Satisfaction with the management of the dying process

At the first point of enquiry, just over two-thirds of the 59 sets of parents (40, 68%) were entirely satisfied with the way in which this part of the process was handled. For a further 14 families (24%) it was mostly or partially satisfactory, but certain aspects of it were not, and for 5 (8%) it was unsatisfactory.

When asked again 13 months after the event to reflect on the way in which things were handled, 72% of the families (36/50) felt satisfied that the management of their case was as good as it could have been under these tragic circumstances. Indeed, some singled out specific factors for positive commendation – for example, the consultant choosing to keep the baby in his care rather than handing the case on to a colleague, essentially futile treatment being continued long enough to give the parents extra time with their baby, and direct and honest information being supplied. But just over a quarter of families (14, 28%) expressed some dissatisfaction or reservations.

When the results at both time points were compared, it emerged that six sets of parents who felt dissatisfied early on, a year later no longer had regrets about the way in which things were handled. Three couples who expressed reservations at first interview were not available for comment at 13 months. However, five sets of parents were less satisfied on mature reflection than they had been initially.

# Helpful elements of the dying process

All except one set of parents could identify factors which they had perceived as helpful during the management of the dying. In the case of this one couple, the baby had died before they got to the hospital, and they just regretted their lack of involvement while he was still alive.

No attempt was made to check exhaustively parents' responses against any preconceived list during the interview. Rather, parents were simply asked what they had found helpful at this time. In this way the main features for each parent were identified, although it is perfectly possible that they omitted to state the obvious (to them), or that they forgot some elements of this intense experience. Given the open-ended question which prompted these responses, it is of little value to provide raw numbers and percentages. Therefore only a general sense of the prevalence of each category is given. Examples of idiosyncratic or specific actions are provided where they give a feel for the types of factors which were supportive.

Inevitably, supportive actions spilled over into different theoretical categories of support.[103] Reporting has taken this reality into account. The comments in this section fell broadly into seven main areas.

## Opportunities to do things with the baby

Almost all of the parents wanted to be physically involved with the baby at this time, and cited this as a helpful part of the management of the dying.

> I'm glad we had that period [of time with the baby] because . . . we've met parents who've lost their babies within an hour of birth and they haven't ever had any time with their babies. And I'm sure it would have felt like that for us if she had have died very soon after we were told the bad news. But because we had that good time with her, she had a little life and we've got all these memories.
>
> (P 51: father of baby with congenital anomalies)

This was a special time for them during which they were simultaneously trying to accept the impending death and build up a lifetime of memories. As one mother put it, it was a time for 'absorbing the reality of his existence.'

In general, both parents appreciated all of the things which facilitated their involvement with the baby, whether it was guiding them (e.g. staff steering them gently through the experience, suggesting options and pro-viding opportunities), being sensitive to their needs (e.g. people knowing when to withdraw and give them privacy, assisting them when their cour-age flagged) or in practical ways (e.g. being given new clothes to choose for the baby, helping them to bath the baby). Sometimes they had decided against certain activities, but were grateful to the staff who anticipated a later change of mind and took appropriate action. Many parents volun-teered gratefully that they would not have thought of all the mementoes or memories they now treasured if staff had not suggested them. For exam-ple, one mother singled out an unwashed blanket which still smelled of her baby as a special treasure. Two sets of parents had not wanted photographs at the time, but were very glad to have them when they were delivered after the death.

> The nurse came and she took the photos. She asked at first if we wanted any photos taken and I said, 'No.' But she just went ahead and took them and we're glad now that she did. Well, obviously they've experienced it before. We were glad that she did do it.
>
> (P 24: father of preterm baby)

Being given time to decide just what they wanted to do, and not being hurried, was identified as a particular help, and parents spoke warmly of the staff who encouraged them to take control in this way. This practice carried a number of benefits. It reinforced their unique status as parents of this baby, it gave them time to think about what they wanted to do and what felt right for them, and it minimised the risk of later long-term regrets. Knowing that they could choose what was right for them spurred them on to identify activities which were important to them, such as undressing the baby, introducing the child to different people or places, or taking him or her home. One mother cited the staff allowing her to go home even though she had just had a Caesarean Section as an example of the kind of empowering which parents found warming and supportive. By being able to escape to the comfort of her own home she could better cope with the pain of visiting the baby in the Unit and his impending death. After about seven hours with the dead baby, another mother knew instinctively how to relinquish the child.

> We just popped her into a cot that was in [the room] and we said our goodbyes and *we* left *her*. Because I think – in retrospect – I do find it much easier to cope with that than the thought of watching somebody take her away.
>
> (P 51: mother of baby with congenital anomalies)

Although close involvement was helpful for the majority of the parents, it must not be forgotten that for a small number of others, performing

parenting tasks was so acutely painful and daunting that it was unhelpful to attempt them. Although they knew that the baby's hours were
numbered, the events leading up to death were initially unknown, and in
reality they were frightening and intensely upsetting. Several fathers commented on a sense of unreality – they could not believe that they were sitting there waiting for their own baby to die. As we have seen, a few opted
out of parts of the process and required encouragement to get involved or
to hold the baby. Parents who thought that they might want to bath the
dead infant found that they could not face doing so when they felt the
baby's cold and lifeless body. Collecting mementoes was too much for
another father. Parents valued a sensitive approach which was responsive to their own cues.

## Sensitive support of nurses

The nurses in the Unit occupied a key place in this part of the process. All
of the parents spoke positively of the warmth and compassion which the
majority of the nurses showed.

> The nurses that came in [to say they were sorry] held him as well . . .
> They must get attached. I know they're not supposed to, but they
> must. They *do*. It was nice to see that. It wasn't just a job for them. To be
> honest I don't think any one of them came across that way, as though it
> was just a job.
>
> (P19: parents of preterm twins)

> It was nice, the nurse, she was crying as well. You always think nurses
> don't cry. It's a no-no for nurses . . . It was a human touch. It was an emo-
> tion that was showing, it wasn't simply a cry for us. A child had died.
>
> (P35: father of preterm triplets)

Male nurses working in the Unit were singled out for special mention by
two families who found them especially sensitive and 'genuine.' Although
many spoke positively of the value of one nurse accompanying them
through the process, one family said that they had appreciated the sense
of team effort during this time of crucial decision making and management of the decision. The whole staff had been alongside them, speaking
with one voice; they could not all be wrong.

It was particularly comforting for them to know that the staff valued the
baby as a unique and irreplaceable person, and the parents as special people
who were crucially important to this baby. However, one family commented
that they did not know whether staff were normally supportive, but in their

case they suspected that the nurses were only being kind to them because they felt guilty about getting the diagnosis wrong at an earlier stage.

The experience of one mother merits special mention. This couple had elected not to stay for the actual death. Walking back into the nursery when staff thought she had left, the mother was amazed to find a nurse cradling her dying baby in her arms. This could not have been to impress anyone, she concluded, since the nurse did not expect her to return. It could only have been a measure of her personal involvement and caring.

> Sometimes people do things just because you're there. You never know what they do when you're not there . . . But that gesture – when she was holding the baby – has left such a profound impact on me. It was only at that time that I thought what incredibly caring, *truly* caring and loving people these are. OK, they do care for these babies in their incubators. They cared for ours. But she did not have to do that. She could have gone and had a cup of tea or something like that.
>
> (P33: mother of preterm twins)

Such thoughtful gestures were greatly appreciated by the grieving parents.

Against this background of compassion and sensitivity, the parents identified a range of aspects of support from the nursing staff which they had valued:

• respect and caring for the baby as an individual

> There was one nurse in particular – she's left now – you'd phone up and if she was on she'd say, 'Tchh, I've just been changing his bed. Did you *see* the colour of the sheets that so and so had put on? [Your baby] doesn't like those colours.' And she'd just take the whole lot out. 'Och, he doesn't suit these colours.' To me that was great.
>
> (P9: mother of preterm twins)

• genuine caring and interest in the parents
• support and guidance through each phase
• reassurance that the parents were making the right choices

> I felt a great comfort from the fact that [the neonatal nurse] who was with me that day – she'd nursed him day in, day out . . . she said to me 'I think you're doing the right thing [letting him go]. He's fought so hard.' And that really meant a lot to me, because *I* hadn't looked after my baby, *they* had looked after my baby. And I just felt that someone who was as close to him as she was . . . she backed me up. They all backed us up 100%.
>
> (P6: mother of baby with congenital anomalies)

- continuity, with one person seeing them through the process

> We were really lucky with the nurse that was there. It just worked that she was on shifts the whole time [the three days we were in the Unit]. And she was lovely... the continuity was really helpful. I would have found it incredibly difficult without that continuity, particularly given that we actually took [the baby] home with us and took him back to the hospital on the Friday morning for the post-mortem and it was the same nurse that I gave [him] to and I actually found that incredibly difficult. I was really distressed. But I would have found it ten times more difficult if it had been somebody that I didn't know.
>
> (P49: mother of baby with asphyxia)

- flexibility in line with parental wishes
- facilitation of memory and memento gathering
- information
- provision of privacy whilst remaining available
- sensitivity when dealing with other family members
- encouragement of sibling involvement.

Alongside these general categories were specific activities which demonstrated the types of things that parents found helpful. They are reported here in detail to provide indicators for clinicians:

- offering to arrange (and in some cases the hospital offering to pay for) the funeral
- arranging transport of the baby's body over long distances
- coming to say goodbye to the baby even when they were employed elsewhere
- encouraging the parents to record each detail of their experience
- suggesting that twins exchange gifts
- encouraging the mother to express milk for the dying baby as something only she could do
- obtaining a take-away meal for the family
- maintaining humour alongside the sympathy
- reassuring the parents that someone would pop in to see the baby after his or her death
- testing the temperature of the water and adding fragrant oil before bathing the dead baby
- selecting new clothes for the baby for the dying process, and then giving them to the mother to keep after the death
- promising personally to pop in and out to see the dead baby after the parents had left the hospital at night.

# Sensitive compassion of consultants

Consultants were seen to play a special role in this part of the process. Again the parents identified their genuine compassion as crucially important.

> He treated us like we were the only people there. He has all these parents and patients and everything but made us feel that he was just ours, *our* consultant, [*our baby's*] consultant.
>
> 　　　　　　(P48: mother of preterm baby with congenital anomalies)

> It was so sad. [The neonatologist] came over and he held her hand and he said, 'I'm sorry, [Baby's name].' I thought, 'He was like a grandad to her. He really looked after her, and really thought a lot of her.' And like he said to us, 'I have so much respect for these wee babies,' he said, 'because they're just such fighters.' And he has and he just apologised to her. And I thought, 'God, he cared.' That really got to me as well – and it always will. It touched my heart, it really did.
>
> 　　　　　　　　　　　　　　(P10: mother of preterm twins)

Parents looked up to the consultants as the experts, and the source of knowledge and often guidance. They were perceived as extremely busy people with many preoccupations and responsibilities. It was expected that they should be the ones to impart the serious news of a grave diagnosis or a bleak prognosis. However, when they showed a personal interest and concern in the actual dying process, when they themselves carried the child to the parents, hugged the mother in sympathy, or comforted a grieving grandmother, the parents felt very privileged and singled out for special attention. This seemed to demonstrate a genuine compassion and caring which went beyond the boundaries of a mere job.

Several consultants were said to have had tears in their eyes as they delivered bad news, stayed with the parents during the death, or pronounced the child dead. To have this 'important' or 'high-up' man, who 'teaches all the rest of them' personally saddened by their baby's loss, and so moved as to express his emotion openly, accorded a value to the child which was immeasurable. Parents were deeply touched by these gestures, and spoke of the consultant with warmth and affection. Many referred to him by his first name and described him as 'like one of the family,' 'a lovely man,' 'fantastic,' 'such a kind person.' A number of parents, contemplating the job of the consultant, marvelled at his ability to make this set of parents, and this baby, feel uniquely important when he must have to repeat this process time after time. They were grateful that he gave so much to so many. However, a few parents retained a sense that it was exceptional for the consultant to demonstrate this level of interest, and that their family had touched a special chord.

Both the consultants especially seemed very upset, concerned. [Our baby had] been there quite a long time and everyone knew him . . . particularly this consultant. He did make us feel as though we were very special. He probably does that to everyone. Good on him. But it was important at that time to us. I thought both [consultants] came over as if he meant something to them, as if he was a special baby. Whether they can portray that to everyone I don't know but . . .

(P6: parents of baby with congenital anomalies)

More specifically they cited the following:

- holding daily meetings to discuss their case to be sure that they were doing what was right, and were not missing anything which would indicate they had taken a wrong turning
- changing the death certificate to a later 'viable' gestation so that the child's birth and death could be officially recognised
- providing guidance and reassurance that the parents were choosing wisely – that they were making the right decision, this was the right time to move on to the next step, the baby was not suffering, the dying process would not be much longer, and the parents themselves were providing essential but special love and tenderness
- sensitivity to the parents' needs
- respect for the baby as an individual of real value
- information
- continuity, with one consultant retaining contact throughout
- respect for parents as equals on the team. Those fathers who cited this factor were all professional men who held positions of responsibility in their working lives. A sense of mutual respect helped them to feel involved and valued, and added to their feeling that they were important contributors to the decisions made on behalf of their children.

# Other professional support

## *Other healthcare professionals*
Comments included the following:

- expressing or conveying sympathy and understanding
- making sure that the parents were fed
- coming to see the parents and/or the baby
- checking that the parents were coping
- organising reimbursement of expenses.

## *Chaplains*

Four parents mentioned the chaplain's contribution as being of value at this time. His ongoing interest and concern, and his very presence, reassured them. Knowing that he supported the decision and actions helped to still their doubts or anxieties. In one case he could also give them guidance and practical advice about a funeral. In one family the mother cultivated the chaplain's involvement quite deliberately so that she had someone to take the funeral, although her partner did not like the involvement of a minister of religion at this time.

> *Mother*: He was nice so we couldn't say, 'No, don't do it.' But then when he came up with this thing about giving [the baby] a blessing, I didn't like it, but we went along with it because we would need somebody to do the service for us and we didn't know anybody... and I didn't want to hurt [the neonatal nurse's] feelings because she's known him for a long time [and she suggested getting him] and we got to know her personally.
> *Father*: [My wife] seemed quite happy to go along with it, and my mother and my father, but to me it seemed not right.
>
> (P 39: parents of baby with brain damage)

# Family support

For the most part couples elected to be alone for this part of the process. Indeed, they sometimes felt isolated even from each other.

> I read in a book about it: we're in this together but we're in it alone. And we have been ... Even at the hospital, he was ours – he belonged to nobody else – but at the same time I sometimes felt *we* were so far apart. We both knew we were losing him, but neither of us could give each other any support or anything to cling on to, because we were both so desperately lost with everything that had gone on. We were by each other's side every day, 24 hours a day, but *he* wasn't making [the baby] better and neither was *I*. And forasmuch as we should have been there for each other – which we were – we weren't either, I think because we were both so completely devastated because *his* individual hopes and dreams, and *mine* – being a father and being a mother – were shattered.
>
> (P 20: mother of baby with asphyxia)

> For me, all I wanted to do in those last hours – and I didn't know how long it was going to be – was just to try to give him a lifetime of love in that time. So I was just really blinkered on [the baby]. In fact I didn't even

know at one point that [my husband] had left the room and apparently was in the corridor crying uncontrollably and I had no idea that had happened.

(P2: mother of baby with cardiac anomaly)

Family members might have been involved at earlier stages, but the actual dying was usually a very private experience exclusively in the province of the parents. Nevertheless, a few parents cited family members as offering helpful support at this time by:

• staying around to be there for them as needed
• taking their cue from the parents about the nature and/or extent of their involvement
• taking other children away
• being uncritical of the decision to stop treatment.

Special mention must be made of the support of the parents' own children at this time. About half of the mothers (51%, 30 of 59) and 63% of the fathers (34 of 54) had other living children. The siblings were variously involved in the experience relating to their new brother or sister. Some were not exposed to the experience at all. Some of these children were taken away to or by relatives or friends (on occasion even out of the country) and excluded from the whole event. For others, involvement was managed according to the parents' assessment of the limits of their understanding or tolerance. Some children stayed in the Unit both day and night with the parents, some were taken into the Unit and involved in most parts of the process of dying, and others were taken in periodically. Some were involved in the dying process itself, while others were brought in especially at critical stages so that they were part of the family experience, but did not have to experience the tedium of being cooped up in a confined space for prolonged periods.

Many parents found it comforting to have other children present to keep them 'sane' and to introduce some normality into an otherwise 'surreal' life, although one parent recalled having to tell a sibling about the death as one of the most stressful parts of the process. Other parents felt that the children helped to lessen the sense of 'failure' because here was living proof that they (the parents) *could* produce and keep normal healthy children. However, for a few the stark contrast between the abilities of and future outlook for the siblings and those for the new baby with all of his or her problems was too great, and they found it difficult to relate to the other children without strong negative feelings being generated. Guilt, anger, a sense of injustice, resentment and a profound sorrow which distanced the parents from the children were all experienced.

# Privacy

Many parents specifically cited the facilities they were offered as being helpful at this time. In all cases this was a reference to the privacy and comfort of the rooms available to them. Being able to close the door and be alone to grieve and to do whatever felt right for them during the precious minutes or hours with their dying baby was valuable.

> We didn't want that day to end. It was the first time the three of us had been together instead of in the nursery with all the other babies round about. It was us as a family in the room. But when [the neonatologist] came and said, 'I think I should take the tubes out,' I was happy for him to take that over because I just wouldn't have – *couldn't* have said to [do it.] We'd have sat there all night. He knew what we were like.
>                    (P48: mother of preterm baby with congenital anomalies)

One mother who had close relatives abroad appreciated having a telephone installed nearby so that she could receive their calls.

Given the depth of pain parents were experiencing at this time, it was impressive that almost all of them could identify positive features of their experience and gain support and comfort from what was offered.

# Unhelpful elements of the dying process

This was one of the most painful and distressing parts of the experience for parents to recall. It must be remembered, too, that the outcome of this pregnancy and birth was so far removed from what the parents wanted that some powerful negative overtones might be expected to colour their perceptions. Even so, when asked shortly after the experience to identify anything which had been unhelpful at this time, as many as 16 families (27%) were unable to think of anything. For almost three-quarters of the parents (43, 73%), however, there was room for improvement.

It is important to reiterate that the parents themselves stressed the need to set their criticisms in context. The overall quality of the service was impressive, they said, with compassion and sensitivity accompanying the expertise. Furthermore, as one mother pointed out, sometimes they did not know themselves what they wanted or what to ask for. In this spirit we present here those elements which parents found less than optimal in order to offer further insights for clinicians.

There was a notable resonance between the helpful and unhelpful factors, and they can be grouped in parallel ways. Unhelpful factors at this time fell into six main categories.

# Limited opportunities to do things with the baby

Parents regretted lost opportunities to do things with the baby while they had the chance to do so.

> I was still hooked up to drips and I was in a wheelchair ... so it was just a nightmare going up to see him. He survived the night. The [consultant neonatologist] had said that he was dying and that we should spend as much time with him as we could. My husband took me up during the night. There was this nurse there [in the NICU] – I don't even know what her name was – and she was really cold. We held him. We thought we were going up there to spend the night with him. We went up and she took him out and we held him for the first time and then after about half an hour she goes, 'Right, he has to go back in.' And I was really shocked because we had expected to be there all night. She goes, 'You can come back up and see him again.' But we were just so devastated, we just went away. We were really, really angry about it at the time. I mean I hadn't slept [for three days] so I was absolutely shattered – I hadn't had any sleep since the Saturday night [and it was now Wednesday night]. We went back downstairs. And [my husband] is going, 'I can't believe it. He's dying and we can't spend any time with him.' But we [were just so confused and devastated] and we couldn't fight with her. So we just went back downstairs ... I don't think she *stopped* us seeing him. It's just so hard to explain. I mean we had him in our arms and we were all geared up to spend all night with him ... we were just so shocked we just went away. But I don't think it had really sunk in either. Although we had been told he was going to die, I don't think we actually believed it.
>
> (P5: mother of baby with asphyxia)

Missed opportunities included the following:

- limited early involvement with the baby because the parents were unaware of the seriousness of the baby's condition
- delays in bringing the baby to them, or in being taken to the baby
- no whole family photos including small children
- no video of the baby while he or she was still alive
- not bathing the dead baby
- not seeing the dead baby again after death. Two families were fearful of the changes which might ensue, but subsequently regretted missed opportunities to be with the baby and to show him to grandparents. Another couple said that they did not know they could return to

see the baby's body after death. One mother wished she could have had
more time with the baby when she was more rested and mobile

- not seeing the baby's body in its entirety. One mother regretted not
  having undressed the baby to examine each part in detail. She had
  never seen his head without a bonnet so that she could recall its shape
  or hair, or his genitalia so that she could remember him as a boy
- not keeping the baby to themselves. One mother resented having to
  share the baby with relatives at this precious time
- not having certain mementoes. One mother would have liked the cot
  blanket but did not think to ask for it. Another mother asked for but
  was not given the baby's namebands
- not being present when the baby was dying. Insufficient warning of
  impending death led to one couple missing the death and being left
  with a sense of guilt.

It is important to note, however, that for nine families there was an element of *over*-involvement which they regretted. For six of these families
the hurt came when they saw the baby again after death. The physical
changes which they saw preyed on their minds and disturbed them. Finding the body cold and heavy reinforced the finality of death, and they
wished that they had retained in their memories the fresh look of the
child who had simply fallen asleep for the last time. Another family was
upset by being left with the baby at all after death, and wished that the
nurses had taken her away immediately.

The other two families cited specific hurts. One family did not want
the footprints and handprints which the nurses took. In the other case the
mother felt that she was expected to be strong and happy for the surviving twin.

> Everybody had drummed into me, 'You've still got [Twin 1] to think of.'
> And I *knew* that but I still had to grieve for [Twin 2] as well and nobody
> was letting me . . . The nurses kept saying, 'Gosh, where do you get your
> strength from? You're amazing.' [But I was thinking,] 'But I'm *not*. You
> just don't know how I'm feeling inside. I'm tearing apart.' But because
> everybody said to me, 'You have to be strong for Twin 1,' I was doing it
> for everybody. But I shouldn't have. No, definitely not.
>
> (P10: mother of preterm twins)

Other parents with surviving babies also reported the pain of being with
living children whilst mourning dead siblings. Returning to the nursery
to visit other babies brought its own acute sadness. When 'everyone' told
them that they must think of the living children, it seemed to deny their
right to grieve.

## Insensitivity of nurses

Most negative comments were idiosyncratic, but one contextual fact was mentioned by four different families, namely lack of continuity which resulted in unknown nurses being on duty at the time of the death. When the baby had been in the Unit for many weeks and staff had built up a relationship with the family, this was perceived as especially disappointing. Even so, the parents reported that they were not criticising the nurses who had supported them – they had been sensitive and done all that they could. But the parents felt that if they had been surrounded by known faces, things could have been better still.

No more than two sets of parents cited any of the following unhelpful factors, but knowing that the potential exists for any parent to be hurt in these ways is salutary. Hurtful features included:

- resuscitating the baby after it had been agreed to withdraw
- leaving the baby 'bloody and dishevelled'
- bringing the baby to the parents 'dirty' after withdrawal
- calling the baby 'Baby (surname)' instead of by his Christian name
- using the baby's name too loosely and disrespectfully
- getting the baby's name or information wrong on documents or mementoes

> That annoys me that they can make that many mistakes. How *can* he have shrunk three centimetres and put on all that weight (2 lbs in 10 days)?!
>
> (P38: father of baby with congenital anomalies)

- not consulting the mother about things being done with and to the baby
- discussing the funeral while the baby was still alive
- giving parents a photograph of the baby after post-mortem which showed cuts to the head
- not making the baby high priority

> We were left hanging about before we were looked at because it was in the middle of doctors' rounds. And they put her into a little cot, it wasn't in the Intensive Care it was in the Special Nursery part. And they put her in a cot right beside the door. I was standing by the door as well and it was [really] cold ... they said to strip her clothes off and she was left there till they got round to her and I thought maybe that's why she was so hypothermic by the time they came ... That did annoy me, the fact that we had to wait while they were doing the rounds ... It felt like she wasn't important because they knew she was going to die.
>
> (P9: mother of baby with cardiac anomaly)

• being inconsistent

> One thing that annoyed me about [the staff] was [the changing rules]. One day I'd go in when she was fine and I'd get to clean up her mouth and just do things to help [take care of her] because one of the nurses said to me, 'You have to get to know her; she has to get used to your touch,' and everything like that. And then I'd go in the next day and the nurses [would say quite sharply], 'Don't open the incubator door! Just leave her.' And you didn't know whether to go near her or not. That was really confusing . . . You didn't know what to do. It just depends who was on if you went near her or not. It depends which nurse was on. And I felt, 'Well, she's *my* baby.'
>
> (P59: mother of preterm baby)

• not warning a father that the child had died, so he walked in on a distressing scene
• being unyielding about visiting rules, so that key people like siblings or grandparents were excluded from seeing or touching the baby

> If I had known – I would never have taken advantage of any situation. He was my son and I wouldn't allow him to be passed back and forward – but I would have said to [the neonatal nurse], 'Well, can we get him out and give both Mums a wee hold; let the sisters and brothers even just touch his hand; let them see him out [of the incubator]?' But then I didn't know I was allowed to do that.
>
> (P48: mother of preterm baby with congenital anomalies)

• distancing themselves from the parents (although the two nurses who were perceived in this way were said to be excellent with the babies)
• using trite expressions or clichés
• being falsely cheerful
• not escorting the parents to the door of the hospital after the death

> It's farcical now when I think about it. At five o'clock in the morning we walked through [the hospital] – we'd just lost our child – with nobody anywhere near us. We just got left to walk away and that was it.
>
> (P36: parents of preterm baby with brain damage)

• not checking that the parents were fit to drive home after the baby had died

> No support at all. Just sent home – after that horrific experience we had to drive home from that hospital ourselves – they just sent us away. The people in the Neonatal Unit were really wonderful – they really were – but the people that were supposed to be in charge of me – they were just useless – they just avoided us.
>
> (P5: mother of baby with asphyxia)

- requiring parents to go back next day for bereavement packs or to sign autopsy forms.

Two families warrant specific mention here because of the context of their comments. In one case the couple was so resistant to the idea of the baby dying that they did not accept the reality until the child collapsed in the incubator and was bundled out of it into the parents' arms just as she died.

> I couldn't believe it was happening [that the baby was dying]. I was determined she was going to pull through, right to the very end. Because she'd been up and down. So I thought she'd pull back up. She managed to last until the next day. But she was ill all the next day. We had to stay with her – ... All of a sudden the machines started going beep, beep, beep going mental. [The baby] just died. The machines were on when it happened. They didn't take the machines away. All of a sudden the machines were going mental. They were going absolutely crazy. And she just went herself. Afterwards they turned the machines off, but the machines were going absolutely crazy and the noise was worse than anything. All I could hear was everything beeping. You knew then [she was dying]. They were [saying], 'Hold her now.'
>
> (P 59: mother of preterm baby)

This mother recalled as hurtful the staff repeatedly asking the couple before that moment whether they would like to have the baby out of the incubator to cuddle, and if they wanted her christened. They did not do so because it would have signified losing hope in her survival.

> *Father*: The nurses kept on telling us to take her out and hold her. That was a bit annoying as well.
> *Mother*: I couldn't handle that. She kept on saying, 'Take her out and hold her.' And we were [saying], 'No, because the machines are helping her. We don't want to muck up the machines. We always want her to get better. Then I'll have the rest of my life to hold her.' I suppose they knew – they must have known she [wouldn't make it].

The other couple came from a foreign country where other customs and practices obtained. The father was 'very angry' with the nurse who brought the dead baby to him, because she was rocking the extremely preterm infant and talking to him. The father said he 'wanted to hit her' for her insensitivity – the child was dead and it was inappropriate to behave as if he was living. These parents were also shocked to be given a photograph of their dead baby. It was 'not pretty', and to them it was an insensitive action.

These cases highlight the importance of treating each family as unique, with its own needs and wishes. Even though many parents greatly appreciated some guidance through this unknown process, they themselves cautioned against the blanket application of policies and procedures. It was salutary to hear from those parents who did not want things which are commonly thought desirable – for example, to have handprints, or to cradle the baby. Their reactions draw attention to the necessity to check with parents what feels right for them, and to steer a careful course between what most families value and what a given individual or couple prefers.

> [It was supportive] because they read what we needed. They said things to us: we *could* sit all night with her once she had died. But we just didn't [want that]. It's always been my belief that once you're dead your spirit's gone from your body and that's just this little shell there. And I just think that there could have been nothing worse for us than sitting all night with a dead baby. And I think they realised that. They seemed to judge. Because [the consultant] came in and he said that to us and then he went outside saying, 'Right, we're going to let you discuss it. We know you want this over quickly, you want her to stop suffering. We're going to bring her through. You tell us when you want the ventilator out.' But when they went away and they brought her back, and she died – which took about an hour and a half I think – he came in and he said, 'I can see you just want to go home, don't you?'. So they didn't push – they didn't say, 'Well, some people stay with them and maybe you should.' It was just a case of, 'What's good for you.'
>
> (P42: mother of preterm baby)

> *Mother*: They kept her in the counselling room – the bad news room! – they had her in there in a Moses basket. She was wrapped in [her big sister's] shawl.
> *Father*: I requested for a window to be open for fresh air to get in and I requested to keep the light on. I don't know if it stems back from when I was young and I was afraid of the dark and I didn't want her to be left alone in the dark. Small things like that – the nurses went through on the night shift to check on her – I asked them to go through and make sure she . . . I just wanted her checked on. The nurses went through and they did that.
>
> (P35: parents of preterm triplets)

# Insensitivity of the consultant

Only three factors were cited by more than two sets of parents:

- lack of information ($n = 8$ sets of parents). This was seen to be in the domain of the consultant. The parents disliked having to seek out information instead of it being offered proactively, believing that it should be given to them from the outset and then kept updated frequently. As one

couple said, being told things twice in 10 days left a lot of time when they were in limbo. Most recalled specific pieces of information which they believed they were not given – for example, the implications of specific impairments, the fact that there would be time with the living baby after withdrawal, or that the baby might gasp after withdrawal, or that the baby had pneumonia (they found this out from the death certificate), or that morphine depressed respiration
- an insensitive request for an autopsy ($n = 4$). A fifth set of parents had doubts about the doctors' integrity in this matter. When they rang the undertaker they were told that the baby's body could not be released to the parents because of the post-mortem. Since they had refused permission for this procedure to be performed, they questioned this. The answers did not entirely allay their fear that the doctors had overruled them and requisitioned one anyway
- unwillingness actively to end the child's life ($n = 3$).

The rest of the items cited were mentioned by no more than two sets of parents. They included doctors:

- not telling them when the staff had meetings about their baby
- requiring them to wait a whole night to see the baby's named neonatologist after the baby had deteriorated
- ignoring parents
- not treating the baby like a real person
- being unable to meet the parents' eyes
- being inaccessible
- not attending a promised meeting with the parents
- shirking responsibility for being with the parents. In one case, the parents felt that it was inappropriate to leave the matter with the advanced nurse practitioner when they believed it was rightly the doctor's responsibility. In the other case, the consultant discussed withdrawal and then vanished, not to be seen again. The family said that they would like to have been reassured about the rightness of the decision when the baby lingered and seemed to be fighting for life
- making insensitive comments which seemed to devalue the life of the baby or the parents' concerns
- not reassuring the parents that they were doing the right thing
- being too pushy. This set of parents subsequently understood better the need for them to decide more quickly in order for staff to orchestrate a peaceful and calm death, but at the time they felt that the pace was inordinately hasty
- insensitively discussing details of the condition immediately after the death when the parents simply wanted to escape to the sanctuary of their own home and think and feel in privacy.

# Lack of support from other staff

## Other specialists
Other specialists were seen as unhelpful by two families.

- Poor communication. A geneticist was said not to be able to meet the parents' eyes and to have failed to follow through the information he had sketchily provided.
- Poor timing and approach. In this case it was an obstetrician who was perceived as abrupt and quelling, going through the events of pregnancy and labour while the baby was still alive and putting a real fear for the future into the parents' minds.

## Junior doctors
A junior doctor was perceived to be excellent until it was realised that the baby would die. He then became unavailable to the parents.

> It wasn't that he wasn't supportive, because I didn't think of it like that. I just felt sorry for him in a way, really, that he couldn't handle it, that he couldn't speak to us. I didn't feel that I needed him to be able to talk to us or to be strong. I mean he just couldn't cope with it and we accepted that.
>
> (P8: mother of preterm twins)

## Postnatal ward staff
Many parents were housed on postnatal wards for at least part of the time during the dying process. Staff on these wards distressed six couples. Factors cited included the following:

- not being aware of what was happening to the baby
- not knowing about the seriousness of the baby's prognosis
- getting the baby's gender wrong
- lacking sensitivity to the parents' needs. In this context they identified prattling on insensitively when the parents were shocked by events in the nursery, objecting to the father walking through the ward, failing to provide the father with meals, suggesting that it was time for the father to go home, and not telling the mother what facilities were available to her
- being inconsistent in the information they provided.

## Chaplain
As was mentioned earlier, only one family criticised the chaplain. These parents had reservations, but the mother had her own agenda for not dismissing him – he could officiate at the funeral.

*Managers*

One couple objected to an insensitive approach at a time of great vulnerability. (Note that this occurred in a hospital rather than in the study Units.)

> When we were told that she might die and we were told to arrange the funeral, I had asked the question, 'How do we get back to [our home town]? 'And the [manager] she turned round and she said 'Well, that's not our responsibility.' She said, 'You either get a funeral director to transport her back or you can take her in the car, but you need consent from the police to take her in the car.' So could you *imagine* taking a dead baby home [in your car]?! They'd washed [their hands] of responsibility for us if she was going to die – that's the impression I got. That I think should be something to be looked at seriously because that was awful ... *They* had put us down there [in a Unit far from home]. If it's all over, it's up to yourself what you do ... we didn't have a carry-cot, we didn't have anything, at most we might have had a box or something but you just couldn't think that you were going to put your baby in a box and stick it in the back of the car like a piece of luggage or something!
>
> (P9: parents of baby with cardiac anomaly)

*Community staff*

Community staff had caused additional distress to two couples.

- A premature visit to the house by the GP. This doctor had responded to a call from the hospital consultant by going to the parents' home immediately. The mother had not yet returned from the hospital, and the rest of the family did not know of the death. She felt that this reaction had been precipitate and should have been planned more carefully.
- False reassurances from community staff which ran counter to what the parents knew to be the truth.

*Counsellor*

One couple had been put in touch with a counsellor, but felt that she was not the right person for them, since she had not taken the trouble to get her facts straight and she seemed unaware of the extent of the damage suffered by the baby.

# Lack of support from family members

Some parents recognised a degree of isolation in their grief. As the baby's parents, this was their own private sorrow, and no one else could really share it. Indeed, many commented that they wanted no other family members around at this time.

> Some family came in on the Sunday and I said to [my husband], 'I don't want any more visitors now. This time is ours and I don't want them seeing her like this' . . . I didn't want anybody coming in trying to hold her, upsetting her. It was *our* time. Every time anyone came in they would get upset and then we would have to comfort them and it was more stress on us. We didn't want to deal with that.
>
> (P9: parents of baby with cardiac anomaly)

Because they had never experienced such a loss, other relatives could not really support them, and attempts to do so sometimes misfired. Parents cited the following as unhelpful:

- too many telephone calls 'demanding' information
- too much pain from having to give increasingly bad news and deal with people's reactions to it
- relatives not listening, but saying what *they* wanted to hear
- family members holding the dead baby and thereby depriving the parents of this precious contact time
- too many people being around and invading the family's privacy
- the grandmother being so upset and wanting to protect the mother that the mother herself felt rushed through the experience
- the grandparents wishing to apportion blame.

However, one mother felt that she had been deprived of a particular experience of family support she would have liked, namely the grandmothers holding the dying child. She did not know until it was too late that this was possible, or that other relatives could have touched or held the baby out of the incubator in order to say their goodbyes.

# Inadequate facilities or poor use of facilities

The parents cited a range of stressors, including the following:

- lack of privacy ($n = 4$ sets of parents). They objected to bad news being given in a public area in front of many other people. Simply drawing screens across did not really afford privacy, as sounds and some activity could still be overheard and observed. Staff hovering constituted an invasion of their privacy, and parents felt inhibited if they were watched at this time

> We held him for at least half an hour [before disconnection]. People kept saying, 'We'll leave you alone now.' And they never did; they just

> stood there. And I think it was embarrassment. They didn't want to walk away probably, but we felt that was [not good]. I would think, 'Well, go away then!' . . . I don't know if it's possible but I would like to have been in a room – just the two of us and [the baby] and nobody else because there were other babies in there all in the same ward. I might have felt more relaxed. I might have walked about with him . . . or held him up to the window or something like that. I would have liked that.
>
> (P27: parents of baby with cardiac anomaly)

- inappropriate location. It was distressing to the parents closeted in this room to be able to hear other babies crying, or women giving birth, or to have to walk past mothers and babies in order to get to their room

> I think they should have a better room [in the Unit] – they've got a wee telly room – just a few seats in there. And you look in and if there's say a family in there with all their kids running about, folk go, 'I'm not going in there!' That's why I think people don't mix the same up there . . . Not everybody has kids that go up there. The mothers I met, not one of us had family, yet there always seemed to be hundreds of kids in this room and it was like, 'I don't want to sit in there with all these kids and have coffee' . . . You could have a mother's sister and her three kids up, and of course the three kids can't get in [to the nursery] so they're in there and they're throwing toys and I didn't feel that was right. It's not very respectful if you're having a rough time with your baby and you're going in there listening to all these wee kiddies screaming.
>
> (P10: mother of preterm twins)

By contrast, when this mother explained her need for peace to the nurses, they gave her a key to one of the family bedrooms.

> I just sat in there and I broke my heart. I was on my own. I came out of there and I felt a hundred times better. I've released so much, I feel I can go on for the rest of the day now. I'm back. I could never have done that in that room with all those kids, folk running about – I just couldn't have.

- unsuitable decoration. For some the decor was 'cold and impersonal' or 'heavy,' instead of 'light and airy.' But other parents qualified their dislike of the decoration, believing that their own bad associations with it had coloured their perceptions of the room itself
- nowhere to smoke. Having to go outside the building was an additional stressor for one mother. She realised, and had been reassured, that this was not the time to quit her habit, but the words were not backed up by

actions when nowhere could be made available to her to pursue this
source of comfort
- seeing another baby in the parents' own baby's space
- having the dead baby locked in a room alone
- the mortuary being 'unfriendly' and 'dirty'
- antenatal women smoking in the doorway of the hospital
- inadequate parking
- no usable phone

> When I went to try to use the phone – there's a room put aside spe-
> cially for the parents, up the stairs – there were two girls in having a
> coffee and having a blether in the room. And at that point I knew that
> as soon as I was going to go in I was going to burst into tears when I
> was on the phone to my mother. So I obviously didn't want to go in
> where there were two girls sitting having a fag, smoking and chatting.
> I was wandering back and forth trying to find a phone.
>
> (P 58: father of preterm baby)

> [My husband] was on the phone telling folk that [the baby] had died
> and there was folk all just sitting there – the room was packed full
> of folk. And he's breaking his heart down the phone ... It was just
> a total nightmare ... with all these people listening, there was just
> no privacy.
>
> (P10: mother of preterm twins)

- inedible food. When they were much in need of solace it was distressing
  to be confronted with meals which were 'inedible' and to have to waste
  precious time going out to purchase alternatives
- having to pass evidence of happy outcomes of pregnancy.


# Administrative or organisational factors

Two major stressors were identified.

- Registering the birth and death at the same time. This was experienced
  as an extremely upsetting task to have to do. A few parents wondered if
  there might not be some facility for the staff to carry out this task in
  such circumstances in order to spare the parents (usually the fathers)
  this pain.

> The most difficult thing of the whole thing was going to the registry
> office and registering the birth and death at the same time because we
> hadn't had time to register his birth at the time.
>
> (P2: father of baby with cardiac anomaly)

- Registration of multiple birth of very preterm babies if one or more was stillborn before 24 weeks' gestation. The parents were deeply upset when this baby's existence was unrecognised and the other babies were registered as singletons instead of twins, or singletons/twins instead of triplets/quads. When the gestation of all of the babies had been the same it seemed incomprehensible that such an anomaly existed.

## Idiosyncratic factors

As one mother said, parents are so vulnerable at this time that they are less resilient in the face of perceived insensitivity. Simply seeing the world going on much as usual was hurtful to many parents – in the face of something as cataclysmal as their baby dying, things should have ground to a halt. Another mother strongly resented a breach of confidentiality which meant that news of the couple's bereavement leaked out into quarters where she would rather people had not known about it.

# Later regrets about the management of the dying process

It seemed important to find out what elements lingered in the parents' memory and were still sources of dissatisfaction after a period of reflection. At 13 months when they were asked to identify anything in the actual management of their case which they now regretted, very few parents mentioned the small details identified above. Concentration was focused on the speed with which events occurred and the parents' own knowledge of the problems.

## Speed of events

As many as eight sets of parents (16%) regretted the length of time it had taken to decide to stop treatment. They now all wished that the child had died sooner.

> We did ask why they couldn't [just give him a big dose of morphine. They said] they can't do that. They're not allowed to do that. Basically, the way I look at it, euthanasia is against the law... I know people would abuse the situation, but in something like that, when people know there's no hope and the doctors agree with you, then I think it should be [allowed]

> ... the end result is just the same, but it could have been quicker – it wouldn't have been any better but it's another two weeks easier healing.
> (P 39: parents of baby with brain damage)

One couple expressed a more specific wish that their baby 'had been euthanased' early on and that they had been spared the agonising experience they had gone through. On the other hand, four sets of parents now wondered if they should have tried harder and for longer to save their child's life.

# Lack of information

A fifth of the respondent families ($n = 10$) felt that they had been given too little information or that it had not been given soon enough. The fathers were particularly vocal about this issue, seeing it as part of their role to gain the facts in order to be able to decide wisely. Since there was a crucial decision to be made, a paucity of information limited the parents' ability to make an informed choice. For a small number of couples the full truth only emerged when they received a post-mortem report. A further three sets of parents regretted being given false reassurances or wrong information which had misled them and deflected them from an understanding of the gravity of the situation. Fragmentation of care was regarded as a major contributory factor for four mothers and three fathers who felt that, had there been continuity, problems would have been better understood and dealt with. One mother and two fathers commented that they now wished they had been more assertive and pushed for more details.

# Long-term overall regrets

Having given this general overview of their satisfaction with the management of the case, parents were then asked individually if they still personally harboured long-term regrets about anything in relation to the whole experience, aside that was from a powerful regret that the child had died. One or both partners in as many as 31 sets of parents (62%) expressed strong regrets at this time, and a further 6 (12%) had reservations.

# Mothers

## *Delayed detection of problems*
The most commonly cited long-term regret for the mothers (15, 30%) was that problems in pregnancy or labour had not been detected earlier or

tragedy averted by a different form of intervention or management. A few recognised the benefit of hindsight in reaching this conclusion, but for most there was a strong sense that things might have been very different if signs of fetal distress or preterm labour had been taken seriously.

## Limited opportunities to be with the child

The second commonest regret ($n = 11$ mothers, 22%) was a personal sense of having been deprived of precious time with the baby. This was sometimes due to outside influences, such as having had a surgical operation post-natally, or being refused permission to travel with the baby in the ambulance transferring him or her to the study Unit. For others it was due to a lack of awareness on their part of the short time that was left. Several mothers commented that, if they had known the baby would die so soon, they would have spent every available moment with him or her. One mother now wished that she had taken up the offer to have her baby home for a period, but at the time she had been too fearful to agree to this. Linked with the desire for closer involvement was the need for accurate and early information mentioned above. Only one mother expressed regret about her actual involvement. She had found the dying itself 'horrific' and sometimes wished that she had not held the baby during this last part of the process.

## Too few mementoes

When the child died, the parents realised how few mementoes they had of his or her short life. For four mothers (8%) the dearth of photographs, video coverage or diary records was a source of additional and ongoing regret.

## Insensitivity of staff

Six mothers (12%) identified behaviour of staff as still rankling with them. Swearing on the part of an obstetrician during labour, a neonatologist's patronising attitude or slowness in attending to the baby, inappropriate comments from junior paediatricians, a specialist's insensitive manner, and a neonatal nurse's hurtful manner and comments were all cited.

## Personal regrets

For two mothers the regrets were deeply personal. At 13 months after the loss of their babies, both blamed themselves to some extent for developments leading to the tragedy. One mother had declined to have a medical student present at her delivery; the labour ward was very busy when she was admitted, and she had only had a student midwife present. She now felt that had a second person been present, the birth trauma might have been averted. The other mother was haunted by a deep fear that she had inadvertently knocked the endotracheal tube when she had kissed her baby. It was many months before she dared to confide this dread, but despite repeated reassurances to the contrary she said that the fear returned when she was low in spirits.

# Fathers

## Limited involvement

Apart from the wish for more information mentioned above, the commonest long-term regret among fathers was that they had not been involved more in the life and death of their baby ($n = 10$ fathers, 25%). A considerable number had earlier spoken of their personal initial reluctance to get involved and their retrospective gratitude to the mother for pressuring them into doing so.

> It's totally contradictory to my way of managing most problems. [I try to distance myself from them]. But I also felt that if I didn't do it then there was no going back. With other things you can go back if you did something wrong or you think you didn't do something wrong and you can go back and revisit that. But I realised that by giving consent to the post-mortem that we wouldn't see him like that again. That was a driver as well to overcome my normal management technique.
>
> (P50: father of baby with multiple anomalies)

Even so, seven fathers now felt that if they had really appreciated what would happen, how short a time was available to them and the significance of their loss, they would have chosen closer contact with the baby. Some did volunteer that they had taken one step back in order to give the mother maximum contact, but they now wished that for their own satisfaction they had taken a more active role. Two men regretted not taking time off work to be with the baby constantly. Only two fathers saw their lack of inclusion as anything other than their own choice: one man felt that the NICU had excluded the parents during the long delay following admission to the Unit, and the other felt that the paediatric team had done so by taking the baby away from the parents to be resuscitated. And only one father had long-term problems with regard to his actual contact with his baby. He had gone back to see the child after the death, and was now haunted by the ensuing changes which he perceived as 'shocking.' He wished that he had not returned.

### Delayed detection of problems

Nine fathers (22%) had long-term problems with events in pregnancy and labour. They believed that better management or earlier diagnosis or intervention might have saved the baby's life.

### Insensitivity of staff

For six fathers (15%) their regrets hinged on the attitudes and behaviour of staff. An insensitive midwife, a patronising neonatologist, an insensitive neonatologist and a specialist who was poor at communicating were all cited.

### Personal regrets

Personal deficiencies were mentioned by four fathers (10%). Two men regretted not being more sensitive to the needs of their partners. The third father felt a real regret that he as a father had been unable to protect his baby daughter from the worst thing that could befall her. The fourth man now wished that he had taken more responsibility for the funeral arrangements, as he might have been able to prevent a number of serious mistakes being made which gave the parents long-term pain.

### Too few mementoes

Two fathers (5%) wished that they had kept a more detailed record in the form of photographs or video recordings, and one of these lamented the fact that there was no photograph at all of him with the child.

### Absence of literature

Several fathers at various points commented on the uncharted territory they had travelled as fathers of dying babies. One specifically voiced regret about the absence of any literature to describe the emotions he might expect to experience. It would have helped to know whether it was permissible or normal to feel 'mad' or 'upset' with the doctors, he said. He had been furious at one point, 'losing the place' in the nursery, and his conscience still troubled him.

# Remaining negative emotions

It was accepted and acknowledged that parents would strongly regret the death of their child, but it seemed important to establish what specific memories caused particular long-term pain. At the 13-month interview, after reflecting on the experience and its consequences, respondents were asked if any particular memories still generated powerful negative emotions.

# Mothers

The predominant sense conveyed by the mothers was one of overwhelming sorrowful regret. Ten mothers expressed anger and three expressed guilt. The actual events which triggered these powerful emotions are listed below to give a sense of when and in what way they were particularly significant.

### Being told the child would die

The most frequently cited factor for the mothers ($n = 5$) was the moment when they were told that the child would die. It was remembered vividly and with acute pain. They described it as the 'worst experience imaginable,' 'worse than the death itself' and the 'desolation of no hope.' However, one mother qualified her comment, saying that alongside the bitter sorrow was a sense of relief that finally the reality was acknowledged, a decision could be made and the suffering would end. For one couple there was a 'huge sense of sadness' attached to holding the baby for the first time after receiving the information about a bleak outcome.

### Awareness of the suffering

It was a source of great pain to five mothers to remember that their baby had suffered. Some worried about what had been inflicted at delivery, as well as the aggressive treatment of intensive care. One felt that treatment should have been withdrawn sooner in order to limit the burden on the child.

> In retrospect now, if I'd have known what happens to babies when they die, my husband and I wouldn't have resuscitated. We're both pretty sure about that. These things happen so quickly. I thought I might see them for two minutes and that would be the end of it. I didn't even think [about what would happen] after that. But they looked so lovely when they were in one coffin together. They looked so human that I frankly would have preferred that than have to go through the SCBU [trauma]. Because they looked so [abnormal] I couldn't bond with them, and at the funeral when I saw them in their coffin I thought, 'Wow, you look perfectly normal.' They both looked like sleeping babies. Not even blue. Nothing. If I'd known ... Because I could have seen those babies any time – they could have brought them up from the mortuary. I could have spent two days with them – five days. And I would have preferred that.
>
> (P 33: mother of preterm twins)

## *Struggling for breath*
Memories of the baby struggling for breath haunted three mothers.

> When she was struggling [to breathe] that was the worst bit. They actually said were we wanting them to video it and I said, 'No, [not that bit]'. The noise she was making, it was like you were killing her or something – a horrible noise.
>
>                              (P13: mother of baby with cardiac anomaly)

One mother described her overwhelming desire to breathe for her child and her utter desolation at being unable to do so. The actual drawing of the last breath was a moment that was recalled graphically by another mother, and it continued to haunt her more than a year later.

## *Fathers' grief*
For two mothers an abiding sorrow attached to the grief was that they saw their partners suffering. The memory of their distraught faces was a sobering reminder of what they had lost. One mother believed that the grief was compounded by her husband's realisation that he would now never have a son, although he himself strenuously rejected this idea.

# Fathers

The main emotion of the fathers was again one of desolation, coupled with shock and a sense of helplessness. Six fathers made reference to their pent-up anger, which was so great in one case that the father wished he 'could explode.'

## *Powerlessness*
Fathers were angry that their child had 'drawn the short straw,' and that they themselves had been powerless to prevent the tragedy. In cases where others had limited the scope of their involvement, or further curtailed their roles, this increased their sense of frustration.

> I've always gone through my life [believing], as with physical fighting, I could do [anything] – and I could never ever fight for [the baby]. It was more like a mental fighting for him – you're hoping that everything's going to be all right. That's what hurt me more than anything, because you can't *do* anything. If anything's ever happened to me before it's always been something you could do something about. Because I couldn't do anything about it that was worse – it was a strange feeling.
>
>                              (P56: father of preterm baby with congenital anomalies)

## Pressure to decide

Three fathers now had deep negative feelings about the pressure that was put on them to decide. (None of the mothers cited this.) One father believed that in a calm state he would have made a different choice. A fourth father remained angry a year later that he had not been given statistics and guidance on risks in order to enable him to make an informed choice. Without the facts he was utterly dependent on medical guidance.

## Being told that the child would die

Actually being told that the child would die was identified by just one father as a bleak moment which still haunted him. Another father summed up the emotions of that realisation as a 'dreadful sense of hopelessness and helplessness' attached to the experience where he was unable to correct this great wrong.

## Awareness of suffering

One father cited the suffering of the child as his main preoccupation one year later. Now that the child had died, others too pondered the wisdom of treating them at all. It was only after the event that they could reflect on what invasive intensive treatment had involved. Vivid memories of a whole week during which both his partner and his baby lay critically ill haunted another father. Alongside the sorrow of the baby's eventual death was the awareness of what might also have happened to his wife.

## Unpleasant features of the dying process

Three fathers repeatedly recalled the actual dying process and were distressed by it more than a year later. Others spoke of the sights, sounds and smells which remained in their memories and still haunted them. For one father, any sound of computers bleeping or 'smells of cleanliness' still brought powerful feelings flooding back. One observed that 'the end' was 'still vivid in every detail', and the sense of incredulity and devastation was so overwhelming as to seem unreal. Another father was still haunted by the sounds of the baby's stertorous breathing. He even dreamed about that 'horrible sound'. Feelings about the death were so negative for one man that he regretted having been present, and he was adamant that he would not be involved again were the same thing to happen in a subsequent pregnancy.

> If I'd had a choice I wouldn't have been there while he died. I think it's just sort of expected of you that you'll be there. And you don't know what you're going to go through. If it happened ever again then NO!
>
> (P 39: father of baby with brain damage)

## Protracted death

For three fathers the predominant negative feelings were associated with the lingering nature of the dying process. Two of them believed retrospectively that treatment should have been stopped earlier.

## Empty incubator

For one father the sight of the empty incubator after the death remained with him and was a source of deep pain a year later.

## Registration

Having to register the birth and death together was an experience which shook fathers deeply. However, only one mentioned it in this context.

> Having to register his birth and his death at the same time. And I had to do that just hours after. And I thought, 'Why is it so important to have to do it now? Can you not wait?'... At the time you're on automatic pilot and you just go and do it, but I've thought about that quite a lot since and it just makes me quite angry when it's something that, let's be honest about it, is just a bit of bureaucracy. It could have been left for a couple of days. But I think it was a legal requirement that it had to be done within 12 hours or something like that. A lovely happy event when it's a wee boy's birth and you're all happy. But when you're registering his birth and his death at the same time it's different. And I think they could have some kind of understanding that you can get a couple of days' grace on that ... And you're in there with people who are getting marriage licences and other people who are registering happy events. And it's just, 'On you go.' My turn now. And you're at the same wee window: 'How can I help you?' 'I'd like to register my son's birth and death, please.'
>
> (P15: father of preterm baby)

# Discussion

A hundred years ago death was very much a part of everyday life. Tombstones in churchyards bear testament to the prevalence of infant and child death. Nowadays, with our Western society's emphasis on health, and with ever increasing medical capabilities, death in infancy is relatively uncommon and the experience of death in the family has moved increasingly out of the home and into institutions. It was against this background that the families who participated in our study faced the loss of their babies.

# The parents' feelings

Not only did the parents highlight the shock and devastation experienced when a baby dies, and their own lack of preparation for such an event, but they also spoke of a sense of powerlessness and lack of control. The child is taken away from them, and the culture within the NICU limits their responsibility for decision making on his or her behalf.[12,138,139] This is uncharted territory, and they are reliant on others to guide them through it.

> I felt [the baby] was the hospital's responsibility as far as I was concerned. I did what they told me, because they were looking after him ... Even at that last day I still thought of [the neonatal nurse] as being responsible for him. She would say what happened. She would say when he could get out. I didn't feel I had any [responsibility to manage things or state a preference]. It didn't bother me, because they were caring for him and that was all that mattered. It wasn't till later that [the neonatal nurse] said, 'I've mentioned to your mum that maybe she can get a wee hold of him later. Is that all right?'. *She* was asking *me*! I was [taken aback]. I said, 'Of course!'
>
> (P48: mother of preterm baby with congenital anomalies)

Fears may be unspoken but are nevertheless deep-seated. Emotions are turbulent and often ambivalent.

However, in providing insights into their personal experiences these parents illuminate our understanding of what it feels like to be on the receiving end of 'compassionate care.' Some of their perceptions shed new light on practice. Other suggestions have been heard before,[78,104,140–143] but the fact that these parents found their own management deficient in these ways indicates that the messages have not been universally received and adopted. They therefore bear reiteration.

# Parents want to be actively involved in the dying process

Although the dying process is a profoundly distressing experience for parents, they give a clear message that it is essential that they have the opportunity to be actively involved in it: 'a cup of tea and an aseptic look at the body does not serve.'[144] Indeed, it has been suggested that *not* being involved is one of the markers for being at risk of developing later problems.[45,145] For these families, not only is this a time to love the child and accumulate memories, but it is also an opportunity to assimilate the reality of the baby's death and his or her inability to sustain life unaided, and to obtain confirmation of the rightness of the decision to stop treatment.

Even where parents do participate, it is evident that lost opportunities to be with the child bring additional pain. It is sobering to find substantial numbers of mothers expressing a lasting regret that they had been deprived of precious time with the child, and the fathers regretting not having been more involved. Although it has to be acknowledged that sometimes the parents themselves choose to distance themselves at certain points in the process, nevertheless these families identified external constraints which sometimes limit the range of parental experiences. The potential for such restrictions must be noted – delays in taking them to see the baby, a lack of information about what they can do until it is too late to do it, or rules which are too inflexible. Their accounts of such limitations ring warning bells.

It was clear from our findings that in most families it is the women who play the dominant role in caretaking during the actual dying process. Some fathers deliberately stand back to allow the mother to take on the main role. This reflects a number of factors – their underlying reluctance to stay for the dying, their belief that it is predominantly a female-orien-tated role, or a need to keep themselves distant until the decision to stop is made, lest parental emotions jeopardise a wise choice. If they have held back at all, there may then be a greater sense of urgency to engage with the baby while they can still do so. This reality is not always recognised.

However, although the overwhelming majority did want to participate fully, the minority who found performing any task with the baby too dis-tressing must also be heard. A perceived expectation that they should change a nappy or bath a dead baby adds to their stress and may be bur-densome. For 15% of parents there was an element of over-involvement which they subsequently regretted. Significantly, in all cases these regrets related to events which occurred after the death, and for six of these nine families, the hurt came from seeing the baby again after death. The unpleasant changes which they saw returned to haunt them, and they wished that they could retain the picture of the newly dead child who appeared simply to be sleeping. It seems relevant to note that during field-work, nurses volunteered that many of them never saw the babies after they had left the nursery, and they had no knowledge of what happened subsequently. When they encouraged families to return to see the body, they did not understand the implications involved if parents did so.

## Management must be individually tailored

Needs and preferences vary widely. The experience of the families from dif-ferent cultures whom we interviewed highlights this variety dramatically.

Even at a fairly basic level, perceptions and reactions may not fit with our ideas of what is desirable in these circumstances.[146–147] Their stories sound a note of caution against others assuming what is best for them.[148] 'Each death is unique and requires its own response from professionals.'[149]

Our findings show that parents are deeply grateful for a sensitive service which is responsive to their personal needs and wishes. Since they have no precedents to guide them, most welcome some steering by experienced staff, but they also value their freedom to adopt only those suggestions which fit with their own preferences. Some writers have offered check-lists to professionals, with up to 70 instructions on how to approach grieving parents,[150,151] but a 'protocol cannot generate empathy if the practitioner lacks the capacity for it.'[152] Rules and other people's priorities must not be permitted to replace responsive listening. In reality, relationships are forged through this powerful experience, facilitating a tailoring of care which is of more benefit than adherence to a blanket protocol.

It is important to recognise that the process is an interactive one. Each individual takes their cues from the other as they negotiate a way forward which is sensitive to the possibilities and preferences of the family. This dialogue is perhaps best illustrated by reference to a specific family. The couple concerned, on hearing that their child had a rare and fatal syndrome, decided that it was best to stop treatment as there was no hope of any quality of life. For two days they spent time with the baby, the night being passed in the family room with the baby and his sibling. On the third day the mother indicated to an advanced nurse practitioner that she thought the right time to withdraw treatment might be imminent. In response, the nurse suggested that she should stop the oxygen at a set time later that day. Knowing how long they had before that moment, the parents felt able to leave the grandparents with the baby while they took a break. They returned in good time for the rest of the process, the short break from the scene having fortified them for what was to come.

# Elements in the dying process may be particularly traumatic

From the parents' own accounts of the management of dying, certain aspects of the process emerged as particularly significant, warranting further scrutiny and discussion. It has to be remembered that these were parents speaking with the benefit of hindsight. It is much easier to state after the event that some other experience would have been better, or the limited time available better utilised. We fully appreciate that at the time there are many unknowns and many sensitivities to consider.

## Protracted deaths

It is clear from our study that parents expect the child to die soon after treatment withdrawal, and that medical predictions are not always accurate. In cases which involve a decision to withdraw treatment, a lingering death has special significance. It raises doubts about the wisdom of the decision to stop, the severity of the illness and the baby's own wishes.

Our findings also suggest that parents are not always well prepared for what might happen. In order to cope with the pain of the dying, they have a number of requirements which our respondents have highlighted. First, they need full information which includes, where possible, some idea of what to expect. Second, they need an honest admission of uncertainty rather than inappropriate estimates of the time that it will take for death to occur. It helps them if they are given the reasons for possible delays so that they are not left questioning the rightness of the decision to stop. Third, they need the messages to be consistent. If it becomes necessary to deviate from an agreed plan, they need to know clear reasons for that change of direction, so that it is not perceived as inconsistency or doubt about the wisdom of the decision to stop treatment.

Parents are also giving a message that where death is the expected and desired outcome, there is no point in allowing prolonged suffering. Some have advocated active measures to end life in hopeless situations. However, this finding raises more fundamental global questions. The law in this country prohibits active killing of human beings, even out of mercy. Professional medical guidelines[9,10] as well as government reports[153,154] uphold this position. Yet the courts have demanded compassionate care and have decreed that children should not suffer unnecessarily.[155] Even though the exact measurement of pain is a difficult estimation for neonates, clinicians do make efforts to limit pain and to reassure parents on this point. But when death is inevitable and compassionate terminal care is required, not only the baby's comfort but also the minimisation of the parents' distress becomes a priority. Our findings clearly show that parents are traumatised by a protracted dying process. So, too, are the staff.[12] What then should be done with the severely asphyxiated child who requires no medical intervention, or the severely damaged baby who lingers long after treatment withdrawal? Current guidelines offer little direction, and these extremely sensitive clinical dilemmas require renewed scrutiny and further debate.

## Autopsy

Of the families in our study who were asked to consent to autopsy, 62% did so. This falls some way short of the UK target of 75% set by the medical colleges, Royal College of Paediatrics and Child Health (RCPCH) and

Royal College of Obstetrics and Gynaecologists (RCOG), but the number of perinatal autopsies has decreased nationally.[156]

Although high autopsy rates do not necessarily reflect excellence of service,[157] the multifactorial value of autopsy remains undisputed.[158–160] Reported rates of consent for babies range from 48% to 79%,[160–166] but there is documented evidence that rates are falling world-wide.[156,159,160,167]

Correlation with a range of factors such as maternal age, race, marital status, employment, socio-economic influences, parity, gestation, birth weight, age of the baby, length of stay in a NICU, and status of the requester has been examined,[161,165,168] but no associations have been found for most of these factors. However, it has been suggested that parents are less likely to agree to autopsy if the baby is extremely preterm.[163] Staff may apply less pressure for an autopsy in these circumstances, but there is no evidence that post-mortem examination is less likely to give new information in this group of infants.[163]

Objectively it might be expected that for the parents themselves the autopsy would appear to have special significance.[169,170] Our study identified many of the cited advantages as those which parents appreciate. It provides information about what actually happened in their child's case. Even in cases where a clear diagnosis has been established, totally new or important information is found in a significant number of autopsies.[156,164,171] It gives confirmation and reassurance or otherwise of the accuracy of the diagnosis and the appropriateness of the treatment given. And importantly it may provide information about genetic or obstetric risk. Apart from these personal benefits, parents gain comfort from knowing that information obtained from the autopsy may be used to help others, thus bringing good out of their tragedy. When children die after treatment withdrawal there is an added dimension: the autopsy may provide confirmation of the wisdom of the decision to stop treatment.

Knowing the statistics for consent and the demographic details associated with consent or refusal, however, provides only a partial picture. An important element in consent may be parental perception. A number of factors may influence their responses, and our study adds weight to some of these.

The literature suggests that the single commonest reason for not obtaining a post-mortem examination is failure to ask for one.[170] Our study shows that this is not the case in the Neonatal Units in the east of Scotland, where all except one of the families we studied *were* asked. It has also been suggested that a request for a post-mortem examination may shock the mother.[172–174] Some of our respondents expressed such an emotion, and it was evident from our findings that both the timing and the approach are critically important.

We have no objective information about how much pressure consultants exerted for consent, but the data suggest that, in line with clinical expectation, more parents agreed to autopsy where the deaths were unexpected, unexplained or might have carried a significant genetic component. Where the causes appear to be obvious, there may seem to be less need to conduct a post-mortem examination. However, it must be remembered that when post-mortem findings have been compared with ante-mortem diagnoses for the total perinatal population, errors in up to 45% of cases have been reported.[171]

There is inconclusive evidence as to whether or not the identity of the person seeking consent matters.[163,167,168] In our study Units, normal practice is for the consultant to ask this question. Furthermore, in almost all cases it is the same consultant who sees the parents at the follow-up meeting when the post-mortem findings are given. This was the case for all except one couple in our study. Disturbing results have emerged from previous surveys where relatives never received autopsy findings, were given them over the telephone, or had no opportunity to discuss them with a doctor.[170,175] The parents whom we interviewed not only identified a need to have face-to-face discussion and interpretation of the meaning of the findings with someone knowledgeable, but more than that, they wished for the person undertaking this task to be someone known and trusted, continuity being an important adjunct to trust. This is often difficult information to receive, and the support of those who shared the life and death of the baby is crucial at this time.

Concerns about disfigurement are known to loom large in the minds of relatives contemplating autopsy, especially where children are concerned,[60,170,173,175] and our results confirm this as a major preoccupation among parents. If a baby has already suffered much in the parents' perceptions, the idea of further mutilation or invasion is abhorrent to many. Although, as we have seen, there is little to suggest that either epidemiological or demographic factors influence consent to autopsy, our study suggests that parental attitudes and beliefs do. Intuitively, it might be thought that parents might be more eager to have autopsy confirmation of a poor prognosis in cases where treatment was withdrawn. In reality, we found that only two parents cited this as an overt reason for consenting to a post-mortem examination. Rather, where the parents themselves still have unanswered questions, they need facts which can be obtained after death to help to complete the picture of what went wrong. Conversely, however, if they are personally satisfied with their current knowledge of the circumstances, but the medical team still has unanswered questions, there may be resistance to any further procedures being performed on the child.

There are, then, many reasons why parents may decline to consent to autopsy, but the fact remains that they may later regret that decision. A recent survey of parental experience following loss of a pregnancy or baby found that one in 18 women who consented to autopsy subsequently regretted doing so, and three in 10 women who had not consented regretted their decision.[176] Our findings at 13 months show that no one expressed such a regret, but a larger, more structured and focused study is needed to establish the facts. Furthermore, doubt may not surface until future pregnancies, even those a generation later, are in question, and there is no available genetic baseline to guide decisions.

### Registering births and deaths

We found the necessity to register the birth and death simultaneously to be a traumatic experience for parents. It is a task which appears to fall mainly to the fathers, and some were clearly distressed by the memory more than a year later. Having to verbalise this tragedy in a public place to an official who is a complete stranger so soon after the event is uniquely stressful, and they strongly recommend that a change should be made to the legal requirements.

The lack of official recognition of infants stillborn before 24 weeks' gestation is a source of acute distress to parents who then have the remaining siblings registered as singletons, twins or triplets when they are in reality part of a larger set of children. This discrepancy persists for the rest of their lives and is a source of ongoing sorrow. When so much else is done to confirm the reality of the child's short existence, and to encourage the parents to mourn a real baby, it seems incongruous that officialdom should not recognise these births.

# It is possible to facilitate a good dying process

Even though parents were describing a grief beyond expression, all except one couple were able to identify some factors which helped them through the experience. Many of these are not new ideas, but they bear repetition. In drawing attention to the key elements which constitute good practice we also note that there were exceptional cases which serve to remind clinicians that every family is unique, and there are no blanket rules which can be applied in these delicate situations.

### Respect and value

Signs of respect for both the parents and the baby are appreciated, and their absence is regretted. Being listened to attentively, having their preferences remembered and being treated as equals are all indicators of respect for them as uniquely important individuals in this process. Providing extra comfort measures for the baby, speaking to them sensitively and ensuring that the child's body is handled with reverence; these are outward manifestations to the parents of the value staff accord to neo-nates, no matter how short their lives may be.[93]

## Compassion

Our study indicates that compassion is a crucial part of effective process when it comes to the management of dying babies and their families. The compassion of the nursing staff appears to be expected, whereas that of the consultant is considered to be an unexpected privilege. Open expressions of sadness are especially valued. The right of doctors to show emotion, and the desirability of their doing so, have been both called into question[177,178] and explored.[179] Our findings reveal overwhelming approval by the parents of a doctor showing emotion when a baby dies. The fact that he has experienced this phenomenon so often and still grieves for this individual baby speaks to them of a depth of caring and an engagement with the family which confirms their worth and comforts them in their sorrow.

## Dignity

When invasive treatment is being or has been withdrawn, dignity both in life and in death is an important factor. There seems to be little value to the parents in persisting with procedures which appear to compromise that state. As the mother of a child with trisomy 18 wrote:

> The doctors were prepared to do invasive dialysis, but we felt our little daughter had been picked and squeezed, transfused, dripped so much that if life couldn't be sustained without this shock treatment, it wasn't worth sustaining. We wanted to let Rachel go before she lost her last vestige of dignity.[93]

## Sensitive approach

As has been said, the dying process is a time for 'extreme responsibility, extraordinary sensitivity, and heroic compassion.'[138] Our study shows that overall care in these NICUs is of a high standard, and that the sensitivity of individuals is impressive in the view of the parents. However, it is an undisputed reality that a chain is only as strong as its weakest link, and the strength of the NICU team is no exception to this rule. The accounts of the parents described above give insights into some of the potential weak links. Parents do notice. As one mother, speaking of a young doctor, put it:

> He was well-meaning though brusque, and his manner reflected the strait-jacket of his training. I wondered, as I watched his brittle approach, how long it would be before he discovered his humility.[129]

By contrast, she described the paediatric consultant as someone who 'radiated a compassion which was personal and approachable. He was so very human that with him there was no sense of "them and us," there was only "us".' Although it is common practice to limit the team to a few key people at this time, the effect of everyone else must be borne in mind.

## Privacy

In moments of intense grief, it can be extremely inhibiting to be watched and to feel obliged to conform to other people's expectations.[144] Insights from our study show that privacy involves more than being given access to a room. It is about respecting the parents' need for space and the freedom to act in ways that express their emotions or needs. The fact that some parents felt they could not do simple things which they wanted to do with their baby bears testament to the sense of inhibition they feel in the presence of others, no matter how benign and encouraging the staff may feel themselves to be. Moreover, simply providing a private room is not in itself enough to ensure that that need is met. If the parents, once in the room, are subjected to the sounds of crying babies or happy parents, or have to spend precious time looking for telephones or food or parking spaces, their limited parenting opportunities are further eroded.

## Continuity

At a time of great distress parents find it unhelpful to have to work repeatedly at establishing new relationships. One couple who had had a baby in the study Unit for many weeks, and had built up strong friendships, were saddened to be surrounded by new faces on the day of her death when a completely new (to them) team of staff took over. Kind and efficient though they were, something was missing. It is clear that changes at this time should be kept to a minimum.

## Providing mementoes

Parents clearly treasure mementoes of their baby's life, and the gathering of these tokens represents an important part of the dying process.[67,78] Photographs, in particular, play a significant role in sharing the life of the child with others and preserving the reality of his or her short existence, although videos appear to be a form of remembering which parents initially find extremely distressing, so vivid is the re-living of the experience.

## Setting

The experience of parents in our study shows that their need at the time when the baby is dying is to be protected from the hurt others may inflict, in order to concentrate on being with the baby while they can. There is time enough subsequently to focus on the reality of their loss and their own status as bereaved parents. They endorse the value of a family room which provides such a sanctuary.[180] Some ambivalence is to be found in the literature with regard to the appropriate setting for providing care for a bereaved mother.[67] The importance of not denying the reality of the loss has to be offset against the pain of seeing and hearing other mothers with healthy babies. The support which other mothers can give has to be gauged alongside the damage they may unwittingly do by random comments. The risk of feelings of isolation and rejection must be considered as well as the harm which may accrue from accentuating the mothers' 'differentness'.

## Support

It was very evident that every one of the parents in our study looked principally to the consultant and the nursing staff for support at this time. Inexperienced family members and friends cannot offer what these parents need, but doctors and nurses who have trodden this path before can guide and support them, empowering them to do the things which create memories and which emphasise their parenthood. Furthermore, parents recognise that the staff who are most intimately involved with the baby are often grieving themselves, and this shared sorrow is supportive in itself. True support comes from understanding the pain, and is shown not only by optimising parental contact, but also by the sensitive touches which empathy generates – for example, encouraging a reluctant father to be involved within his level of tolerance, promising to check on the baby periodically after the death, and escorting parents to the door rather than leaving them to wander through the empty corridors at night feeling empty and bereft.

As the Health Service Commissioner and Ombudsman, Michael Buckley, has observed:

> At each extremity of our lives we are at our most helpless. We depend on others for how those events, and what surrounds them, are managed. In both cases we often depend on professional carers. In consequence, the people closest to us may feel disempowered, even alienated, by the process.[149]

This chapter has included a wide range of issues and covered many facets of parental experience and perceptions during the management of the dying process. The detail serves to highlight the breadth and depth of the insights parents provided. It draws attention to the need for clinicians to be aware of the potential either to facilitate their healthy progress or to debilitate them at any stage of that process.

# Conclusion

- The majority of parents want to be actively involved in the dying process.
- The management of that process should be sensitively tailored to their individual needs and preferences, but should always ensure the provision of respect, compassion, dignity, privacy and support.
- Parents need to be adequately prepared for what might happen once treatment is withdrawn, but no false assurances should be given.
- Lingering deaths are acutely distressing for parents, and we suggest that the best way of managing such cases should be debated openly and carefully.
- Parental attitudes and opinions play an important role in gaining consent for autopsy, and emphasis may need to be placed on the importance of genetic implications and the delicacy of the procedure, in order to overcome preconceived ideas.
- The registration by the parents of the birth and death simultaneously is a traumatic experience, and we recommend that the necessity for it should be re-examined.
- The lack of official recognition of stillborn infants below 24 weeks in multiple births where one or more siblings survive is a source of ongoing pain to parents, and we suggest that this matter should also be examined with a view to finding viable alternatives.

# CHAPTER 9

# The funeral

Burying or cremating one's own child is a traumatic experience for which few parents have preparation. Parents recalled these events with great pain.

## The organisation

The parents took responsibility for the organisation of the funeral in most cases (49 of 59 families, 83%), although a considerable number pointed out that it was the first time they had ever had to do such a thing. Ministers and funeral directors provided guidance. Eleven sets of parents (19%) had assistance from their own parents, and in four cases (7%) other family members undertook this task. The parents appreciated it when those who helped took their cues from them in relation to the form and detail of the day. In six cases (10%) the hospital staff made the arrangements. One other mother wished that she had left it to the hospital when a serious mistake was made by the undertaker, believing that the staff would have ensured everything was handled correctly.

> I feel the hospital should have taken on that responsibility because I had never got her home. They belonged to the hospital – my girls.
>
> (P10: mother of preterm twins)

## The setting

Two couples did not want a service at all, but most (97%) combined some form of ceremony (usually based within a religious framework, but occasionally entirely secular) with the burial or cremation, and drew comfort from it. Almost all of the families chose to go to local churches, graveyards or crematoria, but two elected to have the child buried in the home town of the baby's grandparents. Three sets of parents held the service in the home of the grandparents.

# The officiating person

Several couples pointed out the difficulty of someone taking a service for a baby whom they had not known. It was more meaningful if the officiating person had at least seen the child and knew something of the circumstances. Twenty families (34%) asked the chaplain in the NICU to officiate at the funeral. They drew strength from his presence, and he was regarded as an obvious choice for two reasons: he had met the baby and knew what had happened, and he was also acquainted with the parents to some extent. Many parents commented very positively on the contribution that the chaplain had made through his sensitivity to their pain and need, several couples referring to him as 'a lovely person' 'a special kind of person.' Three families employed the services of the chaplains from their local hospitals rather than the NICUs.

A quarter of the families (15, 25%) chose church officials whom they already knew to conduct the service. These included their own church minister ($n = 10$), minister friends ($n = 2$), the grandparents' minister ($n = 1$), a work padre ($n = 1$) and an old schoolfriend priest ($n = 1$). However, it was a local minister not really known to them who undertook this task for 20 sets of parents (34%). In two cases relatives led the mourners in the service (the baby's grandmother and a great-uncle). (Note that the numbers add up to 62 because three families nominated more than one person.)

# The mourners

The size of the event varied greatly, with some families holding it exclusively for themselves and the grandparents, while others opened the doors to reportedly 'hundreds' of friends, acquaintances and local people.

> We just wanted immediate family there. The reason for that was we just wanted people who [the baby] really meant something to; in other words, not people who were grieving for us, but people who were grieving for [him]. And although it sounds strange, we didn't want aunts and uncles there, but we were quite happy for the two nurses to be there because we could see that [he] did mean something to them and they were very sad.
>
> (P27: father of baby with cardiac anomaly)

Parents were moved by the sympathy which was demonstrated when staff from the NICU who had known the baby attended the funeral. There was something special about busy professional people who encountered death so often caring about a specific family enough to come, sometimes apparently in their own time, to such an event.

One of the nurses came . . . I hadn't spoken to her that day, but I was just focusing on what I had to get through, so I did write to her afterwards. But I appreciated that very much. I think that's quite important for somebody to be there at the service and somebody who'd looked after him. Because realistically, of all the people who were there, there was maybe ourselves and grandparents who had seen him for a bit, and effectively that's it. All the other people there didn't know him and had never met him, so she was probably next to us and knew him best.

(P6: parents of baby with congenital anomaly)

Half of the parents (30, 51%) cited neonatal nurses and two (3%) stated that doctors from the Unit had also been present. One mother said that the consultant had specifically asked her when the funeral would take place; she had looked for him on the day, but he did not himself attend. It was noteworthy that nine other families (15%) specifically mentioned that no one from the Unit had been there.

I did remember thinking that I hope somebody from the hospital comes. I felt that. Because I'd asked [the chaplain] would he mind actually phoning the Unit and letting them know . . . I remember thinking somebody's got to come from the hospital.

(P47: mother of baby with brain damage)

Midwives from other areas also came to support the families in 12 cases (20%). These included the labour ward staff who had attended the birth ($n = 3$), postnatal ward midwives ($n = 8$) and a foreign language-speaking midwife who had supported a couple from another country ($n = 1$).

When other parents came, the bereaved parents spoke admiringly of their courage in doing so. In one case the mourners were parents from the NICU, and in two cases they were parents whom they had met during their time in the hospital, but whose babies were not in the Unit.

# Support

The funeral was a difficult event for all parents, although a number of parents volunteered that it was actually less traumatic than their previous experiences in the NICU. However, there was an element of relief in having the baby's suffering over and the decision making behind them, and for some the anticipation was worse than the reality. Reaction to the events set in later for a small number of parents who got through the day itself on 'autopilot.' But for some there were other burdens in addition to the emotional trauma. One family reported that the funeral cost them

£2000 and they were now in debt. Others borrowed money from relatives. One couple postponed their wedding, using money saved for that to defray the funeral expenses.

There were many decisions to be made, but the consequences of different options were not always recognised. Some parents lived to regret their choices.

> Perhaps we would have wished for a nicer grave for the baby. We don't know exactly where it is. There is no name, there is no [anything].
>
> (P17: father of preterm baby)

> The only reason I was getting her buried was for [her twin's] sake. In case she decided in years to come that she just felt that there was something missing ... she could go and visit her sister in the rose garden, which was fine because she was beside all the wee babies ... But she was in this big hole where [her Dad] and his family had to stretch down and practically drop her in, it was that deep. That was devastating in itself ... If I had known she wasn't going in the rose garden I wouldn't have got her buried, I would have got her cremated. Because I don't want her in a big hole like that, nowhere near the rose garden with any other babies. It was absolutely horrendous – it was the worst experience that I ever had in my life ... we've never been back [to visit the grave] because we were so upset and disgusted by it.
>
> (P10: mother of preterm twins)

In one sense the parents felt that no one could really help them at this time. Their grief was so profound that it tended to isolate them, and 23 parents (39%) specifically volunteered that the only person who could really support them was their partner who shared the same enormous loss. Furthermore, a few parents said that other family members had been so demanding in their own grief that they, the parents, had had an additional drain on their resources supporting them. However, they were comforted by the care and concern others demonstrated, and by their attendance at the funeral. The actions which were regarded as supportive are listed below in order to give a general sense of what was helpful, to augment the findings presented above.

# Staff from the study hospital

At the time of the baby's death the parents were helped by the staff gently steering them through the process of preparing for and arranging the funeral. Sometimes special arrangements had to be made either to transfer the body to the burial town, or to allow the parents to take the child home before the funeral, and the parents appreciated help with this task. As we have seen, the presence of known staff at the funeral was of special importance and significance. These were people with whom the parents could share memories and emotion, and talk and laughter without apology or explanation. Their own sadness at the loss of the child was perceived as genuine. Where particular individuals were unable to attend but sent flowers or messages, these were valued because they came from people who had known and grieved for the child. In one case a midwife brought flowers to the graveside – a gesture greatly valued by the parents, because they had not thought to do so themselves. Another couple was helped by midwives coming in each day until the funeral, giving an opportunity to talk, so that the parents were calmer for the funeral itself.

The hospital taking responsibility for arranging the funeral was regarded as a kindness by some couples, but sometimes things went wrong and parents were left with lasting regrets.

> We had no communication with the undertaker at all so they don't know us and we don't know them. And if they don't know us then they wouldn't have known how important it was to us [that the babies were buried as we left them]. We're obviously very grateful for the fact that [the hospital] made all the arrangements ... but – there's a *big* but – they made a spelling mistake ... that doesn't make up for the money [saved]. The fact that it's taken care of is great, but if it's made a mess of you wish, well, I wish I'd taken care of it myself. If I'd had all the communication I'd have made sure it was right.
>
> (P44: mother of preterm quads)

# Chaplain/minister

Ministers of religion usually officiated at funeral services, and parents relied on them for guidance. Families were appreciative of efforts to get to know them and their wishes in order to arrange a sensitive service in tune with their beliefs. Some ministers devised a unique compilation of hymns, songs, poems, readings, prayers and thoughts which the parents treasured as much for the compassion it demonstrated as for the sensitivity of the words at the time. As one mother said, 'He stayed up most of the night before working on it,' and that effort was perceived as having been made for the baby. What was said varied, but parents' main priority was to have the baby's short life valued. Some parents designed contributions themselves, and others made special requests. For example, one couple asked that the minister should request the congregation not to walk by, but to stop and speak to the bereaved parents. They felt that this helped everyone to know the parents' preferences.

Some ministers carried out other tasks as well as arranging the ceremony. By organising transfer of the baby's body, or contacting the funeral director with details to spare parents having to recount the story themselves, they saved the family from a harrowing task.

# Funeral directors

The practicalities of arranging funerals, burials or cremations were largely overseen by funeral directors. Most parents appreciated their sensitivity and careful steering through the decisions. A significant number of companies did not charge for their services for babies or children, and this was seen as a compassionate act. In some cases where transfer over long distances was involved, parents were especially grateful to have experienced people organising the travel and legalities.

However, for a small number of parents these events were far from sensitively handled. Cars were lost from the funeral cortège, unsuitable vehicles were provided as hearses, no privacy was offered in the cars, and burial sites were mixed up. Parents were extremely distressed by finding that the name was wrong, being told that the funeral director could not tell them where the ashes had been scattered, being confronted with unpleasant or hostile reactions when they registered a complaint, or being given their child's ashes in a cardboard box.

> People in this situation don't want to receive the last remains of their child in a cardboard box. It just wasn't fitting.
>
> (P2: father of baby with cardiac anomaly)

# Family members

As well as the love and concern family members expressed, helpful support from this source included assistance with the arrangements – taking responsibility for the organisation themselves, steering the parents through the procedures, or transporting the parents everywhere while they organised the event. Practical support was offered by loaning them money for the expenses, supplying treasures to go in the coffin, having the baby's body at their house before the funeral, and carrying the coffin on the day. For one couple the help had been in the form of the family taking care of all the practical tasks, thereby freeing them to be together to both feel and express their emotions. Too much emotion displayed by others could be problematic, and parents appreciated family members taking their cue from them about how far to go.

A small number of couples were hurt by the responses of family members at this time. Where they made no attempt to contact the parents or to attend the funeral, they denied the value of the child's life as well as the importance of the parents' welfare. Other relatives were so distraught themselves that they were unavailable to the parents, and indeed in some cases they made additional unwelcome demands on them. But some couples were sympathetic, recognising that the grandparents were grieving simultaneously for their own lost babies or other significant loved ones.

# Friends

Friends' support came from their sensitivity to the parents' needs. Knowing when to leave them in peace and when to telephone or call round or provide a meal was a mark of their awareness of the parents' need. This was a testing time, and whilst some relationships were scarred by inappropriate responses, others were cemented. Practical support was provided in a variety of ways, including taking care of other children, hosting the funeral wake, singing well at the funeral, and helping to raise money to meet expenses. Some close friends substituted for the parents by carrying the coffin. Other friends helped collectively – for example, providing money for a headstone, or arranging for a memorial shrub or seat.

# Work colleagues

Dealing with work colleagues at this time was not always easy, as the parents were to all intents and purposes inhabiting a different world during this traumatic experience. They were greatly comforted when colleagues showed their concern by helping in practical ways or arranging a tribute or a memorial. One firm closed on the day of the funeral as a mark of respect. Colleagues of a father in the RAF arranged a fly-past. As one mother said, colleagues could sometimes be more supportive than family, as they were not so emotionally involved and they were geographically closer.

However, one mother recalled colleagues being particularly hurtful. They said cruel things which dismissed the baby as being of no real importance, and the mother's grief as insignificant, and they did not speak to her. At a low point when any mother would be feeling particularly vulnerable, this behaviour was deeply wounding and made a return to work even more difficult.

## Other bereaved parents

At this sad time parents welcomed the genuine sympathy someone else who had been in the same position could offer. The empathy of other bereaved parents was of a higher calibre.

## The parents themselves

Parents also derived strength and help to move on in the grieving process from things they themselves could do. Having the baby's body at home before the funeral, or returning to see the child in the coffin, allowed a few parents to savour the child's existence while they still could. Designing the service, composing songs or poems, and themselves speaking or singing during the service all represented ways in which they could do something special for their baby and make the event meaningful and significant. For example, one father used the opportunity to encourage everyone who attended the service to view the tragedy positively so that the child's short life would not have been in vain, but he also found that doing this helped him and his partner to move on. It was evident that parents felt a need to do things well for the sake of the child. Whether this was reflected in their smart attire, steeling themselves to carry and/or lower the coffin, throwing a party-like celebration of the child's life, or taking drugs or strong drink to help them cope on the day, the impression conveyed was that they were doing things for the child and that they wanted to feel that he or she would have been proud of them. Several couples spoke movingly of the pain of sitting with the coffin on their knees, or the moment of lowering it into the ground, but their resolve held because they were doing it for the child. However, even in the midst of their own grief, a few parents felt responsible for others, such as grieving grandparents or their own children. More than one mother said that she was too busy watching out for others to really feel the horror of what they were doing.

Making decisions at such a time was not easy, and parents found some aspects more difficult than they had expected, leaving them wondering if they should have handled things differently.

> I saw her the day of the funeral and I wish I hadn't. She was horrendous. She was terrible. [My husband] didn't think so but I did. She wasn't my wee girl any more. The day she died I mean she went bright yellow and she went blue quite quickly, all the bruising just came all over her face . . . even then she didn't look like my wee girl. I felt like she was away now and I wish that I hadn't seen her the day of the funeral.
>
> (P10: mother of preterm twins)

Others regretted that they had not taken the baby's body to a place where other family members were (and had thereby excluded them from the funeral), having to drive a long distance by car to the graveside, carrying the coffin on their knees, denying the grandparents a more lavish funeral, having a cremation instead of a burial (and consequently now having nowhere to visit), having no facility to have a stone erected at the crematorium, and denying others the opportunity to join in scattering the ashes.

For a small number ($n = 4$ sets of parents), differences between the parents themselves had been an additional source of difficulty at this time. These tensions related to differences in religious conviction, the extent of the parents' own active involvement in the service, who arranged the funeral, the location of the funeral, and the choice of burial or cremation.

A small number of children were buried outside the area where the parents lived, and the families were sometimes shocked to find that they had to pay extra for such a service. Two other families were traumatised by problems with their burial sites. In one case the site was tampered with, and in the other the delays in getting a headstone erected meant that the site became indistinct.

# Discussion

It has been said that the ritual of a funeral 'gives a focus to parents' grief and helps family and friends to acknowledge the baby's existence.'[173] Our findings support this view. All of the families in our study chose to observe this ritual in some form, and it was clearly an important step in the grieving process. In a small study conducted in 1981, the importance of seeing the baby and arranging a proper funeral was emphasised by mothers who had lost two babies but who had only had this experience the second time around.[92] In our own research, this difference was seen in the case of a couple who had twins. One was stillborn and the other died in the neonatal period. The mother graphically recalled the comparison:

> [The two funerals were in the same crematorium]. The first time [for the twin who was stillborn] there was only [my husband] and me, my sister and brother-in-law and my Dad. With [Twin 2] they were standing, there wasn't enough seats. There was loads of people – there was family, friends, nurses, people from my work ... Nobody knew about [Twin 1's funeral]. Nobody really mentioned him. It's terrible. I think because they thought that I had [Twin 2] that it didn't really matter that I had lost another one.
>
> (P8: mother of preterm twins)

Alhough it is clearly a significant ritual, arranging a funeral for a baby is nevertheless a poignant experience. It is not infrequently associated with additional complications such as having to transport the baby's body from a Unit far from the parents' home. However, despite the obstacles and the pain, the majority of parents appear to want to undertake at least part of the organisation themselves. They convey a strong sense that this is the last chance they have to do something for their baby, and it therefore behoves them to do what is needed with dignity and pride, whatever the emotional cost to themselves. The significance of their contribution is captured by harrowing accounts of travelling for miles with a tiny white coffin on their knees, burying an engagement ring with the child, and standing alone at the grave's edge looking down at the coffin they have just lowered. Some indeed need the help of drugs or alcohol to get through the occasion, but they seem compelled to endure this final act. Satisfaction and comfort are derived from ensuring that everything about the funeral is as good as it can be.

The fact that the parents do this should not blind us to the cost however. It is a profoundly sad moment in a painful experience. Parents are grateful when others help to take some of the strain. As well as the psychological and emotional toll, there can be the added burden of the financial cost. Our study provides examples of such burdens, including extra fees charged for transferring the body out of the area, couples having to borrow money from relatives to pay for the event, and one mother deferring her own wedding in order to pay the funeral bills. The fact that a considerable number of undertakers waive expenses for babies' and children's funerals draws attention to the injustice of a two-tiered system, and highlights an opportunity to ease one strain for grieving parents.

It might be thought that in cases where the hospital staff arrange everything the parents will be spared some of the burden. Our findings show that this is not necessarily the case. Where parents are not closely involved in the choices, special vigilance is necessary. Not knowing where a child's remains are, having errors made in the spelling of the baby's name, or in the place of burial, or fearing that bodies have been tampered with against their wishes are all heavy concerns for parents to have to carry for the rest of their lives.

Undertakers have special responsibilities. This is often the first funeral the parents have organised, and they look to these individuals to help steer them through the choices available to them. Although most undertakers appear to be sensitive to parental vulnerability, clearly errors are sometimes made which add to the family's hurt – for example, in the choice of cars, the disposal of ashes or the conduct of the occasion. It is also salutary to hear the reactions of parents to events which an undertaker might well take for granted. One couple had a family friend who was a funeral director, and they were glad to leave the arrangements to him. However, on the day they were unprepared for the sight of a small white coffin. Had they been consulted, they felt that they would have preferred something less exceptional and heartrending, such as an ordinary wooden coffin.

The second person who plays a significant role is the NICU chaplain or the minister. Parents appreciate a service being taken by someone who can speak with knowledge and conviction about the baby, and the hospital chaplain has an advantage in those circumstances where the baby has never left the Unit. But even his acquaintance with the family is often only brief. We found that, irrespective of their religious commitments, parents had two principal needs – to have the reality and the value of the baby's life acknowledged, and to have the depth of the parents' love and grief recognised. By being sensitive to the parents' preferences and tolerances, and arranging an individually tailored service in tune with their beliefs and circumstances, the minister provides comfort and support.

Our study has highlighted the value of NICU staff attending the baby's funeral. When so few people ever met the child, the parents are grateful to staff who did know him being present, showing that they personally cared and that their grief is genuine. It appears that, despite the trauma of attending their own child's funeral, they do notice the gap if no one from the Unit attends. The staff offer the parents an opportunity to share memories at this time which other relatives and friends often cannot. They also make no demands on the parents' resources, and with them the parents feel that they can be themselves and express their emotions freely without fear of being misunderstood.

Once the funeral is over, the parents must then adjust to life after the child. Our findings clearly show that an identifiable place which marks the child's body is an important part in the grieving of many parents, and they may be further traumatised by the discovery that no such clearly defined spot exists. If the child has been cremated and the ashes scattered they know not where, or the burial is in a general area rather than in a clearly demarcated plot, they are denied this focus. It is important that parents, many of whom have no experience of the death of a close relative, should be made aware of the implications of different forms of disposal. We found that the majority of those who did have a grave to visit were keen to set it apart quickly, and they catalogued many objects – gravestones, treasures, toys, flowers and plants – which identified it as theirs. Solace came from spending time there, talking to the baby or simply remembering. Tidying the spot became a way of doing something to care for their baby. Our finding of the ongoing significance of these events in the lives of these families draws attention to the importance of helping parents to make wise choices at the time of arranging the child's funeral.

# Conclusion

- Care must be taken to ensure that all details are correct when arrangements are made for babies' funerals.
- Parents should have the opportunity to arrange and contribute to the funeral service in ways which meet their needs, irrespective of their beliefs.
- Funeral directors and ministers/chaplains have an important role to play in organising an event which parents will find meaningful and tasteful, and in ensuring that the parents understand the consequences of different options.
- Staff who knew the family should be encouraged to attend the funeral, as they are uniquely placed to mourn sincerely with the parents.
- The particular difficulties that family, friends and colleagues experience in supporting bereaved couples following the death of a baby must be recognised, and wherever possible appropriate support must be facilitated.

# CHAPTER 10

# Follow-up

After being the centre of attention while their critically ill and dying baby was in the Unit, it could be something of an anticlimax for parents to go home to a community which had not shared this profound and traumatic experience. Many families expressed their eagerness to meet up again with people who had known them and the baby during this time. To understand the adequacy and value of follow-up contacts, it is important to obtain an overall picture of follow-up meetings over many months. Information obtained from both interviews with the parents has therefore been amalgamated for this chapter.

## Attendance at a follow-up bereavement appointment

Before looking at the respondent families, it should be noted by way of context that six eligible families were not recruited to the study because they declined all follow-up by the hospital team. It will be remembered that the bereavement clinic visit was the time selected at which neonatologists would seek permission to pass their basic contact information to the principal researcher. These families were therefore unavailable for recruitment.

Of the 59 respondent families, during the whole period of the research five sets of parents (8%) were not seen at a bereavement follow-up visit by the NICU staff. In these cases they were identified as eligible for inclusion in the study in the course of periodic checks for the purposes of recruitment, and their permission was sought by telephone or letter. The reasons for their exclusion from follow-up bereavement care varied. In one case the parents themselves elected not to return to the hospital because they had no further questions to ask and they considered that there was nothing more to discuss.

In two cases no appointment had been offered. One of these couples concluded that they had fallen between two stools – being looked after by a local hospital and the study centre – and they assumed that each thought the other had taken on responsibility for follow-up, but in reality neither had done so. The other couple from an island community had not been seen because, rather than requiring them to travel huge distances at great inconvenience, an arrangement had been made for the parents to see a specialist who visited their remote area periodically, and that visit had not yet taken place.

In the remaining two cases, attempts had been made to set up an appointment. In one instance, the father worked such long and erratic hours that he found himself unable to keep appointments which were made, but the mother did not wish to attend without him. The other couple attended at the agreed time, but the consultant concerned did not appear. The parents considered that it would not be helpful to see someone who knew nothing of their case, so they left without seeing anyone. They subsequently wrote to say that even though they had no specific questions, they would like to see the neonatologist, but they reported that they had received no reply to their letter.

In total, 54 of the 59 sets of parents (92%) did attend a follow-up appointment at some point. In order to avoid distorting the figures, percentage values are given for 59 families unless otherwise specified.

# How appointments were made

First appointments were commonly arranged routinely by the hospital (45, 73%), whereas subsequent appointments were more often made at the instigation of the parents. Six sets of parents (10%) reported that they took steps to bring first appointments forward because they were unwilling to wait any longer for the hospital to contact them. However, in two cases (3%) the mother deferred the proffered appointment on the grounds that she was not yet ready to hear hard facts about what had happened. Parents of multiple births where one or more of the babies had survived fell into a slightly different category, since they maintained contact with the NICU. It was during such regular visits to see their living babies that parents from three of these families were invited to go for a chat with the consultant about the child who had died.

# Timing of follow-up visits

The stated policy within the three study Units was to schedule first bereavement visits for about 6 weeks after the death. In reality, only

13 couples (22%) were seen by the neonatologists during the first six weeks (see Figure 10.1). For a further quarter (14, 24%), the first visit took place during weeks 7 or 8. However, by four months as many as 48 families had been seen for the first time, and of these three couples had been seen twice ($n = 2$) or three times ($n = 1$). The first follow-up visit for the remaining six families (10%) occurred between 6 to 11 months after the baby had died.

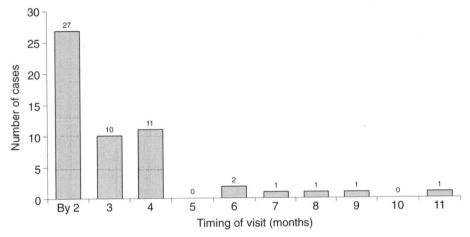

**Figure 10.1:**   Timing of first follow-up visit to neonatologist ($n = 54$).

Most parents simply stated the time at which they were seen, but seven gave an explanation for the delays in their cases. Five parents cited family factors. One appointment was delayed until more than 8 months had elapsed because the mother was ill and unable to attend an earlier appointment. Two mothers simply could not face going back when they were first contacted, and requested a delay – they were subsequently seen at 11 weeks and 4 months, respectively. Another couple forgot their first appointment, but were seen at 4 months. Postponement resulted for one couple when it proved difficult to find a date convenient to both the parents and the consultant neonatologist involved. Hospital factors caused delays for two families. One couple slipped through the follow-up net and received an apology from the consultant neonatologist – they were not seen for 6 months. In the other case, the parents reported that it had taken almost a year to get the results for their baby, who had had a rare abnormality, and the consultant had postponed arranging their follow-up visit until 11 months after the death, when he finally had all of the facts at his disposal.

When the three study Units were compared, important differences emerged. Only 30% of the parents in Unit 3 were seen within 8 weeks of the death. By contrast, 50% of those in Unit 2 were seen during this period, and 66% of those in Unit 1.

# Those in attendance

In the majority of cases (at least 42 of the 54 families; exact figures are not available because parents were talking about all of their follow-up visits, and tended to single out certain visits for more detailed comment), parents went together to follow-up meetings with the neonatologist. However, for visits to the obstetrician a number of mothers attended without their partners. Only one mother reported being upset that her partner had consistently refused to attend with her. Occasionally other family members accompanied the parents. These included the baby's grandparents ($n = 5$), another relative ($n = 1$) or a friend ($n = 1$).

Sometimes partners came to meetings with different expectations and agendas. For example, in one family the mother came away feeling that she had learned a lot, but the father said that he already knew all the facts because of discussions he had had with the doctors at the time. In four cases, the mothers were dissatisfied with their management, had challenging questions to ask, or wanted to register complaints, while all four of the fathers in these cases thought that the matter should just be laid to rest. One mother did not like the obstetrician she went to see, whereas the father found nothing to object to in his approach.

# Who they saw

All except one set of parents who attended for follow-up saw the named neonatologist who had cared for their baby. Most (48, 81%) had been back just once to see him. Twenty-four families (41%) reported also having seen an obstetrician at some point between 3 weeks and 9 months after the death of the baby. Seven sets of parents (12%) had had joint meetings with the neonatologist and obstetrician together at some point.

Many parents commented that they had been told that they could return any time to see the neonatologist if they wished to do so. In fact, only five families (8%) did so. In two cases a return visit was arranged in order to allow the parents to meet with the neonatologist and obstetrician together. One mother who had been alone on the first occasion was keen to have her husband present to hear what the neonatologist had said, so a second visit was arranged although, for domestic reasons, in the event he also missed the second appointment. Two mothers elected to return several weeks later to register complaints about the conduct of staff during their Caesarean Sections. In a sixth case, the named neonatologist was not present when the couple presented for their first appointment, so they had to go back a second time in order to see him.

A few parents commented that it was burdensome to have to attend repeatedly for follow-up visits, and said that they would have welcomed joint appointments. A small minority had kept three ($n = 1$) or four ($n = 3$) separate appointments within the first 3 months following the death of the baby.

Eight sets of parents (14%) also saw a geneticist at some point – four within the first 3 months, two at 4 months, one at 6 months and one at 8 months. One mother received a follow-up telephone call from the geneticist at 3 months after a consultation at 6 weeks. It was 'a high-risk specialist' who saw another couple (at 13 weeks), and yet another couple also saw a social worker (at 8 weeks).

In addition to the consultant, other healthcare staff were sometimes present. Some consultants make it their practice to take to the bereavement appointment the neonatal nurse who cared for the baby during the dying process, but only 18 sets of parents (31%) remembered the nurse being present. Others recalled a junior doctor or medical student ($n = 6$), a midwife ($n = 3$) or a biochemist ($n = 1$) attending.

# Setting for appointments

Two couples (3%) were seen in their local hospitals. Where neonatologists and geneticists or other specialists had travelled considerable distances to see them they expressed appreciation for their sensitivity and effort. However, the majority of the parents (52, 88%) visited the neonatologist exclusively in the study hospital. Of these, almost all (48 of 52 families, 92%) were taken to a small room away from the nursery. Two others were seen in the out-patient clinic in the hospital, and two were actually seen in the NICU. One mother felt so distressed about entering the hospital where her baby had died that for her first visit the neonatologist went out to meet her in her car, and they sat there talking about the events and facts of the case. She expressed great gratitude towards him for his understanding. For another family, three visits to three different people were arranged sequentially so that they had to make only one trip to the hospital, and they were grateful for the careful planning which made this possible. By contrast, another couple had requested that their meeting be held away from the actual nursery, but were told that this was not possible.

# Length of meetings

The parents found out information about the birth, life and death of their child from different sources; information was obtained from visits to obstetricians, neonatologists and other specialists. Data for this section includes all visits. The parents remembered meetings lasting from a few minutes to more than 2 hours. Appointments with the neonatologists tended to be considerably longer than those held with obstetricians, and many families commented on the unhurried approach of the doctor which made it easy to talk about everything they wanted to raise.

> In his office there was stuff piled all over the floor – he obviously had loads to do. But he never once looked at his watch or gave any indication that he had anywhere else to go. You would have thought it was his day off or something.
>
> (P25: mother of preterm baby with asphyxia)

# Discussion of the autopsy

On this point, data from one couple were missing. In 23 cases (39%) no post-mortem examination was carried out. Of the 36 cases in which an autopsy had been performed, 34 sets of parents (92%) reported having a discussion with the consultant about the results. One couple recalled the consultant neonatologist telling them that they would not understand what the report said. Another couple who did not have such a discussion before the first research interview intended to return to see the neonatologist subsequently. However, they were not available for the second interview, so it is not known whether they did eventually receive the post-mortem results.

# Later follow-up

Most of the 54 sets of parents (37, 69%) who attended a first follow-up visit did not expect to return for any further sessions. A number of parents mentioned the fact that they knew they could if they wished to do so, but that it was unnecessary in their case. Some families planned to stay in touch with the staff for other reasons, however, to share the development of surviving infants, to take gifts or money raised, or to show off future children.

Fifteen sets of parents (28%) did intend to have a further consultation – with a geneticist ($n = 8$), the neonatologist ($n = 7$), an obstetrician ($n = 3$) or a cardiologist ($n = 1$). These numbers total more than 15 because four families planned to see two doctors together. Three of these 15 families were not available for a second interview, so no information is available as to whether or not they did return. Of the remaining

12 famililes, only three were actually followed up during the 13 months after the death of the child, although one couple had received a letter instead. Non-existent appointments were with the neonatologist ($n = 2$), a geneticist ($n = 3$), an obstetrician ($n = 2$) and a cardiologist ($n = 1$). When the parents were interviewed over a year later, most had given up expecting further communication.

Although this section deals with follow-up visits to doctors, it is important to recognise that parents sought support and information from other sources, too. One mother had selected the community midwife as the person she might talk to about future pregnancies, and another had made her own private arrangements to see a bereavement counsellor. One couple had plans to seek out other bereaved families who had had a baby with similar problems incompatible with life.

# New information learned at follow-up

The follow-up visit was clearly an important milestone for parents, but several commented that they had approached the date with some trepidation. Going back to the hospital which had been the scene of so much pain would be difficult, it would be hard to hear facts about serious damage so soon after the death of their baby, and it would be troubling to find out that if things had been managed differently the child might still be alive and healthy. On the other hand, receiving reassurance about an accurate diagnosis or prognosis, or confirmation that nothing more could have been done, might be helpful.

In a small number of cases the consultant had telephoned the parents at home prior to the meeting just to tell them that there would be no new revelations. Those who were in receipt of such disclosures expressed gratitude to the doctors for understanding their feelings so well, recognising that it would be an anticlimax to come away knowing no more, and taking sensitive action to prepare them so that they did not experience a strong sense of disappointment.

The parents were asked specifically whether they had found out anything new at the follow-up visit. For 14 of the 54 sets of parents (26%) the information simply confirmed what they already knew, but there was a degree of comfort in that. Having concrete evidence of an accurate diagnosis was reassuring.

For other parents, new information was given at the first visit. The parents' perceptions of what they were told are reported in some detail here in order to give experienced clinicians insights into the kind of information that parents assimilate and recall. This includes the following:

- new details about the illness/damage the baby had sustained ($n = 33$ sets of parents)
- future risks and implications ($n = 17$)
- further details of the complications, filling in gaps in the parents' understanding ($n = 15$)
- the tragic outcome could not have been prevented, and management was appropriate ($n = 9$)
- the child was congenitally perfectly normal ($n = 8$)
- no chromosomal or genetic factor was involved ($n = 7$)
- the parents were not to blame for what had happened ($n = 5$)
- the hospital was not to blame ($n = 5$)
- the problem might have been detected earlier ($n = 4$)
- problems had occurred earlier and the baby had been resuscitated ($n = 4$)
- if the problem recurred with another pregnancy, it could be detected and action taken earlier ($n = 2$)
- test results were inconclusive ($n = 1$)
- staff were shocked and saddened by what had happened ($n = 1$)
- care had been suboptimal and this had contributed to subsequent complications ($n = 1$).

At subsequent visits, often much later on, the parents learned principally about genetic findings and the future obstetric risk. Included were the following:

- the risk of a recurrence ($n = 7$)
- no conclusive chromosomal evidence or recognisable syndrome had been identified ($n = 4$)
- a specific chromosomal abnormality had been found ($n = 3$)
- the geneticist was still seeking answers ($n = 2$)
- a specific cause for the tragedy had been discovered which had not been known previously ($n = 2$)
- other babies with the same condition who had initially survived had since deteriorated and died ($n = 2$)
- earlier detection might have averted the tragedy ($n = 2$)
- colleagues had behaved inappropriately ($n = 2$)
- there had been a degree of negligence on the part of the hospital ($n = 1$)
- subsequent pregnancies would be carefully monitored ($n = 1$).

A small number of families stated that they now knew that the hospital had been negligent (in all cases this related to the time of labour and/or delivery). For most that admission was sufficient, and they now felt free to grieve. Five families had seriously considered taking legal action, but one year later only one couple was actually doing so. That mother was so traumatised by the horror of endlessly rehearsing her story that she felt she could not participate in a second interview for the research study which would require her to talk about the matter yet again. One other mother felt that she had received no satisfactory answers to her grievances, but she was too weak and vulnerable to pursue her case further.

# Helpful factors

Of those parents who attended for follow-up, all except one couple could identify helpful features about the visit. The following list serves as a reminder to professionals of the value of being sensitive to the needs of bereaved families at this critical stage. The numbers of parents who cited different factors would seem to be unimportant, but their identification of the things which they personally found helpful is useful. If all of these catalogued points had been offered to the parents for them to tick the relevant ones, it is likely that more families would have recalled some of these factors as helpful. However, no such attempt was made to obtain comprehensive and specific coverage, but rather parents were left to identify those things which had made an impression on them. Neither have points been prioritised, as distress cannot be measured, and anything which is helpful at any level needs to be noted.

## Shared experience

Many parents commented on how helpful it was to talk about the events surrounding the life and death of their baby with people who had known him or her and shared some of the experiences with them.

> I found it reassuring talking to [the neonatologist] because we had spent seven weeks talking to people that hadn't seen [the baby] ever and here we were speaking to somebody that knew him as a real person.
> (P 27: mother of baby with cardiac anomaly)

The number of people who had personally met the baby was often small, and the parents were keenly aware of the bonds which staff formed with the baby – attachments which gave them a special place in the parents' affections. Having the consultant or named nurse available to talk to was comforting in itself, as they had shared a most profound experience, and they could reminisce or grieve together in a natural way. A small number of parents had received messages of sympathy from other staff who had been closely involved, but whom they did not meet again, and they expressed their appreciation of these tokens of genuine interest and concern.

# Information

This could take different forms, but it was evident that parents had a need to know for themselves exactly what had happened, why, and if there was a risk that it might be repeated in the future.

> I knew it wasn't going to bring her back, but I just wanted to hear somebody say it.
>
> (P1: mother of baby with asphyxia)

Obtaining answers to their questions and clarifying exactly what had happened, was a major component of the follow-up visit. For one couple, the four months they had to wait before being given accurate information were very traumatic. As the weeks passed, the mother convinced herself that she had killed her child and that the prognosis was wrong. It was not until the parents were shown the evidence of severe damage and an expert report stating that the baby could not have lived that her fears and guilt could be allayed. As she said, 'It finally put the pieces back into the jigsaw.'
Frankness was essential.

> [My husband] put [the neonatologist] on the spot: 'How can you assure us that what we're hearing is [the truth]?' And he didn't shirk it. He said, 'Well, I'm a great believer in telling [it as it is]. It's not helping me, it's not helping you, who's it helping to keep all this [hushed up]? All I can do is just tell you as it is.'
>
> (P46: mother of baby with brain damage)

It was important that the information came from those who really knew what had happened. Where events spanned different disciplines, it could sometimes be helpful to have dialogue between the different parties – for example, the neonatologist with the obstetrician, or the geneticist. As one couple explained, listening to different consultants frankly questioning one another about what had happened reassured them that everyone was being honest and open.

> Seeing them both together was very, very helpful – because it happened during the labour. Because they were both there as well, I felt we were getting more in-depth answers from one because the other was there and they were both different specialities. One couldn't hide anything with the other being there. That probably more than anything told me that everything that had been done [was the best that could have been done, and we were just unlucky].
>
> (P46: mother of baby with brain damage)

Subsequently receiving a written account of what had been discussed was a helpful *aide-mémoire*, and it enabled parents to check whether they had heard or understood information correctly. Several families cited receiving a print-out of the autopsy results with an understandable interpretation as being one very helpful factor. Some parents found it helpful themselves to write down questions they wished to have addressed. It was too easy in the emotion of the moment to forget what they wanted to ask, or to lose the thread of the discussion. Pre-prepared questions anchored their thinking. One mother drafted several pages of questions to take to the meeting, and inserted the answers she had received after the session. This provided her with a concrete reminder of what had happened and why.

Another aspect of information-giving related to prediction. Parents were understandably worried about the prospect of future problems, and they found it helpful to have risks and options spelled out. Knowing that they would be carefully monitored next time, or that a particular consultant would take care of them, was reassuring.

If there were still unanswered questions, parents welcomed opportunities to be referred on to other specialists who could help them to piece together the full picture. As one parent said, it was only when the facts were fully slotted into place and they could understand what had happened that they could bring matters to any kind of conclusion. One mother who sought answers over a period of many months found GPs and health visitors helpful in marshalling the facts from notes or reports and passing them on to her. Since, at the time, her husband was not supportive of her endless searching, she was particularly grateful for this help.

# Reassurance

Gaining reassurance from an authoritative source brought comfort. In cases where there was no genetic component to what had gone wrong, parents expressed their relief at finding out that they were 'normal,' and that there was no greater risk either for themselves or for their existing children of a repeat experience. This information freed them to embark on a further pregnancy. But for a few couples there could be no such reassurance, as no answers had been found. Nevertheless, some of them were comforted by hearing that the geneticist or other specialists had kept their baby's file open and the search for clues continued. New tests or understanding might at a future date shed light on what had happened, and tissue or data would then be re-examined.

Reassurance that nothing more or better could have been done was consoling. If it was possible also to reassure the parents that no one was to blame, they appreciated that confirmation. However, they did not want false reassurances. In cases where there was a suggestion of incompetence, negligence or mistakes, the families concerned said that they welcomed, or would have welcomed, an honest admission of error. One family had suspected an obstetric blunder, but were reassured by the neonatologist who stated that he believed in absolute honesty, as in his experience there was nothing to be gained from covering up mistakes because when they later emerged the fault was compounded. His frankness and trustworthiness impressed the couple concerned, and they believed his personal conclusion that the obstetricians could not have predicted what would happen, or have prevented it. A few families mentioned the reassurance they derived from the staff confirming that the best decision had been made. Where this was accompanied by a clear picture of what the alternative would have been, based on post-mortem evidence, the reassurance was even stronger.

Other parents were reassured by confirmation that they themselves were not to blame. One father reported having told his partner many times that it was not her fault that their child had died, but that she needed to hear it from someone with knowledge and experience. The neonatologist's reassurance set her mind at rest because it was rooted in fact and not just a wish to make her feel better.

A few parents found it reassuring to know that they were not alone in their plight. Seeing other parents waiting to talk with the geneticist, and meeting other parents in clinics who faced similar traumas, eased their sense of being singled out for tragedy.

## Consultant sensitivity

Parents greatly appreciated the compassionate approach of the consultants at this time of great pain. Not only were they the source of expert knowledge and opinion, but they offered understanding which stemmed from years of experience of families' tragedies.

> The skills that [Dr B, the named consultant neonatologist] has in explaining these things – he's very much more skilled verbally than [Dr A, the consultant in our first hospital]. Dr A's very nice, very factual. But Dr B is just so totally different – instead of saying, 'You're in a high-risk group,' he would say, 'In future you'll be treated as a VIP and they'll look at you very closely and examine the new baby closely.' There was none of this, '*If* you have a new baby,' it was, '*When* you have another baby.' It was so much more positive, and he very carefully chose his words. And we came out of that meeting feeling so totally different.
>
> (P2: mother of baby with cardiac anomaly)

A variety of practices were singled out for special mention. These included sympathising with a father's reluctance to attend a follow-up appointment, meeting parents at the door of the hospital and escorting them to a quiet room, telephoning to give them results before the meeting so that they had time to think of questions they might want to ask, giving written accounts of verbal communication, not keeping the parents waiting, remembering names and circumstances, and being sympathetic to the parents' concerns. Parents noted these gestures and valued the understanding which prompted them.

> Our meeting was on the Thursday and [the consultant] phoned me on the Monday to tell me that they didn't have any positive answers for us. I wanted to go into that hospital and I wanted to come out with an answer. And the fact that he phoned and told us, I felt was very helpful because I was still very sad coming out of there, but I wasn't as angry as I would have been because he'd said they don't have anything positive. He said, 'I don't want you coming in on Thursday and being dreadfully disappointed, going out thinking, "Well, I still don't have a reason."'
>
> (P6: mother of baby with congenital anomalies)

## Ongoing interest

Personal interest in their progress shown by the staff (both medical and nursing) warmed the parents. When they remembered names, events and circumstances, made a fuss of the children, and enquired after other relatives, it confirmed the parents' sense that they were perceived as real individuals, and that the staff's affection, sorrow and interest were genuine.

> When we went back after we'd lost [the baby], never once did [the neonatologist from the study Unit] look at his notes. His name was [the baby's name], and he knew everything about him. That felt really good ... [The *obstetrician*] hadn't even pulled the file out – it was lying on his desk and he hadn't even looked at it. I thought, 'Well, maybe *you* deal with parents losing their baby every day, but *I* certainly don't.' I was just so angry.
>
> (P56: mother of preterm baby with congenital anomalies)

Sometimes the parents visited the NICU after the follow-up appointment. They gained solace from the neonatal nurses remembering and referring to the dead child or children. Parents who still had surviving babies in the Unit also found it comforting to have staff make appropriate reference to their dead children. Many parents appreciated the consultant leaving the door open for them to make contact at any time in the future if they felt a need for further discussion. Knowing that this avenue was available to them was often all they needed and, as we have seen, very few parents actually did request further appointments.

What I thought was helpful was the fact that it was left open. If I ever had any questions I wasn't to hesitate. Phone him [the geneticist] and he'll make an appointment to see us. He was very [sincere] – phone him any time, it wasn't a problem. . . . It's nice to know you can pick up the phone and say 'Look, I've really got some more questions.' And you know they would see you right away. And they were so nice, so it puts you at ease. You don't feel like you're bothering them.

(P 38: mother of baby with congenital anomaly)

# Support and assistance

Apart from the support of the consultant and neonatal nurses, a few parents had received help from other professionals or knowledgeable relatives in order to gain access to additional information or to speed up a follow-up appointment. In their vulnerable state they found it difficult to fight any more battles, and they appreciated the service of others who contacted the hospital on their behalf or accessed sources of information.

# Mementoes and aids to grieving

A tiny minority of parents collected mementoes at this time which they had not wanted previously. A few others were given books on grieving, or the opportunity to have the babies' names entered into a Book of Remembrance. These all helped them to move forward.

# Opportunity to air a grievance

Parents also found it helpful to have people listening properly to their questions and grievances. Indeed, sometimes merely rehearsing their anger, dissatisfaction or fear was therapeutic.

I wanted them to know that I was very angry and that I did hold them responsible . . . we had a slight disagreement because I regarded it as negligence on their part; [the consultant obstetrician] decided it was human error . . . I said, 'I'm not here today because I'm interested in going to court or anything like that' . . . [in recent court cases] it really irritated me that people are getting money for these things. To me the issue should be that you go to court to find out the answers . . . I don't want to go to court; I just want plain and simple answers.

(P1: mother of baby with asphyxia)

This mother spent months talking to her health visitor and different GPs and SANDS people before she felt ready to go to see the obstetrician to state how unhappy she felt about the management of her delivery. When she eventually felt that she could face him, 8 months after her baby had died, she took precautions:

> I decided that I wanted to go on my own. And what I did was I decided I would put it down on paper in case I went up and came away without saying everything. I put my feelings down in a letter; the things I wasn't happy about and the things I really felt as if I should have had answers but I wasn't happy with my consultant – how he dealt with things. I really just put it all down on paper so that I thought at least if I don't tell him face to face I can leave the letter, just as a statement, not as anything I wanted a reply to. I actually ended up giving him the letter when I went in.
>
> (P1: mother of baby with asphyxia)

The need for a satisfactory resolution and an airing of their own feelings was especially apparent among those parents who had followed up their questions and complaints over a long period of time. A small number of families commented that it was only when all of the facts had fitted into place that they could conclude that no one was to blame and let the matter rest. In one case a mother, after detailed investigations over a period of several months, found that someone *was* to blame, as the hospital had been negligent. She sought legal advice and was told that she did have a case. That was enough for her. She could then start to grieve, and she felt no need to pursue her case through the courts. For one couple a diagnosis of an extremely rare condition had been made. Post-mortem confirmation brought the parents to a realisation of the skill of the neonatologist in identifying the problem on the basis of clinical evidence. They had a new respect for his expertise and a deeper satisfaction with the care that they had received. One mother found it particularly helpful to talk on the telephone with an independent obstetrician with no vested interest in the case, who could listen to her concerns without being defensive.

# Unhelpful factors

Of those parents who attended for follow-up as many as 16 families (30%) could identify nothing unhelpful in the visit. For the reasons stated above, no attempt has been made to prioritise or consistently quantify those factors which were cited as unsatisfactory. Knowing that pain was increased for anyone as a result of what was done is sufficient to alert staff to the need for vigilance and sensitivity with regard to parents' needs at this difficult time.

# Visiting the hospital

Almost half of the parents commented spontaneously on the pain they had experienced on returning to the hospital. It clearly took courage to go back. It was not just the revisiting of the scene of their own tragedy that they had to endure, but also they had to expose themselves to the pain of other healthy pregnancies and babies. It was clearly a problem in some cases to know where to see the parents. If efforts were made to avoid these stressors – for example, waiting in an area adjacent to students working on computers – the parents could feel even more isolated from normality. Particular pain was attached to the NICU; two couples looking for the consultant in a nearby room were distressed to find themselves by mistake in the clinical area where their baby had lived and died.

# Delays in follow-up

As many as 10 sets of parents specifically cited delays in the first follow-up as a cause of hurt.

> I was very disappointed with the follow-up from [the study Unit]. Certainly the *initial* six weeks [follow-up visit] it *was* six weeks; it was exactly when we were told it would be. But following that, I felt that if he said [another] six weeks, it should have been six weeks. Even a 'Well, it's not ready yet, but we are chasing it up' type thing. I was thinking about it a lot, and eventually I followed it up myself – followed it two or three times. And finally there was a phone call to say they hadn't found anything so they were handing it over to the geneticist. No, *I* had phoned *them*. I phoned to chase it and nothing had happened, and then I said, 'What will I do? Will I leave it with you?' It was actually the paediatric secretary at [the study Unit] – who was excellent – and I left it with her. And then again I had to phone, about three or four weeks after that, which really spoiled my [memory of the study Unit] and my last contact with them. I was very disappointed with that. The follow-up was not what was promised.
>
> (P6: mother of baby with congenital anomalies)

As has already been mentioned, other parents took action to bring their appointments forward. When the timing of their visits was examined, it was noteworthy that six of the ten sets of parents had been seen within 3 months of the death, and even these early appointments were too long for them to wait. By contrast, other families whose visits were delayed for many months did not cite this as an unhelpful aspect of the follow-up.

At the 13-month interview, only one mother expressed anger at the delays in subsequent visits. Her dissatisfaction was compounded by her sense that various people were conspiring to prevent her receiving answers to her questions, and she spent months circumventing these blockages to unearth the truth of the tragedy. The persistence required took its toll on her, and the broken promises of other appointments simply added to her frustration and anger.

## Seeing strangers

It was also unsatisfactory from the parents' point of view if the 'wrong' people were present for the follow-up consultation. As one couple said, the problems had arisen during delivery, but the doctors who were present in the labour ward at the time were not there. The neonatologist could only refer to the notes, but was unable to give confident answers to the parents' questions. One mother also resented the presence of unknown faces at a subsequent follow-up visit with consultants whom she did know.

Even on a social level it was reassuring to see familiar faces. One set of parents found it discouraging to go to the Unit to hand in a donation and find no one on duty there who knew them.

## Consultant insensitivity

Not only what the consultants said, but how they said it and how they came across to the parents mattered a great deal. Parents tended to regard them with some awe because of their undisputed knowledge and experience, but this could be disempowering. As one mother commented, non-medical parents would not think of arguing with them.

> I felt myself that there's a barrier [in] saying what you want to say to a consultant – there's a barrier there, even though they've been very helpful in telling you to come and speak to them. It took me until the second visit to [the consultant obstetrician] to actually say, 'Is there anything else that you could have done?' The barrier was there in the beginning. I could find myself wanting to ask questions but couldn't . . . This is your consultant - you don't want to ask any awkward questions.
>
> (P1: mother of baby with asphyxia)

It was rare for parents to convey their dissatisfaction directly, but on occasion consultants did not meet parents' expectations. All consultants have been grouped together in this subsection, in line with the researcher's responsibility to protect identities, but it should be noted that complaints about obstetricians were more numerous than complaints about neonatologists. It must also be remembered that things went very wrong for all of these parents, and memories of their labour and delivery were potentially coloured by this fact, a possibility which some of them acknowledged. Nevertheless, there were consistently bad reports about certain individuals, with several sets of parents perceiving serious deficiencies in their approach, which make sobering reading.

> The [consultant obstetrician] didn't communicate to us on a human level, there's no emotional level and people kept on saying, 'Oh this doctor, it's a cultural thing ... he doesn't mean to sound the way he does, but it's just his way.' And I've been quite angry about this, and I felt that every time I went to see him I could never ask him the questions I wanted, and I was always sidelined.
>
> (P1: mother of baby with asphyxia)

Singled out for mention were factors as diverse as dismissal of a parent's concerns as 'silly', a patronising or 'bullying' approach, obvious reliance on notes to remember what had happened, getting information wrong, failing to turn up for an appointment, neglecting to enquire how the parents were coping, failing to refer parents as promised, inappropriate 'giggling', evasiveness and lack of eye contact.

> [The consultant obstetrician] doesn't communicate well ... the social graces – just tiny little things – a lot of people might think them trivial but they do help. Another thing that struck me when I went and sat with [the first obstetric consultant], there was a table and he sat [on the far side from us]. When I went into [the different obstetrician's] room, that time when I was just myself, I just sat down and he pulled his chair over and he sat down. And then he realised he was quite far away so he drew himself in. We were sitting together in a room and we were going to sit and chat. That's what we were there for, and we didn't have this barrier in between us ... I actually felt I could say what I wanted to say and not feel uncomfortable.
>
> (P1: mother of baby with asphyxia)

Broken promises caused hurt and were seen to demonstrate a lack of real caring. During the first 2 months after the babies had died, three families had been promised a follow-up letter, but it had still not materialised more than a year later.

In situations where there was a perceived lack of compassion or under-standing, the parents felt diminished and just part of a vast impersonal group who were of no consequence to the doctor. As one young father put it, for himself and his girlfriend it was an important day when they learned exactly what had gone wrong for their baby, whereas for the neo-natologist it had been 'just another day.' They rarely pursued matters, but rather went away not only dissatisfied with the specific meeting, but with their confidence in the whole healthcare system undermined.

## Inadequate information

Lack of pertinent information caused unease. Efforts to unravel the facts could be baulked at the level of GPs as well as of hospital staff, and parents found it difficult to battle to overcome obstacles. On a few occasions the parents reported that results and information were not available when they went for their hospital appointments. If, as a consequence of this, they were unable to discuss future risks they were left in limbo and very troubled. One couple had travelled well over 100 miles only to find that their baby's notes were missing. Without the facts it was difficult for the consultant to tell them what they had gone to find out. In another case basic information in the notes was inaccurate and gave rise to considerable misgivings in the parents – if these details were wrong, what else might not be correct? Sometimes the results were available but there were no answers in the form of reasons why things had gone wrong. Although parents understood at an intellectual level that medical knowledge is finite, they still regretted that they would now never know the cause of their baby's death. In their search for the truth it was also unhelpful to be given facts without any explanation of their meaning or significance, especially where this related to future risks with regard to fertility or childbearing.

Perceived poor communication arose from several sources. A small number of consultants seemed unable to pitch their language at an appro-priate level for parents. Medical terms, jargon and complicated statistics could all be disempowering. Non-verbal cues could convey discomfort and tension. Strong accents, even British ones, which were difficult to understand were problematic to parents who were already struggling to understand what had happened. Evasion was regarded as another source of deficient communication. For example, one consultant obstetri-cian declined to comment on what had happened during labour in a local hospital, advising the parents to look forward not back, but the parents found this attitude unhelpful. Until they had answers to their questions about what had happened during labour, they could not move forward.

Erroneous or conflicting information was also very unhelpful, and gave rise to doubt and mistrust. One couple referred to 'lies' and 'errors', demonstrating the strength of feeling aroused. Since all of the consultants were acknowledged experts in their field, if they conveyed different messages, which one were the parents to believe?

> All I've [been told] is, yes, they think they've repaired [my uterus] and that's been it. There's been no aftercare on that whatsoever. I had to ask what the future held – for future pregnancies. Should I wait and give it time to heal? And [the consultant obstetrician] said, 'Just go home and start trying tomorrow.' But I don't believe a word that comes out that man's mouth any more. Because I've got a friend that's a sister at [another hospital] and she's saying there's scar tissue that needs time to heal before it could even stretch and withstand another pregnancy. So I've had to ask my GP if I could see a consultant gynaecologist [at another hospital] because I couldn't go through this again. I need to know a hundred per cent that it'll never rupture or burst.
>
> (P5: mother of baby with asphyxia)

Sometimes the parents did receive the information they had gone to obtain, but they perceived it negatively because it was so hard to hear. Included in this category were those who learned very painful facts about the events surrounding the death, the extent of the damage, too much detail about the exact problems from which the baby suffered, and the violence or probable suffering associated with the actual dying.

> [The consultant] discussed the risks of a future occurrence of this happening again, because it was such a rare thing, and we spent a lot of time discussing statistics and facts and figures about the chances of these things happening again and the fact that we were in a high-risk group. Although we were aware of it, it hadn't been put to us so bluntly before, and we came out of that meeting feeling very angry and upset that we had gone through all this and the chances were now – we were in a high-risk group although he kept trying to stress that the chances of having a healthy baby are higher ... To us 1 in 20 seemed absolutely a very high chance of something happening from being 1 in 3000 and being the one person that it happened to, to say 1 in 20 you just think there's no way this *can't* happen to us again.
>
> (P2: father of baby with cardiac anomaly)

Simply having the autopsy results read out could be difficult to listen to – a cold dispassionate catalogue of problems which they did not want to relate to their own child.

For a small number of parents it was also painful to learn that the baby would have been perfectly normal but for the trauma of birth. Finding out that chromosomal anomalies were involved associated with one or both of the parents presented them with difficult choices with regard to future pregnancies, sometimes compounded by a sense of guilt.

It was especially painful to hear that if things had been managed differently the baby might still be alive. Two sets of parents were given this information at follow-up, and although they appreciated the honesty of the disclosure, they rated this aspect of the visit as unhelpful because it was unpalatable to learn that the death could have been prevented.

> It was just a formality [getting the results of the post-mortem]. He was just perfectly structurally normal. I think we always knew he was normal, but actually hearing it confirmed and that he should never have died, it was just horrific.
>
> (P5: mother of baby with asphyxia)

# Lack of reassurance

Where there were no real answers and there could be no reassurances, some parents were left feeling uneasy. A few of them did acknowledge that such comfort was not in the power of the consultant to give in their case, and they did not want to hear hollow platitudes, but nevertheless they came away feeling unsupported.

# Missed postnatal checks

It was a source of irritation to a number of women that they had had appointments with the obstetric consultant at around 6 weeks after delivery but he did not carry out their postnatal examination. They subsequently had to go to see another doctor for this service, sometimes even having to arrange the appointment themselves. When they had travelled considerable distances to visit the consultant, it had taken courage to go at all, the consultation had been very brief and they had learned nothing new, it was unsatisfactory to come away feeling that the time and effort had been wasted. At least if the physical examination was performed it had not been entirely unhelpful. Furthermore, the postnatal check confirmed the birth. As one mother said, 'It's like you don't have a baby because it's dead.'

# Carelessness

Notes or records being mislaid, specimens being damaged and results being unavailable were all factors which contributed to a sense of dissatisfaction.

In one case a mother reported that because a portion of the baby's tissue had been damaged in the laboratory, they would now never have answers to some of their questions or know exactly what had gone wrong. This was a bitter pill to swallow when these parents had been ambivalent about agreeing to samples being taken after death in the first place. Another couple who had already had several problem pregnancies was upset to find out at follow-up that they had not been given the recommended treatment for their situation.

# Insensitivity

A small number of families perceived that they had been treated insensitively when they presented for follow-up. Being mistaken for an antenatal couple, or being the butt of tactless or cheerful banter was hurtful and made parents question whether there was any indication in their notes to alert ancillary as well as professional staff to what had happened. It was difficult for many parents to return to the hospital and these types of experiences further increased their discomfort and tension.

> It was maybe a month and a half or two months [after my baby had died] but that [follow-up visit] was actually terrible because [the consultant obstetrician] was still in the maternity unit. When I went in and they got my notes out, the nurse came up and asked for a urine sample. I was just too upset to say, 'No,' so I would have done it if it hadn't have been for the fact that there was a nurse from my ward who saw me getting up and walking forward, and [she] came running forward. I would just have given her it because I just couldn't have explained to her why I *shouldn't* give her it. That was quite horrible . . . it never even occurred to me . . . that they would do that. I thought they would have some kind of red dot on my files to say – some way of letting them know that you've had your baby and that they've [died].
>
> (P42: mother of preterm baby)

# Need to be proactive

Parents found it difficult to go out and seek help for themselves, and a number of them recommended routine support being offered to obviate this necessity. One very articulate, professional mother found that although she was normally very much in control and well able to express her needs and wishes, at this stage in her grieving she felt too fragile to approach strangers for help.

There was a leaflet in the package for bereavement counselling. I don't think that's enough. I had no follow-up after that whatsoever. Because sometimes it's a little bit [difficult to make the first move]. Some people just don't like picking up the phone to say, 'Excuse me, my babies have died, I want to come along and speak to someone.' I think, quite soon after – let things die down a little bit maybe, maybe after about a month – I'd have loved to have talked to somebody... I think it should actually be part of [the service provided]. I should have had an appointment handed to me because if I'd had the appointment I'd have gone to it if I wanted to and not if I didn't.

(P 33: mother of preterm twins)

## Environmental factors

When emotions are already running high, perceived limitations in amenities can cause irritation or distress. Limited parking facilities, and a poor telephone system in the hospital which meant it took a long time to track someone down, both fell into this category. Injustices or perceived incongruities could rankle. Several couples drew attention to the strong feelings aroused by seeing other mothers standing in the doorway of the hospital smoking. When their own babies had died despite the fact that they had taken every care in pregnancy, it felt unjust that these other women should be deliberately doing something which could be harmful, but that they would probably deliver healthy babies. One family felt that it had been incongruous to be offered refreshments at the follow-up meeting when the purpose of the appointment was so grave.

## Visits for other purposes

Many parents had also attended the hospital for reasons other than to talk with the consultant. Some had returned to deliver donations, to attend fundraising events or simply to say hello. A considerable number had returned for a memorial service. This powerful experience had one of two effects. For some it offered real solace in enabling them to share personal grief with so many others who were suffering in the same way and who really understood, and it affirmed the significance of their own child's life. However, for a considerable number it was too painful and distressing an event, which put them back a stage in their grieving. They spoke of it being a 'nightmare,' 'dreadful,' a 'fanatical raking over of old stories' and 'torture hearing another father speaking of his lost dreams.'

# Information obtained from other sources

Some parents had independently obtained information from sources other than the hospital staff responsible for the care of themselves and their baby, or the specialists to whom they were referred. A small number of parents searched the Internet for additional information on the specific conditions relating to their experience, read books on the subject or sent off to societies specialising in given conditions. A number of parents had found discussion with their GP useful for clarifying their understanding, but only one mother learned anything new via this route. Two mothers obtained evidence of perceived negligence in labour through other avenues, one via a solicitor and the other by looking at her own notes copied for her by community staff. One couple was helped by a knowledgeable medical relative who could provide general information about their baby's condition.

# Discussion

This study has highlighted several potential loopholes in a system for recalling bereaved families for a follow-up visit. Parents may be overlooked for a number of reasons. They may simply slip through the administrative net. Where babies are transferred out of the area, each hospital may assume that care will be offered by the other. Where one or more siblings survive in multiple births, notes may not get into the system for bereavement follow-up. We identified missed families because periodic checks were made to ensure that eligible parents were not excluded from the study, but are such safety measures in place in clinical practice?

It is evident from our findings that recall practices vary, but what must be set alongside these overt differences are the variations in consultant loads and available resources. The consultant who referred 17 families to the study clearly carried a heavier bereavement support load during the study period than the four consultants who only referred one family. What is possible for any given individual may be influenced by a range of factors, including the willingness and availability of colleagues to cover the NICU while a neonatologist gives bereaved families protected time, the number of consultants who are prepared to deal with cases of treatment withdrawal, the efficiency of information exchange, and other commitments. But this study has shown that follow-up care is crucially important for these vulnerable families: from their perspective, appointments need to be scheduled at the appropriate time irrespective of such constraints. Vigilance is essential.

The timing of appointments is another important issue highlighted by this research. It is sobering to find that a considerable number of parents wait for many months before they are seen. A few parents are unready to hear information soon after the baby's death, but for the majority any delays in being recalled add to their distress. Having to expedite their own appointments is a painful process. The traditional 'postnatal check' time of 6 weeks has been widely adopted as the stated time for recalling bereaved parents, but it appears to be based on no firm evidence, and our findings indicate that even 6 weeks is too long for some parents to wait. Preliminary autopsy results can usually be available within 2 weeks, and it has been suggested that this represents a more suitable point for recalling such parents.[181] In more complex cases, post-mortem tests will inevitably be protracted, but it is evident from our research that early contact is desirable, even in the absence of a full picture. However, when our data were analysed for causes of dissatisfaction, it was clear that the timing of interviews was not of itself the sole key to good practice. Some parents who waited many months did not express regret about the timing, while others who were seen within 3 months did. A negative feeling was found to be associated with the absence of essential information. Parents needed to have enough information to enable them to piece together a coherent picture of what had happened, in order to make progress in their grieving, to assess the risks of recurrence or the genetic implications, and to contemplate another pregnancy. We may conclude that parents should know when they will be seen, and staff should make every effort to honour that arrangement. Until such time as rigorous, focused studies have produced more precise parameters, it seems desirable that such interviews should be offered soon after the death, and certainly within 6 weeks of it, with parents being given the opportunity to defer the visit if this seems too early for them.

> The only frustrating thing is having to wait so long for [the results of] genetics testing, but that's science and you can't rush science. That's the only down side – that we are having to wait. Because until we find out that information, our lives are on hold, because we can't plan what we're going to do.
>
> (P51: mother of baby with congenital anomalies)

Our findings demonstrate that follow-up visits have two main purposes, namely obtaining information and talking with people who have known their child, and both must be borne in mind when arranging appointments.

> Personally I would have said, 'Look, there's a bit of outstanding information. We want to do this research, but in general terms . . .' because we want to get on with our lives, I would have still had us in earlier and said, 'Look, it's OK if you want to go ahead and have another attempt at a

family, and we could leave that bit out rather than wait for every single bit of information to be available. It was such a key role for us – putting things to bed almost – that that could have been sealed on the information that was available and then anything resulting from any studies could have been conveyed to us – as it still would be – at a later time.

(P 50: father of baby with congenital anomalies)

Where delays in obtaining results are unavoidable, realistic time-scales can be negotiated with the parents in order to reach satisfactory compromises. As one mother advised, in their case, instead of telling them that they would be recalled in 6 weeks, and their anxiety mounting over the ensuing weeks when no appointment came, the staff might have said, 'Realistically because it's going to be complicated this might take 3 or 4 months, or 4 or 5 months', and then I think if you have that kind of time-scale you don't get as anxious.

Our respondents have highlighted the desirability of providing full and frank information. Information is of crucial importance to bereaved parents. As the SANDS literature puts it: 'It is impossible to over-emphasize the importance of information to parents. At a time of crisis, information gives strength and understanding, whereas to be deprived of information is disempowering and adds to parents' distress'.[78] Even with all of the facts available, it can be hard for parents to accept that things have gone so wrong; they re-live events and search for causes. The truth itself may sometimes be painful, but concealment hurts more and undermines trust in both the healthcare system and professionals within it.[78,128] What parents are looking for is an account which fits the facts they have seen and heard, and which provides a cohesive explanation of what happened, which they can understand and learn to accept. This is essential if they are to move forward healthily and contemplate another pregnancy. Consistency is an important factor in this process. It is deeply troubling for parents when they are given conflicting information from different consultants. To be told by an obstetrician that the child's brain was damaged antenatally, and by the neonatologist that the damage occurred during birth, raises doubts about both the management of the case and the integrity of the staff. Where such facts relate to future risks, the parents are especially vulnerable. If both are 'experts', whom are they to believe?

It is important to remember, however, that some truths are difficult to hear and accept. For example, clinicians have suggested that detailed descriptions of the infant's structure in the post-mortem report aid the grieving process.[182] Yet insights from our research show that some parents find such a catalogue of problems or impairments extremely distressing. The enormity of what has happened feels too stark to bear. They may need to put the written report away and read it later, or speak to the consultant more than once in order to piece the story together in bearable instalments. Nevertheless, the consistent message which parents give is that they do not want sanitised versions of the truth. Reassurance is welcomed when it comes from an authoritative source, especially if it confirms the wisdom of their decisions, the bleakness of the prognosis, the absence of blame, or hope for the future. However, false reassurance is unacceptable, as at all times the parents ask for honest and open information, and if confirmation with regard to decisions or actions cannot be given truthfully, they prefer to be told honestly of the impossibility of reassurance about these matters.

The parents in our study gave a clear message that they understand that staff are fallible and that mistakes will sometimes be made. However, covering up errors is counter-productive. Concealment undermines trust. Most families are seeking the truth about what happened, not redress through the courts. Their view reflects what has already been concluded: 'in the small number of cases where the evidence suggests that the medical profession were at fault, doctors are doing parents a disservice by not accepting blame where it is due.'[93]

The second component of follow-up care is emotional support. When the parents leave the hospital after the death of their baby, they are leaving behind those who formed their intimate group. Often there is no one outside who even met the child. There are friends who quickly grow weary of the story, family members who find it too painful to hear, and acquaintances who dismiss the loss. The professional team who shared the life and death experience with them can offer a unique form of support. They remember the child and understand the significance of the event, and they can also supply medical facts and explanations, bear strong emotion and listen actively. These functions are highly valued by parents. Meeting after the death, talking about the child and reflecting together all provide comfort and confirmation.

Clearly therefore these two aspects of support must be balanced and the timing of appointments chosen to reflect the importance of each. Some negotiation may be necessary. The obvious corollary to earlier appointments is that already busy consultants might be overloaded with additional bereavement care work. We found that currently very few families take up an open-ended invitation to come back at any time after the first scheduled bereavement clinic visit (only 8% did so). It thus seems possible that if early intervention is effective, burdens on neonatologists might not be significantly increased. Not all parents would need to come back to see the consultant in person to obtain test results, unless they carry significant implications, although it is acknowledged that consultants may prefer to communicate all such information face to face. If so, the implications of a number of visits for these families will need to be carefully considered.

Ongoing monitoring of any changes would be necessary to determine whether the balance of needs, responsibilities and priorities is a healthy one for both medical teams and parents.

In arranging and conducting follow-up meetings, it is important that staff respect the pressures and needs of the parents themselves. Their importance is diminished if the neonatologist is not available as promised, they are kept waiting for long periods, they are repeatedly called back across long distances to meet different consultants, notes are missing, or their fears and concerns are belittled. Their priorities are not those of experienced clinicians. The power balance is perceived as unequal. Their need to know and to share their experience helps parents to overcome a reluctance to return to the scene of so much pain, but it takes courage to do so. Their vulnerability must be accepted, and their criticisms as well as their questions must be heard.

As part of this sensitivity to the parents' needs, careful thought needs to be given to the setting for follow-up visits. Revisiting the hospital where their child died is a painful journey for all parents, as those in our study have eloquently explained. Encountering the evidence of other successful pregnancies highlights their own loss,[78,183] and seeing hospital doorways crowded with women smoking compounds their sense of life's injustice. Obstetricians have suggested that their distress is sufficient justification for domiciliary visits,[181] but such a practice would have major resource implications. However, if parents are to be expected to summon up the courage to return to the hospital, great care is needed not to compound their pain when they get there. Being mistaken for an antenatal couple, or being the butt of tactless or cheerful banter is deeply hurtful. It is essential that a reliable system of marking the notes of bereaved parents is adopted to avoid such errors.[78] Our research supports the guidance from SANDS on choosing a meeting place away from antenatal clinics or the Neonatal Unit, and using dedicated time outside clinic schedules for their visit,[78] but it also indicates that this advice is not always heeded.

Enormous sums of money and a high quality of compassionate and skilled care are devoted to families in our NICUs. This study has highlighted deficiencies in the aftercare of parents whose babies die following treatment withdrawal. The Royal College of Paediatrics and Child Health framework which deals with treatment withdrawal gives only a brief mention of this part of the process.[9] It advocates that 'the consultant in charge and the nurse most involved should offer to see the parents, to discuss the death and the result of the post-mortem examination if it is available,' with other arrangements being made if the parents wish to meet with other members of the clinical team. Our findings demonstrate that to parents this is a crucial part of their management, and it merits strong emphasis.

Until now follow-up bereavement care has largely been predicated on an intuitive response to a perceived need. In revealing what the parents themselves find helpful, our research has provided empirical support for some of these intuitive practices, but it has also highlighted areas in need of improvement. NICU staff play a highly valued role in the experience of these families who live through the trauma of treatment withdrawal and death. Resources must be drafted into supporting them in the completion of their task.

# Conclusion

- Vigilance is needed to ensure that no families slip through the net and are omitted from follow-up care.
- Parents should be given appointments soon after the death of their child, and certainly within 6 weeks, unless they choose to defer the visit.
- Any changes that are made to existing systems of recalling parents should be carefully monitored to determine those practices which best meet parental need.
- The meeting should be with the named neonatologist who is known to the parents, in order to provide continuity and an opportunity to share memories and experiences.
- If specific issues arise, parents should be given the opportunity to discuss the labour and delivery with those obstetric/midwifery staff who were involved at the time.
- All information given should be full, frank and honest.
- Visits should be arranged in a setting and style which respects the parents' priorities and vulnerabilities.

# CHAPTER 11

# The effect of the death on the family

After the funeral the family face the adjustments which follow bereavement. The loss of any close relationship can leave a person feeling bereft, but as we have seen from the background literature, the loss of a child strikes 'even more deeply into the very being and integrity of the mourner.'[59]

> I don't think anybody could ever tell you how hard [it's going to be]. I wouldn't presume to tell anybody else who goes through the same thing as us, what it's going to be like for them. I don't think you *could* adequately warn them really. It's just a nightmare. For so long – for months and months and months – you just wake up and it's right in your face every morning. It really is terrible.
>
> (P15: father of preterm baby)

Although studies have yielded varying and conflicting findings about the effect of such a loss on family relationships, what emerges from the literature is that it does strain the couple's own relationship.[57,71] The *shared* loss creates a profound and deep bond between them, but their *individual* loss may create a deep sense of estrangement.[57] Both parents are mourning and may be unavailable to each other. Furthermore, fathers and mothers mourn differently and, in general, maternal grief reactions are more intense and more prolonged than paternal reactions.[43,60,89,184–186]

However, rather than singling out the relationship between the couple, we have tried to set the effects of this bereavement within a wider context. It is important to remember not only that the couple does not exist in isolation, but also that the death of a baby does not take place in a vacuum. Although this event is of cataclysmic proportions, other things are still going on in the parents' lives.

# Other major stressors

A considerable number of the families whom we studied were grappling with other major life events either immediately before, during or just after the tragedy of losing their baby. During the ensuing year the majority of parents could identify major events which were stressful in themselves.

# Death and illness

Other deaths or life-threatening illnesses were cited by a number of parents. At the time of the first interviews, one young father had died, and in four other families (7%) close relatives or very close friends had died. In one family the mother's father and grandmother had both died during her pregnancy. One mother and one father themselves had serious and potentially fatal illnesses. Three respondents (5%) had a parent fighting cancer. By 13 months, the health of the parents' own parents was giving cause for concern in eight families (16%). Three more had died, and six were suffering from serious illnesses.

The parents' own health caused unease in other cases. In addition to the two cases mentioned above, who already had serious illnesses at the time of the first interview, two fathers and one mother had had mental breakdowns, and two mothers underwent major surgery. One father and one mother developed a drink problem in both their own and their spouses' estimation. One mother resorted to taking illegal drugs for a time.

# Infertility and subsequent pregnancies

As has already been noted, a number of these families had a history of infertility. Additional pain was attached to the loss of babies who had been conceived only after a prolonged period of stressful treatment and considerable monetary expense (in one case a family used an inheritance to fund fertility treatment abroad). Several mothers spoke of the 'horror' they felt about facing further fertility treatment and potential disappointments. Problems of infertility continued to haunt three couples, but two mothers who had previously had treatment found themselves unexpectedly pregnant soon after the death of the study baby. Both expressed their delight at avoiding the stressful processes this time.

However, for some families the issue of having another baby was not straightforward. Where the risk of problems was higher then normal, some parents were reluctant to embark on another pregnancy. Several fathers in this category observed that they could not themselves face going through this trauma a second time, or they feared what it might do to their partners, or to their relationship. In one case the couple had deemed it 'irresponsible' to have another child, but the mother accidentally became pregnant. She was very ambivalent about this, agonising over a decision while routine antenatal screening was carried out. She miscarried soon after an amniocentesis. Another couple interviewed at 13 months still could not agree whether or not to have another child: the mother was keen to try again, but the father deemed it too risky.

Just over half of the mothers (26 of 50, 52%) became pregnant again in the year following the baby's death. Of these five had delivered safely and had living babies at the time of the second interview at 13 months. A strong impression was conveyed that the new pregnancy had helped them to move on. Many stressed the fact that the new baby would be no replacement for the one who had died, but represented renewed hope for the future. However, for more than a quarter of the couples (7 of 26, 27%) the outcome of the new pregnancy was not a happy one. Three of the pregnancies were lost through early miscarriages, and a further one was lost at 20 weeks. There was added poignancy in one case when the fetus lost this time was found to be normally formed, whereas the one who had earlier died had been congenitally abnormal. For two families tragedy was repeated when they delivered another baby which also subsequently died. Another infant lived but was found to have serious congenital anomalies.

# Relocation

As many as ten families (20%) moved house during the year following the loss of the baby. A number of others contemplated doing so, but in the end decided that the time was not right for such a radical change. Most of them instead concentrated on renovating or altering their present homes.

# Work changes

A considerable number of individual parents had been involved in major changes at work. These included redundancy (one mother and two fathers), change of employment (seven mothers and four fathers), return to work (three mothers), withdrawal from paid employment (five mothers and one father) and retraining (two fathers). Major changes within their existing workplace were mentioned by seven other parents. These included a slump (one father), promotion (four fathers and one mother) and greatly increased pressure (one father).

## Other stressors

A few families were coping with momentous events apart from those related to health or location. Two were pursuing legal action (these were in addition to the mother who declined to take part in a second interview because she was suing the hospital), one mother had resorted to crime herself, one father had been involved in a serious car accident, and one couple had been burgled.

As some respondents pointed out, when a number of major life events occur close together, it is difficult to separate out the effect of single stressful events. Nevertheless parents were encouraged to talk about the effect of the death of the child in so far as they felt it had changed their own thinking and influenced their relationships, at least in part.


# Personal changes

Several parents observed that they were now different people, and it was not to be wondered at that their relationship had been affected. The experience had changed them fundamentally. Some felt that they were now more mature, wise and solemn. Some of the very young parents regretted the passing of their carefree youth before they had had time to really enjoy it.

> Obviously through these tragic experiences you *have* to mature, you can't kid about. [My experiences] have speeded up the process [of maturing]. It's made me realise how lucky I am to be here and to be healthy. I don't want to wallow in the past and the tragic things that have happened – that would be sad or morbid or something – but it happened and nobody will ever forget [the babies*]. But you can't just live life [in that shadow] . . . I don't want to be dragged down into a depressive sad [state]. The only thing you can do is to move on and try to be happy in some way . . . I keep on getting told I'm far too serious for my age. To be honest in one sense of the word, I wish I was immature. Of course I'd rather be mature than immature, but at the same time I'm only 21 and I want to be 21. But because I've had all these things in life, you can't joke about it, just laugh . . . it's just matured me too quickly.
> (P28: father of preterm baby)*

Many parents spoke movingly of the profound effect of becoming a parent. It had been a revelation to find that parental love was so strong. However, experiencing something major going wrong in their lives, often for the first

---

* This couple had lost a baby previously.

time, forced the parents to take stock of their lives. As a result, many said
that they had acquired depth and maturity.

> I do think she's changed me for the better in a way as well ... I think
> before [the baby] I was quite shallow inasmuch as I just went out and
> had drinks and went for dinner. I think I think about things a lot more
> now. I think it's made me a bit deeper.
>
> (P45: father of preterm baby)

The majority of parents reported that their priorities had changed. Life
itself was now extremely precious, family life had a high priority, and
work and material possessions were of less importance to them. Things
which had seemed important before, and things they had worried about,
now seemed so trivial when placed alongside this momentous event.

> *Mother*: Before when I was at work ... there were three or four girls
> there that really gave me a hard time, and it got to the stage where
> I nearly quit my job because I just wasn't emotionally or mentally up
> [to dealing with it] ... I've gone back to work now and I couldn't give a
> [tinker's curse] what they throw at me – after what we've been through.
> *Father*: I'm like that now. Life's too precious ... There's nothing can
> bother me at work now. It's so immaterial. It doesn't matter.
>
> (P9: parents of baby with cardiac anomaly)

They spoke of being less argumentative, less selfish, a 'better person,' more
inclined to charitable work, more tolerant, less judgemental and more assertive. They were now also more appreciative. Parents with other children
valued in a new way the health and normality of their existing family.
They no longer took reproduction for granted as most had done before.
In valuing the life of the baby they had lost, they appreciated the blessing
of parenthood and this recognition made two couples with underlying
fertility problems even more determined to have another child so that the
dead babies 'would not have died in vain.'

On the other hand, the parents could identify some changes which were
less positive. It had been a shock to a number of parents that something so
painful could happen to them: they had been 'totally happy' before, they
were 'good people,' and they had taken care during pregnancy. They now
felt that they were the victims of injustice.

> I just thought, 'Wait a minute. I've been on bedrest for four months.
> These are IVF* babies.' Everybody who loses a child is devastated, but
> I felt IVF, bedrest – having gone through all that – [this is more devas-
> tating than ever].
>
> (P33: mother of preterm twins)

---

* *In-vitro* fertilisation.

In the beginning you feel as if a thief has come and stolen away your most prized possession ... this had been after [a series of tragedies with previous pregnancies which had gone wrong], you're saying to yourself, 'We're in the labour ward! We're home and dry.' You're within touching distance of the finishing line, and then it's all snatched away. I think that made it ten times worse.

(P 20: father of baby with asphyxia)

This feeling was compounded when the parents saw other people who were careless of the health and welfare of the mother and the baby, or who were irresponsible parents, but who none the less had healthy normal babies. They were aware of feelings of anger and jealousy.

Many of the parents were now less optimistic about life. They felt insecure, realising that they were not in control of the major events in their lives, and they were more anxious and more inclined to dwell on the negative side of things.

I don't go on now thinking there's a tomorrow, it's all today.

(P 38: mother of baby with congenital anomalies)

A young girl at my work has just fallen pregnant and she was scared to tell me because we're really quite close. She's fallen pregnant by accident. She said, 'I'm so sorry. The timing's just so bad.' I said, 'Don't be so silly,' and I put my arms around her. And she said, 'And I'm so scared.' I said, 'Nothing's going to go wrong.' And I thought, 'How can I say nothing's going to go wrong?' I said, 'The chances of anything like that happening are a million to one. I was just unlucky, very unlucky.' I said, 'You'll be fine.' And all the while I'm saying it I'm thinking, 'There's no guarantees in this world.' But you can't say that. You can't.

(P 9: mother of preterm twins)

Since this appalling thing had happened, they could have no confidence that other even worse things might not happen to them – for example, older children or partners dying or having terrible accidents. Some parents admitted that they had become very over-protective or over-indulgent and this had produced tensions within the family and strained hitherto happy relationships.

With their own changing priorities there arose irritation with other people, concerned as they often were with trivial things. Although it was only a few weeks since these were the very same preoccupations which they themselves had shared, their view of what was important had changed fundamentally and irrevocably. Not only so but they were also more sensitive to other people's tragedies. They were now aware of the burdens others, too, carried, some worse than their own, and some of them hidden from view. This awareness made parents look at people and behaviours differently. They felt they were now more sensitive and less judgemental of others because 'you never know what they're really dealing with.' It made them more circumspect and careful in their dealings with others.

The actual experience of having a baby in a NICU had affected parents, too. Several of them spoke of the new respect they had for people who worked in such places. They were amazed by the depth of kindness and compassion that staff provided alongside the high level of technical expertise. One father who had a high-powered job said that he had previously felt stressed by work pressures, but he now saw his own stresses as 'nothing' compared to those with which the neonatal staff were grappling. This changed perspective gave the parents a different approach to tensions and stresses.

The encounter with death itself had changed some people's views. Some said that they were now no longer scared of death. Others reflected on the brevity and uncertainty of life and resolved to do what they wanted to do now, rather than defer things for a future which might not materialise.

# The parents' relationship

Matters associated with personal intimate relationships are sensitive issues, and the courage of the parents in addressing these questions in discussion with the interviewer was impressive. They spoke with feeling of the strain that this profound experience had placed on their relationship. It had the potential to either strengthen or break it, and a number of couples whose own relationship survived the first year said that it could easily have gone the other way.

Actually voicing their feelings and expressing their difficulties was seen to be therapeutic, and many couples added at the end of the interview that this was the first time they had heard just how their partner felt. Sharing their feelings through a third party had helped them to express their own emotions and better understand their partner's reactions and needs. The interview freed them to talk more openly together subsequently, too. It is noteworthy that in a few families the mothers had not expected the fathers to participate in the study at all. They were amazed that not only did their partners agree to take part, but also they contributed during the interviews. Significantly, too, several fathers who had left or were in the process of separating from their partners came back into the maternal home for the purposes of the second interview, and both partners expressed their feelings openly to the interviewer in the presence of the other.

Three mothers were not in touch with the baby's father at all, and one other mother saw the father only occasionally. Ninety-one per cent of the other couples (that is, all except five) said that the death of the baby had had an effect on their relationship, although one couple could not actually identify the resulting effect – they just knew that all such experiences changed people and they concluded that since they had been profoundly affected by this event, it must have impinged on their relationship in some way.

In the early days after the death the parents were usually united in their shared grief. Indeed, some reported that at this point they were closer than they had ever been, communicating at a level they had not experienced before, and sharing thoughts and emotions in a new way. It was like a 'honeymoon' period.

> We were a bit *too* nice with each other to begin with. We can argue with each other now and say things to each other we want to without [fearing we're upsetting them].
>
> (P 56: mother of preterm baby with congenital anomalies)

However, as time went on this initial effect tended to diminish to varying degrees. When other people had returned to their normal lives, and the reality of their own changed circumstances impinged on their lives, difficulties sometimes arose as each parent tried to cope with their loss and profound emotions.

We shall look first at what seemed to be happening, before considering the implications for the relationship. Since both parents were sad and grieving, it appeared to be common for them to hide their own emotions. There were many other reasons for this – for example, to protect their vulnerable partners, in self-defence, because they felt emotionally distant from their partner, or because they felt guilty, or because they were advised to do so.

> If I was down and I spoke to [my husband] it didn't help me because it would upset [him].
>
> (P18: mother of preterm baby)

> That's what everybody was saying, 'You need to be strong for [partner]'. So I was doing it for [her] and doing it for everyone else and for myself. [I did cry] but not in front of [her] and she doesn't know I got upset.
>
> (P22: father of baby with asphyxia)

> The trouble was we were finding it difficult to speak [to each other about our feelings]. It's much easier to speak to people you're not close to. I think that was the most hurtful thing, because we are really close but sometimes it was just too acute. If I was feeling really, really bad, [my husband] just couldn't listen, and I think in some ways I was probably the same – not realising you're doing it. It's self-defence. And you don't want to say something hasty and hurt the other.
>
> (P1: parents of baby with asphyxia)

Some parents recognised that there were different levels of sharing, and they were conscious of a dividing line beyond which they did not go.

> I think there's talking and there's talking. There's talking that's just remembering, you're going back to events that happened . . . you're talk-ing about *those memories* as opposed to talking about *you* [and how you feel]. Obviously if I'm upset, I don't always go to [my husband and talk about how bad I'm feeling], but you can talk about your baby to-gether, remember the good times, remember the smiles. That's the sort of things that can help bring you through . . . that's what puts a bond there. Talking about how you're grieving is something different, and how you're coping.
>
> (P23: mother of preterm baby with congenital anomalies)

Others were aware of different agendas which prevented them from com-municating all of their feelings. One mother spent months seeking answers, which involved going to various doctors, meetings and hospitals. The father never asked her about her progress, only finding out what she had discov-ered when she told the researcher at the second interview. He then became upset and acknowledged that for all that time he had been carrying a great burden of guilt, believing that he was to blame for the death, because he had not intervened and challenged the midwives when things went wrong during labour.

> [The sense of guilt] is there. I'll never get rid of it because there's always the 'but if . . .' I'll never get rid of that. It was my daughter. Anything you can do you would do. [Maybe I should have said something]. But I didn't.
>
> (P1: father of baby with asphyxia)

Sometimes the parents came to realise that the tactics they had adopted had not been beneficial to their relationship. One young father was bewil-dered by the complexity of the emotions and demands surrounding him. His relatives all exhorted him to be strong for his girlfriend and support her. He did his best to suppress his own feelings and do what was 'expected' of him, but his girlfiend had still left him.

An attempt was made to explore the specific ways in which the death had impinged on the parents' relationship. Communication was strained at times, with each partner reluctant to say anything to upset the other, each grieving in their own way but not fully understanding the other's way of dealing with the pain. Tensions mounted, and the principal source of such tension in the mothers' perceptions was the fathers' unwillingness to talk about their feelings. The men in these families acknowledged that this was a fair comment. They cited two reasons for not expressing their feelings: they did not want to cause the mother additional hurt, and they did not find talking about their grief helpful, preferring instead to keep their feelings to themselves and get on with living.

> Trying to deal with [my wife's] way of coping – wanting me to discuss it – is bad for me. Maybe it's that I'm selfish enough [not to want to invite that sort of pain]. The other aspect to it is that I'm not good at what [she] needed to do. I know I'm not good at it. I'm not a touchy-feely person who's good at sitting listening and understanding somebody else. I'm afraid my kind of perspective on things is: 'Oh, get a grip!' That's just the attitude I have. I'm the person least suited to be a counsellor! So in a way not only was it bad for me because I had to deal with things for myself, but also I didn't feel that I was able to offer the kind of help that [my wife] wanted.
>
> (P18: father of preterm baby)

The mothers not infrequently construed the man's silence as evidence that he had moved on and was not now feeling the pain. During interviews it was often a revelation for them to hear the father describing his own ongoing sense of loss and grief and the things he did to try to cope, things of which the mother had known nothing. However, even occasional glimpses behind the coping exterior could be helpful to the mothers. For example, one father only ever got upset at memorial services or in the rose garden.

> Those [memorial] services have been good for me because they've let me see that [my husband's] still grieving. The fact that [he] does cry in those situations makes me feel so much better and then, of course, I have to go through the guilt of, 'Oh my goodness, I'm so happy because my husband's upset!' . . . it's knowing it's there even though it's not showing all the time.
>
> (P18: mother of preterm baby)

For their part, a number of fathers found themselves edgy because their partners were so easily provoked to tears and so preoccupied with the death, instead of trying to take an interest in other things. To them it seemed unhealthy to spend time alone 'brooding' over the death for such long periods: being busy and thinking about other things was a better way.

> I remember coming home from work quite often and [her asking something like], 'Why haven't you [thought about the baby or remembered something special about him]?' – more or less saying, 'Well, what *have* you been spending your time thinking about?' And I think the reality was I was jumping in the car, and on the way home from work, when [my wife] thought perhaps I should have been thinking about things

[like the baby], turning the radio on and enjoying the music or whatever and just blanking my mind out. It's not too exciting driving the same road every day, so you don't really think too deeply during that time.

(P16: father of preterm baby)

The overall effect of these strains varied from couple to couple, and it also varied over time for a given couple. For only three families did the strain have a detrimental effect on the parents' own relationship in the first 3 months. However, during the whole year after the death of the baby almost half of the 48 couples (23, 48%) had struggled to maintain their relationship, with many of them wondering whether they should separate.

I've met couples at the hospital – two of them have split up because . . . just because the pressures are incredible. You've got all the grief and all the anger. It's just a horrible experience. If there are cracks there they're just going to go even further.

(P12: mother of preterm triplets)

By 13 months, four couples (8%) had actually separated and a further four (8%) were seriously contemplating doing so.

When those parents who, in their own estimation, had real relationship difficulties were compared with those who did not, the presence of children in the family appeared to show a negative correlation with problems between the parents. Sixty-one per cent of those who felt secure in their relationship were childless (that is, they had no living children), compared to only 26% of those who were unhappy in their relationship.


## Perceived positive effects

By the time of the first interview, as many as 34 of the 55 couples (62%) felt that they had grown closer since the tragedy. The initial intensity of their closeness usually lessened, but the effect was still of a stronger bond. However, for a small minority ($n = 2$ couples) the intensity persisted for more than a year, and they were now totally wrapped up in each other, choosing to spend all of their free time together, and in some cases cutting themselves off from previous pursuits and other company.

By 13 months on, this overall figure of 62% had dropped to 33%, and only 16 of the 48 available couples now considered that the tragedy had brought them closer. Of these, a small number felt that the dying experience itself had been so profound that it had forged a bond which was very special. As one mother said, having lived through this experience together, neither she nor her husband could ever contemplate a future without the other parent of this baby they had created together and lost together. But for most, the impression was given that it was the whole shared experience which had brought them closer. This was confirmed in many ways. In descending order of frequency of citation the parents mentioned the following effects which the experience had had on their relationship.

### Changed values and perspectives

It had made them appreciate one another and what they had, so that they no longer took such things for granted. For some there had been a recognition of new strengths in their partner. Several parents commented that since they were now much less materialistic, they attached greater value to each other and to family life, and appreciated healthy developing children or a new pregnancy in a deeper way.

### Strengthened relationships

The strength of their feeling for each other had been tested and found to be strong. Some partners now acknowledged a greater dependence on each other.

### Maturing effect

With a new maturity of outlook they felt that they were more considerate and sensitive. Little things they had once worried about or argued over now seemed trivial and not worth conflict. Some couples specified that they were now much less argumentative.

### Improved communication

The depth of their communication had improved. They could now talk about things more, and were more ready to actually express their feelings.

## Perceived negative effects

As has been reported above, by 13 months eight of the 48 couples (17%) had either separated or were seriously contemplating doing so. Data are not available for seven of the 55 couples. Of the eight who had split up or were close to it, all of them considered that the baby's death had precipitated this crisis. Respondents not infrequently remarked on the changes of personality which they saw in themselves or in their partners – for example, 'he used to be fun-loving but is now withdrawn and empty,' 'he is so immature – just a mental bully,' 'we used to laugh together, we were good together – but not now.'

Different consequences of the tragedy impinged on the relationship and affected it adversely. For a few couples the effect was a general sense that something just was not right, or that vital ingredients were missing. However, of the total of 55 couples, as many as 31 (56%) could identify specific negative effects accruing from this experience.

## Emotional separation in grief

This was the commonest effect. Parents described a mounting of tension as they each went their separate ways in grieving, each excluding the other. Silences simply grew longer, and resentments mounted as the fathers continued to hide their feelings and the women continued to weep.

## Depression

Three families reported that one or both partners had been 'very depressed' in the first 3 months after the death of the baby, and as many as 33 couples (66%) reported having felt depressed during the year following the loss. Low spirits day after day strained relationships.

## Guilt

Guilt related partly to the problems associated with the baby and partly to the need to get on with life afterwards. Three couples worried that they might have passed on faulty genes. One father felt responsible for having taken his partner to hospital and leaving her there, trusting the staff to care for her well, only to have that trust apparently betrayed. One mother reported that she felt guilty if she was happy because it was disloyal to the baby, and she also felt guilty if she was sad because it was not fair on her other children. Her husband could not understand why she remained so wrapped up in the family instead of going out more and getting things into a better perspective. Another mother felt guilty because after initially being strong she was now not coping well, and this added to her husband's pressures.

## Unavailability

Some parents found that their partners had no space for them now. When mothers became absorbed in their grief or in their other children to the exclusion of the father, tension built up. When each parent grieved in their own way – ways with which the partner could not sympathise or empathise – they could easily feel excluded and rejected or unloved.

## Insecurity

The death of their child rocked the security of parents. As one mother succinctly put it, she now had 'no confidence in a tomorrow.' If, as it had, 'the unthinkable' had already happened, what else might next hit them?

Several parents described worrying obsessively about the safety of partners or other children. However, sometimes their fears irritated their partners, who saw only over-indulgence or over-protection of the baby's siblings. Fathers felt sidelined, and households were disrupted as children went undisciplined and stress built up.

### Uncertainty about the future
In one family the couple could not agree about the wisdom of having another child, given the risks involved, and this had a negative effect on their relationship.

### Personality change
A number of parents reported having lost their happy approach to life and their optimism, and felt that this had changed them as individuals, making them less attractive to be with. Mothers acknowledged that they cried a lot. Fathers were sometimes reluctant to return home to face all the tears and the fear of upsetting them again. Two parents (one mother and one father) lost confidence after the tragedy and felt unable to go out. These changes imposed strains on all of their relationships.

### Blame
Only one set of parents blamed each other, but this had a corrosive effect on an already difficult relationship.

### Dependence
For some parents there was an additional strain in having their partner so dependent on them now. It could feel oppressive to be together too much when they were both grieving so profoundly.

### Anger
Five families reported that stormy arguments characterised this time after the death of the child. On occasion things were said in the heat of the moment which vulnerable partners found hurtful.

### Role change
When a baby did not come home, expected roles could be lost or revised. Parents who had arranged to take time off to be at home looking after the baby now had to revisit their plans.

> I don't think I'm grieving any more [than my husband] but my grief's different because I'm a mother. It's the mother's role to be at home with the baby. Although we both came home from hospital and [the baby]

isn't with us, in an ideal world [my husband] was going to go straight back to his work anyway − or have a week off or two weeks off with me and the baby anyway, then go right back to his work. His role was going to be at work and come home to the baby at night. My role was going to be coming home from the hospital and being with that baby for 24 hours a day. And to begin with [he] couldn't quite grasp what I was trying to explain to him that, although we both came home to nothing, that his way in life is still going the same way as it should have done, whereas mine was going in a different way. I was coming home, I wasn't ready to go back to work, but I was just sitting here on my own all day. And no matter what you did, no matter where you went, there was always somebody either pregnant or pushing a baby − there was always something to remind you that, well, *I* should be doing that or *I* should be doing that. And even when I went back to my work, it was − I shouldn't be here.

(P23: mother of preterm baby with congenital anomalies)

Some fathers found it hard to return to spouses who had been at home all day but who appeared to be unproductive and demanding.

### Breakdown in communication

When it was so easy to trigger tears, some parents found it easiest simply to stay out of the way or keep quiet. Lost in their own grief, they were often unaware of the effect that their silence had on their partner.

# Other children

Just over half of the sets of parents who participated in the second interview (28 of 50 families, 56%) had living children. A number of parents observed that they had become more possessive or protective of their remaining children, fearing that some tragedy would befall them, too. This anxiety could be manifested in several ways, including crushing adventurous tendencies, keeping the children close, getting cross with them, and limiting the time they spent with other people.

Some siblings were too young to really understand what had happened, but almost all parents reported that, whatever their age, the children seemed to have coped well with the loss. Parents themselves were helped by the youngsters talking naturally about the baby, as this reinforced the reality of his or her existence and the significance of his or her life for the whole family. Some parents commented that death had become part of life in the family's experience, and they now all talked about it in a matter-of-fact and healthy way. Two sets of parents had noted a temporary disturbance when a new pregnancy aroused anxiety in the siblings, but they found that the situation improved dramatically once the next baby was at home.

For just under a quarter of the families (6 of 28, 21%) the effects of the death on the children were more worrying. They reported depression, regressive behaviours, withdrawal, anger and preoccupation with death. When the children would not or could not talk about the baby, the parents felt powerless to help them to come to terms with the loss. The parents themselves found it disturbing when the children endlessly re-enacted death scenes during play, or expressed deep fears about health or death. Four children had become badly behaved, but the parents were unsure whether this was a response to the death or a manifestation of other stresses in the child's life. Subsequent deaths of other relatives or child friends, tensions between separated parents, and reactions to other aberrant behaviours were all cited as possible causes.

# The parents' approach to other people

The altered perspectives of the parents themselves seemed likely to influence their perceptions of and reactions to other people. Where parents felt that they themselves were more sympathetic and understanding, there was a potential for improved relationships. But for a few the effect of this tragedy was more likely to be negative. Some found that it had driven the parents in on themselves, so that only *their* feelings really mattered and they felt it appropriate to be entirely 'selfish', concentrating on their own needs in their struggle to deal with their great loss. In these cases, all other relationships were affected to some extent by their withdrawal. A minority did indeed withdraw from the social scene altogether. In other cases a reappraisal of their priorities had a knock-on effect. Careers and the acquisition of material possessions were no longer important goals to achieve. In families where home became more important than a career, some parents found that they were not as favoured by their employers and were less likely to be promoted than before.

Before we examine the parents' perceptions of other relationships, however, it is important to draw attention to the feeling which prevailed among them. They believed that, since they were the ones who were most profoundly affected by this death, other people should take their cues from them.

> That's one of the hardest things. When you're at your lowest point you're having to guide people through [how to handle grief].
>
> (P1: mother of baby with asphyxia)

> I did try to talk to [a work colleague] one day, but he didn't want to know so I just thought, 'Well, if that's the way it is . . . that's it.' I did find it hurt a bit. One day he was drunk and *he* was wanting to speak about it, but I thought, 'No, if you don't want to speak when you're sober . . .' I just closed it.
>
> (P13: father of baby with cardiac anomaly)

> Even now my friends will say, 'How's [my wife] keeping? Is everything all right? Is she still thinking about the baby?' *You're* trying to move on, but folk can bring you back . . . You never ever forget about him, we can always talk about him, but that just keeps bringing it back.
>
> (P 56: father of preterm baby with congenital anomalies)

However, interpreting parents' cues was inevitably complicated in some instances, since by their own admission some of them disguised their real feelings.

> People have said to me, 'Oh, you're coping amazingly well.' And you think, 'You don't *know* how I'm coping.' 'You're so strong,' and 'I admire the way you've handled it,' and what not. And I think, 'How do people know the way you've handled it?'. They're not there at night-time when all the lights go out, and you're on your own and you sit and look back on it all. I mean there are mornings that I have woken up and I've thought, 'Oh, I just don't want to get up today.' But I don't have any choice in the matter. But people don't understand that you've got no choice in the matter. [But I'm someone who appears in control of my emotions]. I am that kind of person, I know I am. Sometimes I get annoyed with myself because I'm like that.
>
> (P 6: mother of baby with congenital anomalies)

It is against this background of changed personalities and mixed cues that we shall address the issue of the effect that the death of the child seemed to have, in the parents' estimation, on other relationships.

# Other relationships

Many parents commented that it was hard to deal with the shallowness and trivial preoccupations of others at this time. If others were unable to bear strong emotion or distress, this limited their availability to parents who were grieving and absorbed in the tragedy which had overtaken them. One additional couple commented that they themselves had tried to be the same with everyone else, but others now treated them differently.

As many as 80% of the parents (40 of 50) felt that the death of the baby had had an effect on other relationships outside their own intimate family.

The changes reported were both positive and negative, and to some extent they were situation specific. Details of those actions which parents found helpful or unhelpful are given in the following chapter, but here we shall address the relationships which parents felt were altered by this experience.

# People who shared the life and death of the child

When a baby dies there are few memories and only a select body of individuals with whom those memories are shared. These people were clearly potentially important to the parents in that they could talk with authority and feeling about the child's characteristics and about different aspects of the experience. By doing so they helped to reinforce the reality of the child's life and death, giving them meaning and significance. These relationships acquired special significance.

## The parents' own parents

For most couples, relationships with their own parents were strengthened as they all grieved for the loss of the baby. The emotional bonds which made this grandchild so precious were strong, and the parents were comforted by the manifestations of the significance of the baby to their own parents. Previously undemonstrative grandfathers showed their love and concern more openly. Single mothers sharing a home with their own parents found that the experience brought them all closer together. Fathers noted that they had grown closer to the maternal grandmother, as she had shown herself to be particularly sensitive to and very supportive of their need. Two mothers found that they had grown closer to their husband's parents as a result of this tragedy. They had shown sensitivity and real understanding which strengthened the existing bonds.

Sometimes, however, the grandparents swamped the parents by the intensity of their response. More than one couple either unplugged their telephone or went out in the car to escape the excessive demands the family made on them. In other cases the grandparents appeared to be so wrapped up in their own grieving that they were unavailable to the parents. A small number of parents reported that the family members had been competing in the grieving stakes, each trying to outdo the other. This was a damaging experience for parents who had little space or inclination to referee family battles. In one family the two sets of grandparents had clearly had some kind of difference of opinion. The parents knew nothing of its origins, but they were very aware of a new coolness between them. In the face of such a major disaster as the death of a child, these 'petty' differences seemed to the parents to be immature responses.

In a small number of cases the mothers observed that they no longer confided in their own mothers. This was not necessarily a feature of a breakdown in their relationship, but rather it symbolised a change in themselves – a form of maturing. They had now had an experience out-with that of their own parents. They had themselves been the principal decision makers in the life and death of this baby. They had given birth, borne the bad news, lived through the death, buried their own child, and they were now coping with life after that loss. They had demonstrated that they were mature adults in their own right who were able to accept responsibility without reference to others. Alongside this growing up was an awareness of the vulnerability of grandparents. It was evident that they were deeply pained by the experience, and parents became protective of them subsequently, in some instances shielding them from a full knowledge of what had gone wrong, or the enormity of the choices, or the potential for future problems. Some parents did not tell them about new pregnancies for many months in case things went wrong and they were again disappointed.

For three families there had been a real breakdown in relationships with the grandparents, and in all of these cases the paternal grandmother was cited as the principal cause of the rift. In two cases she was perceived as unsympathetic and cruel, making derogatory comments about the mother's capacity to produce a child. In the third case she had publicly disgraced the parents and 'disgusted' and 'angered' them greatly by her preoccupation with her own feelings and her total disregard for theirs. But in another family it was the father's relationship with the maternal grandparents, already a poor one, which had become even less tolerable.

In two cases the father's family had made no contact at all since the baby had died, and the parents were angry and hurt by this insensitivity. One mother tried to establish contact, but her efforts were spurned. However, in another case a couple from a minority culture reported that such an experience was an intensely private one, and not something to be shared with their own parents. Their perspective serves to highlight the importance of recognising the need for individually tailored systems of support.

## The parents' siblings

Many parents spoke of the strengthening of relationships with their own siblings at this time. Closeness seemed to be related to the willingness of their relatives to be with them in their grief, to speak openly about the baby and the tragedy, and to bear with their strong emotion. They valued those who made it clear that they were willing and available, but who took their cues from the parents themselves. Those who were in tune with the parents' needs and who visited often became closer and more involved, and the parents felt the benefits of a deepening relationship as a consequence. For some couples there had been surprises. Sisters or sisters-in-law who had known tragedy themselves proved unsympathetic or were even perceived as 'cruel.' Childless sisters who had been thought shallow and self-centred revealed hidden depths of compassion, were readily available and did not tire of lending an listening ear.

Parents were conscious of the awkwardness on both sides where there were other children, especially when there were striking similarities in age, looks or names to the dead child. Knowing when to visit and how much access parents wanted to their nephews and nieces was a delicate matter. Sometimes such circumstances influenced the contact the families maintained, and that in turn affected relationships.

# Friends

During the first year of bereavement, friends were singled out for commendation more than any other single group. Some parents commented that friends were of more value than family in these circumstances because they were not so emotionally involved. The parents could voice their grief, anger or doubts without worrying about the effect on the listener's own personal sorrow. Those who had shared the parents' experience or had themselves experienced the loss of a child were especially valued, and relationships developed and deepened over the year as they supported and reassured the parents.

If friends were able to be with the parents in their distress, listen to their grief without judging or offering platitudes, and continue to be real friends, those friendships were cemented. Some parents singled out for mention those who had shown such characteristics against expectation. For example, 'macho' men had shown a soft side, and apparently frivolous, fun-loving, single friends had been patient, caring listeners.

Where so-called friends appeared to ignore the parents, relationships cooled and were sometimes severed. The sensitivity of their responses could promote acquaintances to the rank of friends or demote friends to mere acquaintances. In one case, neighbours rallied and offered such sympathetic help that they became friends. However, friends of one mother angered her greatly by asking either her husband or her friend how she was, instead of consulting her directly. This woman who had now lost two children, relinquished a number of friends during the first year following the death because of their inability to understand what she wanted and needed. Several parents observed that it was inappropriate for people to expect the grieving parents to do the running to preserve these friendships; they were not prepared to do so. Parents were saddened, too, when friends did not visit as before, although a few did appreciate the awkwardness involved for those with children exposing the grieving parents to potentially upsetting experiences. Young parents found the immaturity and care-free approach to life of their peers suddenly incongruous. It served to highlight the loss of their own youth and innocence and set them apart.

# Work colleagues

Two mothers cited changes in relationships with work colleagues. In one case the mother found that her workmates became 'softer and nicer' to everyone following the tragedy. But in the other instance the staff avoided the mother after the baby had died. As a consequence of this, when she lost a subsequent pregnancy she could not face working with them and moved to a different office. This mother had been so hurt by her previous experience that she did not tell her new colleagues anything of her history.

Having looked at the effects on relationships, it is important to understand something of the balance of factors which made the parents happy or sad. This was explored in order to provide a context for their overall position in terms of coping with the loss 13 months after the death.

# Sources of happiness

Although there were similarities between the things which mothers and fathers identified as sources of pleasure, there were also differences in emphasis, so these factors are listed separately for each partner. This seemed particularly relevant in view of the fact that a number of fathers reported being ignored or overlooked.

> I think a lot of the attention is centred towards the mother. Fathers in this sort of [experience] are forgotten about to some degree ... nine times out of ten the [enquiry] is about the wife: 'How's the wife?'
>
> (P35: father of preterm triplets)

# Mothers

Only four mothers could think of nothing that had made them happy during the year following the death of the baby. Others, however, added a comment to the effect that there was, and would always be, a shadow over their lives which prevented them from ever feeling completely happy again.

> We'll never ever be totally happy again. There's always going to be something missing. Things make you smile and make you laugh, but we'll never be properly happy as in totally happy with life ... You feel as well, if you're enjoying yourself too much, you're always going to have this little nagging guilt as well; that you shouldn't be enjoying yourself that much ... we do go out and we enjoy ourselves, but we don't seem to have the same level of enjoyment as we had before ... we feel we've been robbed. We really have been robbed. There's not a day goes by that we don't think of him.
>
> (P2: parents of baby with cardiac anomaly)

The main triggers of happiness are listed below in descending order of frequency of citation.

## New pregnancy

By far the commonest event to trigger happiness was a new pregnancy. As we have seen, 26 mothers (52%) became pregnant again within the first year. One mother remarked that the new pregnancy gave her a 'sense of achievement and equality with other women.'

> You do feel like you've failed. I don't know why, because obviously you know it's just one of these things. You feel that people [regard you as sort of substandard]. Once you've gone and had another healthy child again it's almost like you're back on an [equal] footing with other people. It's almost like [declaring], 'I can do it!' ... once I was pregnant again, that was enough. You felt like you'd achieved something ... [This idea of people judging us], it's probably totally in my head. It's probably not like that at all [really].
>
> (P43: mother of baby with congenital anomalies)

The new baby kept the mother busy and stopped her dwelling too much on the sadness of her loss.

> I think it was easier around [the baby's] birthday and his anniversary... because we *did* have a [new] baby... I know lots of people have gone on for years after they've lost their child and it's really still awfully painful because they haven't had any more. Whereas my experience is different because I fell pregnant again so quickly. Within the year I've had two

children. Not that [the first one's] loss is any less now, but it's easier to take, I would say, because I have a baby to fill that gaping hole that he left. It doesn't make it any easier to forget, but it makes it easier to deal with. My life's not hollow . . . it's busy, busy, busy.

> (P 20: mother of baby with asphyxia)

Although the overall feeling generated was one of pleasure and hope, many mothers added that they were much more fearful this time around, conscious as they now were of things which could go wrong. To a degree they regretted the loss of innocent excitement, whilst at the same time they marvelled at their earlier naivety.

## Other children

As has already been mentioned, 56% of the mothers had living children. The majority of mothers cited them as key figures in helping to lift them out of their sadness, a considerable number spontaneously commenting that everything would have been harder to bear if it had been a first child who had died. Watching the children develop, feeling their love, and dealing with their chatter and antics helped to restore a sense of normality, and reassured the mothers that they were capable of parenting a child successfully. They gave the parents 'a reason to get up in the morning.'

However, those who had surviving children from the same pregnancy described mixed emotions – pleasure in the developing survivor, but a constant reminder of what should have been. One mother spoke strongly of the existence of a twin as inhibiting her grieving because people expected her to get on with life and appreciate what she had, rather than wallowing in misery. For her there had been no space to grieve for the child she had lost.

Six mothers cited other people's children – their own nephews and nieces or children of close friends – as bringing happiness into their lives since the death of their own baby. They could be glad that others had happy experiences and enjoy the pleasure that they themselves gained from being with children. One additional mother had given articles of her baby's bedding to a friend, and for her there was a bitter-sweet sense of happiness in seeing them in use.

## Holidays

As many as a quarter (13 mothers) cited a holiday as bringing some happiness. Planning the break, getting away from the scene of so much sadness, being with people who knew nothing of their story, and engaging in different activities all helped to distract them from their sadness for a time.

### Changes in housing

Four mothers found that moving to a new house had been a positive experience in helping them to move forward in their grieving. They threw themselves into the change and planned for the future. Three others invested their energies in substantial changes to their existing homes, and found solace in the improvements obtained as well as the hard work involved.

### Memories and mementoes

For five mothers there was a form of quiet happiness in remembering the dead child. Visiting the grave, choosing a headstone, buying or collecting gifts or laying flowers added to a sense of treasuring the child.

### Work

Three mothers started new jobs which offered distraction and a sense of purpose and helped to return them to a more 'normal' life. Two others cited a return to their previous employment as a cause of happiness. These mothers found that for them it had been counter-productive to sit at home with nothing in particular to do but dwell on the tragedy. Working helped them to get things into a healthier perspective.

### Friendships

Through this traumatic experience strong friendships were forged, and a small number of mothers cited these as a source of deep pleasure. They could share things at a different level and truly value the compassion and caring of others. One mother had joined a new church and enthused over the depth of caring and friendship the congregation provided.

### 'Simple pleasures'

Several mothers found new happiness in what they called the 'simple pleasures' of life. These included being with family members, hobbies, walking, and taking up new pursuits. One couple got married after the death of the baby, and the mother cited this as a major source of happiness for her. Parents also valued their own health more after this experience, and three mothers cited improved health as a source of pleasure.

# Fathers

All except four fathers could identify specific events which had made them happy during the year since the baby had died.

### New pregnancy

Almost half of the fathers (19, 48%) cited their partner becoming pregnant again as a source of real happiness. Two fathers observed that it was a very good experience to see the whole family smiling again.

### Other children

Seventeen fathers found happiness in watching their existing children growing and enjoying life. However, where the children were born at the same time as the dead child, feelings were mixed.

> If I had have had just one [baby] and lost one, that'd have been a damn sight easier. Oh yes, so much easier. Definitely. You go into hospital to have a child, you come out of hospital without that child, yes, it's hard but you can cry right away. You can go straight into the grieving process. I think half the problem with us is that we haven't had the chance to grieve. We haven't had that total breakdown – that you're meant to have, that you usually have when you've lost someone close. Because the day of [the baby's] funeral, we went to her funeral, came home and then went back into the hospital [to visit the survivors].
>
> (P35: father of preterm triplets)

Three men derived pleasure from being with other people's children.

### Holidays

Getting away and having a good time on holiday were sources of pleasure for a quarter of the men (11 fathers). For a limited time they could give the appearance of being a normal happy family enjoying themselves. Some felt that it had been beneficial for the women to get out of the house where they spent so much time 'brooding,' and the men enjoyed this brief respite from their constant sadness.

### Work

Many fathers found that work helped to keep things in perspective but some were aware that they were less efficient or effective for a time.

> My mind wasn't as fit and sharp as it was previously. I think mentally I took a very large knock and it took me a long time to get over that ... it was a confidence dent. It was almost as if a quarter of your brain was shut off and impaired and it took a little bit of time before that was used again.
>
> (P16: father of preterm baby)

Three fathers who had had successes or promotion said that although they had been pleased at the recognition of their efforts, the awards gave only transient pleasure and lacked the sparkle they would have had if their family life had been happy.

> *Mother*: [My partner] got an award for [work achievement]. He felt really happy but he knew [we] weren't as happy as [we] could have been. So I think there's always going to be that. You're going to feel happy about things but not *as* happy. That's why we can't think of something really tremendous [that's made us happy].
> *Father*: What is it? It's money, it's a trophy. You'd give it all back [if you could have the baby again]. If the baby had have been here that would have been [an outstanding thing]. It was a big thing for the company, but I gave the trophy away ... it's nothing [now]. It makes you smile and pretend you're happy for a while, but deep down you just think of the cemetery. That's where your happiness really lies.
>
> (P 38: parents of baby with congenital anomaly)

Two fathers had changed jobs and found pleasure in the improved conditions they now enjoyed.

### Changes in housing

Although two men cited moving house as a good experience during the year, more ($n = 4$ fathers) commented that it had been a source of pleasure to them to find that there was no necessity to uproot themselves. After a period of feeling unsettled they were now content with their present homes. Two of these four men had embarked on fairly major renovation plans and gained pleasure from applying themselves to these practical projects.

### Celebrations

Celebratory functions, including marriages, anniversaries and Christmas, had been sources of happiness for five fathers.

### Commemoration

Three fathers cited commemorative events as providing happiness. In two cases these related to getting a gravestone to mark the plot and visiting the grave, respectively, as satisfying feelings. In the third case the father had engaged in a fundraising event, and described his sense of pride in performing the feat for his dead child, and the happiness he felt when it was accomplished successfully. One other father said that he got a glow of pleasure from remembering his son putting up such a fight to survive – it was as if he was 'thumbing his nose at society' and defying authority.

### *'Simple pleasures'*

Simple domestic pleasures brought a new sense of contentment to a few fathers. They included ordinary family events, football successes, seeing the mother laughing or sharing a joke, and temporarily 'not hurting.' But even these pleasures were less intense than they would have been, as the child would never now attend a sporting fixture, and the sadness would return to the mother's face.

### *Friendship*

Only one father cited a friendship as a source of happiness. He and his partner had forged a new, strong relationship with another bereaved couple, and he commented on the freedom he felt in being able to share intense emotions with someone else who understood that feeling.

# Triggers of sadness

## Mothers

All of the mothers could identify triggers which made them sad. Some commented that it did not take much now to make them miserable, as there was a pervasive sense of sorrow so near the surface of their lives. Even something as simple as a long dark winter night could upset a mother who thought of her baby outside alone in the cold and darkness. Shopping could produce a sense of emptiness because there was one less person to buy for than there should have been. Endings were now times of real sadness as they left work, parted from friends, and lost relatives.

Everywhere the mothers went there were things to remind them of what might have been, several observed sadly. A family resemblance, photographs or video footage, the different stages of a new pregnancy, travelling along the same route they had taken to the hospital, songs, a memorial service, a church service, visiting the graveyard or rose garden, or new furniture which they would never have bought if the baby had lived – all served as painful reminders. Particularly poignant was the existence of surviving siblings from the same pregnancy. Where one child began to smile, there should have been two. Where two babies were discharged home after weeks in hospital, there should have been three.

The women also found that they now took things more to heart and were sad for others as well as themselves. A sad film, or news of tragedies involving children, touched them in a way that they had not previously experienced. When friends, relatives or colleagues faced death or disaster, the mothers felt their pain acutely.

The main factors identified as triggers of sadness are listed below in descending order of frequency of citation.

## Anniversaries

For many mothers the anniversaries of the birth and death of the baby were times of particular sadness. Although they grieved every day, these dates forcefully reminded them of what had been happening a year ago.

> For me I don't think it was his [death] anniversary [that was hard so much] as it was living through that period of his life and death *up to* the anniversary of his funeral. I still remember conversations verbatim. I knew exactly on every day during that period who I was talking to, what was being said, what [the baby's] oxygen levels were – just everything was so vivid, which amazed me because at the time you think when you're going through this, it's all very hazy and you're just stumbling through it. But everything was very vivid. Just the process of going through that again day by day – a year ago at this time on this day this is what was happening – that was a turning point for me going through it. It's hard to describe it, but it was like I could let go of something. But I don't know [what]. It's not as though I'm letting go of my memories because they're there, but it was almost as if I *know* that I remember, therefore I don't have to *try* to remember. I don't have to grip on to these things.
>
> (P18: mother of preterm baby)

However, where there were surviving babies from the same pregnancy, emotions were particularly turbulent at the time of anniversaries.

> That was the worst day because that's when cards came in from nurses, so I found that quite hard. They were lovely but . . . if she hadn't been a twin, if she had just been an individual it would have been so much easier. It's just that when I was opening cards I'm opening birthday cards and then opening these other cards and I'm thinking, 'What am I feeling here?' And the tears were streaming while I'm trying to say to [the surviving] twin, 'This is from your Granny. This is from your Aunty.' My emotions were really [haywire] that day. But I must admit, looking back on that now, it was lovely because she was remembered, people were remembering her for what she was. It was very important to me, because I don't want her to be forgotten.
>
> (P10: mother of preterm twins)

For a few mothers, anticipation proved to be more traumatic than reality. One mother said that for her the anniversary was no worse than any other day, and a further four found that the build-up to the dates was worse than the actual day, and the ensuing week was harder to bear for another mother, producing a real 'crisis of confidence.' Because the dates held such significance for the mothers, they were hurt when others forgot or ignored them, especially if it was the child's father who appeared to be oblivious. One father was amazed to hear his partner's sadness that the expected date of delivery had passed unmarked by him: for him that day had ceased to be important when the baby had a real birth date.

Christmas was cited by 18 mothers as a time of great sadness. Their rejoicing was hollow, and they felt out of tune with the rest of the world. A certain person was absent, and presents were always one too few. New Year celebrations were similarly triggers of sadness for some mothers. Mother's Day and Father's Day were poignant reminders of what they had lost.

## Other children

Many mothers commented on the fact that everywhere they had to face other children or pregnancies, and there was no escaping them. They described feelings of 'anger', 'jealousy' and even 'hatred' of these more fortunate mothers. The birth of children at around the same time as their own held a special significance, each milestone compounding the sense of loss, and each birthday highlighting the absence of celebration in their own lives. Some spoke of a deep sense of injustice, which was exacerbated by stories of abuse, mistreatment or too casual an attitude towards other children.

## Next pregnancy

Although the start of a new pregnancy commonly signalled a change to a more positive and hopeful phase, many women cited it as a time of sadness, too. They were very fearful in case things went wrong again. Some felt a sense of guilt about wanting another child which could be perceived as disloyalty to the dead baby. Comparisons between the two babies, or a realisation that subsequent children would never know one of their siblings, could bring waves of sorrow.

For some mothers there had been new problems with this subsequent pregnancy. In one instance there was a deep sense of injustice when a perfect preterm infant had died while a full-term baby with abnormalities lived. For others, even relatively minor correctable problems could create panic as the parents re-lived the gathering trauma of their previous experience. These new difficulties added to the sense of pervasive sorrow.

For a few mothers, the sadness was compounded by difficulty in conceiving or an inability to conceive again. Older women with a limited potential childbearing time ahead experienced each new menstrual period as a trauma. A younger mother grieved over her own lack of confidence to try again. However, by the time of the second interview some mothers had started to accept the fact that they would never have a surviving child. One such young mother herself had an incurable illness, but although she mourned her state, she spent her time and energy enjoying activities with other people's children. Another described a 'terrible sense of failure and loss of identity,' while yet another spoke sadly of the finality of getting rid of the pram and cradle.

Particular sadness was felt when other people asked the mothers about the size of their family. Full explanations threatened to shock or distance the questioner, while brief inaccurate replies felt disloyal to the baby and resurrected the mother's own pain.

> You know what I find hard? When people ask me if I have a family. I mean what *do* people [like me] say? I don't know how I'll ever get over that one . . . When people ask me I feel very [awkward]. I hate saying, 'No.'
>
> (P8: mother of preterm twins)

> I find it difficult if people ask me how many children I have. I never know how to answer it. If I say I've got one, I feel it's so disloyal because [the baby] is such a big part of my life, although he's not here. But at the same time I don't want to [upset people] – if someone's making casual conversation, it's such a terrible thing, and they're so shocked and then embarrassed and feel awful for bringing it up . . . last week someone asked, 'So which number is this?' And I couldn't say, 'Two.' So I had to explain then, why. That's coming from people innocently asking things. That's difficult because it's a no-win situation.
>
> (P27: mother of baby with cardiac anomaly)

This was a preoccupation of many mothers. Some made a conscious decision to act in a certain way, but their resolve could be challenged by circumstances.

> I don't know quite what to do when I go to the antenatal class . . . one of the first things they say is, 'For how many is this the first? How many the second?' If I turn round and say, 'It's my second,' [they're going to say], 'How old's your first?' So I'm going to be a bit on the spot because we've always said that, even if it upsets other people, even if it's a stranger, if we made out that this was our first, or that no, we haven't got any children, then it's almost like denying that [the baby] was ever there and we can't do that. So if it upsets them and makes people feel awkward, we don't mean to do that, but for our sakes, we feel better saying that, 'Well no, it's actually our second but we lost our first.' But when it comes to the *antenatal clinic* it's slightly different because there's going to be a lot of

anxious first-time Mums in the same position that I was in, thinking
that everything's all hunky-dory... Personally I would rather *say.*

(P51: mother of baby with congenital anomalies)

## Strained relationships

Relatively small things could weaken relationships when parents were so
vulnerable, and a number of mothers cited strained relationships as
sources of additional sadness during the year following the baby's death.
Three mothers included in this the relationship they had with the baby's
father, which was now less robust. However, for others it was events outside the nuclear family setting which saddened them. These included relatives not marking the date of birth but only the death, other family events
eclipsing the anniversary of the baby's death, cruel comments about the
inability to have children, insensitive flaunting of a pregnancy, too casual
an approach to the welfare of a baby, or a demand to hold a party for a
surviving twin against the mother's wishes.

## Other major events

Having lost a baby it was hard to contemplate losing other significant
people as well. Five mothers had a parent either dying or battling a potentially life-threatening illness. The shared grief of a young friend whose husband was terminally ill, or leaving work and friends, were all experiences
which added to their sadness.

For three mothers pain had been caused by desecration of the baby's
memory. A burglar had rifled through their mementoes in one case, a
headstone was moved and the grave area mutilated in another, and in the
third case a vase was stolen from the grave site.

## Memorial service

Memorial services drew mixed reviews, but a number of mothers found
them intensely painful and sad events.

If I had known beforehand I wouldn't have gone.

(P32: mother of preterm baby)

That was dreadful. I honestly thought that it would be full of hope and
talk about the future, but they really dwelled on your baby, and they kept
having silences where you were to think of your baby and it was like...
everybody hurts. Maybe it would be good for some people, but I actually
wanted to go and hear them say, 'Yes, but you really need to look forward.' But it was all dwelling right in the moment of your baby. It was
too upsetting. I was really upset after it and for *days* after it.

(P45: mother of preterm baby)

# Fathers

Only one father could think of nothing in particular which made him sad. However, two men summed up the impression conveyed by many: 'Nothing making you happy makes you sad,' and 'Everything reminds you and the sadness hits you.'

Although the fathers seemed to find it more difficult than the mothers to pin their sadness to specific triggers, they did, none the less, identify certain factors which precipitated or increased feelings of sorrow. Some of the triggers were common to both genders, but the frequency of citation differed, indicating that the reactions of fathers were different from those of mothers.

## Anniversaries

As we have seen, the mothers sometimes felt that their menfolk were less affected by specific dates. However, about half of the men identified anniversaries as particular times of sadness, as they remembered and thought of what should have been. Two men commented that the build-up to these dates had actually been worse than the date itself. Some fathers added wryly that they never could remember dates, so there was nothing sinister in them forgetting this one. One man regretted a relative reminding him of the birth date of the baby who had died: he would have preferred not to have had this association, and it just added to his low spirits.

Other times of celebration were hard for a considerable number of fathers. When everyone around them seemed to be happy at Christmas or New Year, and when 'everyone' expected them to be cheerful, too, their own sense of loss and misery stood in stark contrast. One father spoke movingly of having put money into a savings account over the year, and the pain of withdrawing it knowing that instead of buying special gifts for both of his children, there was now only one to buy for. Mother's Day and Father's Day triggered sadness for two fathers.

## Remembering the baby

For a large number of fathers anything which reminded them of the baby provoked sad feelings during the year following his or her death. Clear associations with the death, such as visiting the cemetery or rose garden, making up the commemorative album, or returning to the same hospital, brought back poignant memories. Fathers were also sometimes surprised by the strength of feeling generated by other associations, such as getting baby things out of the loft for the next child, seeing the same model of pram they had chosen in use by many other parents, being near a plot for stillborn babies in a graveyard, or a certain song.

A song on the telly, somebody saying the wrong thing – makes you sad. You don't expect the sadness to happen, it happens – *big* time. You're sitting with your pals and a song comes on and you just get really deep. Everything seems to remind you of [the baby].

(P38: father of baby with congenital anomaly)

As one man commented, the women folk missed the baby stage, but the men lost out longer term. Some described a powerful feeling of loss when they went to a football match or saw other fathers enjoying family experiences such as feeding animals or playing on the beach together. The realisation washed over them each time that they would now never do these things with the child who had died. One father often felt this sadness when he watched his other child at play: he feared that she might reproach them in the future for having no playmate of her own.

## Memorial service

Several fathers spoke with a shudder of the memorial service. Such concentrated sadness was unhelpful to them, and one described attending it as the 'worst experience of the whole year.'

The worst thing we've encountered in this last year was the memorial [service] at [the study hospital]. That was the Sunday. That was awful; that was really, really bad. We were in two minds whether to go ... because we felt we were coping very well with it and we were moving forward. But I think – whether it was cowardice or fear of cowardice – we thought we would go along. [And] to support [the hospital]. But unfortunately a lot of people found it very difficult. People were crying before it started. It didn't help that we sat next to the couple who cried the most ... it just brought everything back to you. I think we were actually stronger afterwards because we were out for a Chinese [meal] in [the city] after it and we talked quite a lot and I think that was quite good. Once we eventually got home I think we felt it had probably done us some good. But at the time it was, 'We don't want to be here!' ... I think we felt it actually set us back quite a bit ... it was very poignant. We wouldn't go back ... Don't get me wrong – the service itself, it's a beautiful service but it's emotionally charged. I don't think I've ever felt anything like it ... It was just that I think with everyone being there and the symbolism of putting flowers down. It was very intense. I think it was only half an hour or something but it felt like a very long half an hour.

(P32: father of preterm baby)

Another father was amazed and impressed by one parent reading a poem about his baby son at the memorial service. He could not ever envisage himself sharing his own emotion so publicly, and he found the whole experience disturbing.

> Because of the way I am, I find it very difficult to put my emotions on display in front of people you don't know – or even people you *do* know! I thought that took some doing. I came away feeling a great deal of admiration for that man. But the whole ceremony – I just found it quite upsetting. Because for me what it does is it exposes my emotions about the whole business and then I have to go away and cement them over again ... generally speaking these services don't do anything for me in the sense that they don't comfort me because I don't go to them feeling as if I need to be comforted. The way I treat them is there's like a ritualistic thing.
>
> (P18: father of preterm baby)

## Major events

Many families had other major events happening in their lives which added to the fathers' unhappiness. Three lost parents through death, and one lost a grandmother. One father felt a huge sense of loss and grief when his marriage fell apart and he moved out: the loss of both his wife and his living children, coming on top of the death of his daughter, was a profoundly distressing experience. Another father had to deal with separating from the baby's mother and the death of his own mother, as well as losing the baby.

Work pressures and financial problems added to the unhappiness of several fathers. Slumps in trade, being made redundant, or having to move away from the area all added to their stresses. The father's own poor health, and suffering a mental breakdown following the baby's death, were also cited as triggers of additional sadness.

## Other people's pregnancies

News of other pregnancies and births could precipitate a sense of sadness for the fathers, although several volunteered that the feeling was usually short-lived.

> The first six months it didn't matter where you went there was a push-chair.
>
> (P13: father of baby with cardiac anomaly)

The first time he saw a new baby in his own house caught one father unawares. Another found it hurtful when other people thrust their babies at him. The attention of one father was drawn to a family he saw in a restaurant. They had a disabled child, and as he watched that child he realised that his own would have been far more incapacitated, and he felt a huge sense of sadness as this realisation hit him. More lasting sorrow was experienced when the fathers saw other couples being careless about the welfare of the fetus or baby.

### Fathers' own sense of inadequacy or powerlessness

Six fathers spoke movingly of perceived deficiencies within themselves which added to their sense of sorrow. Two of these men were very aware of the difficulty of being a good father. They were under such pressure at work that they found the demands of their small children oppressive, and they quickly became irritated with them, or they were now over-protective of their existing children, thereby limiting the scope of their activity. A young father who, in addition to this bereavement, had been forced to accept family responsibilities from an early age, felt sad about the passing of his youth; he could no longer be carefree, immature and innocently happy like his peers. Another father mourned the loss of his spirit of optimism; if this tragedy could befall his family, anything might happen. The whole experience unsettled these men, and one even concluded that the world was such a troubled place it was questionable whether it was a responsible act to bring more children into it.

### Subsequent pregnancies with their partners

Only four fathers cited elements of the next pregnancy as inducing a sense of sadness. Most of them were relieved and positive about the development. But one father regretted the shadow which lay over this new pregnancy; he and his partner could not be excited and happy as they had been last time. One mother was 'very ill' during the second pregnancy, and this had had a negative effect on her husband. Where there was a history of infertility, fathers found themselves back on the emotional roller-coaster, and one described graphically the effect of being told (falsely as it transpired) that their treatment had been unsuccessful. Coming so soon after the death of an earlier baby, this disappointment was particularly hard to bear. Similarly, when the next pregnancy was lost through miscarriage, it was yet another bereavement. When their partners did not or could not become pregnant again, the fathers faced a source of ongoing sorrow, although they were quick to point out that they suspected it was worse for the mothers to face childlessness.

### Others' sad stories

Being vulnerable in their own personal grief made some fathers more sensitive to others' sadness. They cited the tragedies which befell other parents they had encountered at SANDS group meetings or memorial services, strained or broken relationships within their families, any waste of life in wars, conflicts or acts of violence, and the needless suffering of children.

Having known sorrow themselves they now empathised more closely with the suffering of the victims of such traumas.

### Insensitivity

Just as they felt that they themselves had become more sensitive, the fathers became aware of the insensitivity of others around them. Thoughtless or flippant comments hurt and saddened them, and the actions of other people with new babies further marginalised them.

# Overall happiness/sadness 13 months after the death

In order to obtain some measure of progress, it seemed to be useful to ask parents to rate their overall sense of happiness. They were asked to imagine a scale from 1 to 10, where 1 represented sad all the time and 10 represented happy all the time. Where would they put themselves on that scale now, 13 months after the death?

Only one father rated himself higher now than he had been before this event (7 instead of 6). He said that he now felt 'better in himself', having coped with the loss. It had not adversely affected the parents' relationship, they had shown that they were strong enough to cope with such a tragedy, and they now appreciated the miracle of a healthy normal child. Had he not been suffering from sleepless nights since the birth of a new baby 8 weeks previously, he believed that he would have rated his happiness as 10 out of 10.

Two-thirds of the parents felt that overall they were now more happy than sad. In total, 31 of the 47 mothers who placed themselves on the scale (66%), and 25 of the 38 fathers who did so (66%), rated themselves above 5 out of 10. Given the exact similarity in percentage terms, this might appear to be a feature of both partners in a couple rating themselves the same. However, this was not in fact the case. More than a quarter of the mothers (28%) rated themselves as 8 or 9, while only 11% of the fathers did so. A quarter of the fathers (24%) but only 15% of the mothers rated themselves as neutral at 5. A tenth of the fathers (10%) but nearly twice that percentage of mothers (19%) rated themselves as more sad than happy (4 or below on the scale). The women's ratings appeared to be more extreme than those of the men (*see* Figure 11.1).

Some qualifying comments are needed when interpreting these results. As we have seen, the death of this child was not the only event happening in these parents' lives. Many were grappling with other major stresses in their personal and professional capacities. As one father in the legal business said, work had escalated to such an extent that he had little time even

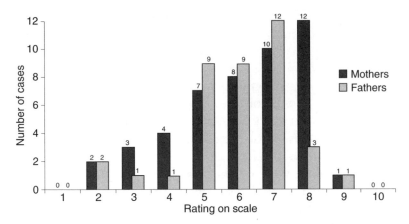

**Figure 11.1:** Parents' rating of their own happiness 13 months after the death of their child.

to think about the baby, and when he did so it was not something that made him feel very unhappy, but none the less he could only rate himself low on the scale because he felt completely swamped by responsibility and work. Where they did not spontaneously volunteer how their present rating would compare with that before the baby had died, most parents were asked how they would have rated themselves beforehand. Almost all of them concluded that they were very happy before tragedy struck, some adding that everything had gone well for them up until that point, and they would have put themselves as high as 9 or even 10 out of 10 on the scale. Some added sadly that they recognised that they could now never be totally happy again.

# Discussion

The death of a child is a profoundly sad experience which alters the lives of parents. Our findings show that it has an effect both on their relationships with family and friends and on their overall happiness for at least a year afterwards. A number of important factors emerge which have implications for the care and support of these vulnerable people.

## The baby's death does not take place in a vacuum

Parents find it difficult if assumptions are made about the baby's death being the only thing in their lives that is preoccupying their thoughts.

A sobering number of our respondents were simultaneously grappling with major life events such as the death of significant people in their family or social circle, the break-up of relationships, moving house, or violation of their property or possessions. Even fairly common events in the ensuing months can generate powerful feelings. For example, contemplation of another pregnancy involves a measure of ambivalence. Parents feel anxious about being seen to try to replace the dead child, or about whether loving one will be a betrayal of the other, or whether history will repeat itself, or whether their own relationship will withstand the strain. Where couples are also dealing with fertility problems, there are additional significant burdens which complicate the mourning process. These other factors must be added to the equation when the effects of the death are being assessed.

# Child bereavement changes parents

Grief changes people. We found that parents were very conscious of changes within themselves, and they were saddened by this 'marking' of them as different. They recognised the potential for these changes to impinge on others and alter their social circle. When they are feeling in low spirits, tearful or withdrawn, they may be less attractive to others, and normal avenues of support may be withdrawn. The world about them can also impinge on the parents and add to their burden of sorrow. They become highly sensitised to the prevalence of pregnant women and babies. Other people's children are an ongoing reminder of what they have lost, especially if their milestones coincide with those which the dead child should have shared. If the baby was one of a multiple pregnancy and there are survivors, constant comparisons will be made with what should have been.

# The loss of the baby strains the parents' relationship

In trying to deal with their profound pain, each parent struggles to get through each day in the best way they can. We found that an initial 'honeymoon' effect was common where in the early days the parents were very close as they shared intense emotions.[68] Consistent with other literature we also found that in some instances the experience served to strengthen the couple's relationship in a more enduring way,[70] but in many cases the early intimacy was followed by a subsequent deterioration in the relationship.[68,69] Their own intense anguish and their wish to spare their partner further hurt could lead each to withdraw from the other to some extent at a time when both were in need of comfort and support. The fact that men and women react differently to events in general as well as to grief explains some of the differences we uncovered. We shall discuss these in some detail, as problems with relationships are clearly common and any illumination of the causes may contribute to a solution.

In his assessment of gender comparisons, Gray has concluded that one of the biggest differences is to be seen in the relative approaches of men and women to stress.[187] 'Men become increasingly focused and with-drawn,' and they 'tend to pull away and silently think about what's bother-ing them.' Women, on the other hand, 'become increasingly overwhelmed and emotionally involved' and they 'feel an instinctive need to talk about what's bothering them.' As a result, 'he feels better by solving problems, while she feels better by talking about problems.'

Tannen has summed up the position slightly differently, but the conclu-sion is essentially the same.[136] In the male world, 'conversations are nego-tiations in which people try to achieve and maintain the upper hand if they can, and protect themselves from others' attempts to put them down and push them around. Life, then, is a contest, a struggle to preserve indepen-dence and avoid failure.' Women, on the other hand, approach the world 'as an individual in a network of connections. In this world, conversations are negotiations for closeness in which people try to seek and give confir-mation and support.' Men are essentially problem-solvers and see little merit in going over and over something which cannot be changed. For women, talking about a problem is a bid for an expression of understand-ing, or is intended to reinforce a sense of identification or a shared experi-ence. When they do not receive this reinforcement they are frustrated and distanced from the person who appears to be saying, 'You have the pro-blems, I have the solutions.' Such behaviours are learned as children and reinforced as young adults: 'for girls, talk is the glue that holds relationships together. Boys' relationships are held together primarily by activities.'

At a time when a man and a woman are each mourning their dead child, each being vulnerable and in need of support, these essential differences may create obstacles. There is ample evidence that parents grieve differ-ently.[36,60,61,63,64,71,188,189] Our findings corroborate these differences. Men tend to hide their grief in order to protect their partners and live up to soci-ety's perceived expectations of them, plunging back into work and appear-ing controlled and strong.[174] Paradoxically, women tend to find it hurtful when their male partners do not share their feelings and emotions.[71] When they need one another most they can find that the other is unavail-able as they each withdraw into their own private world of grief. There is little confirmation or reassurance to be gained from the person closest to the other's grief. Attempts to support the other may increase distress rather than ease it, because each is trying to support the other in the way that they themselves would wish to be supported. For example, presenting the woman with the suggestion that she should get out of the house and go back to work, which the father has found helpful, may merely serve to tell the mother that her partner has forgotten about the baby and is now absorbed in other matters. Well-intentioned efforts on the mother's part to try to get the male partner to share his feelings and thus ease his pain may be counter-productive, as this only upsets him more. However, persisting in these misunderstandings perpetuates the problem: 'the risk of ignoring differences is greater than the danger of naming them. Sweeping something big under the rug doesn't make it go away; it trips you up and sends you sprawling when you venture across the room.'[136] The reality of these gender differences must be acknowledged and the understanding of them used to good effect. A catalyst may be needed to free the parents to express their own emotions and needs without the inhibition produced by the pressure to be supportive of the other parent.

## The loss may also change other relationships

Because they are singled out as different, and because they are now themselves changed people, bereaved parents find that relationships with other people are affected. Much depends on the strength and nature of the existing bonds. We found that parents became less tolerant of trivia and insincerity, and valued the sensitivity which allowed them to grieve in their own way. It is important to note that parents cannot always predict sources of empathic understanding. Just because a person has experienced a similar loss does not necessarily mean that they are more sensitive to others' need. The relationships which blossom in these circumstances are those which arise from a genuine sympathy and response to the parents' own cues.

## A new pregnancy changes the parents' focus

Over half of the parents in our study became pregnant again within the first year. Concern has been expressed about the possible adverse effects of embarking on another pregnancy soon after a perinatal loss.[190] Vulnerability to depression and anxiety has been seen to be a potential problem. However, there may be overriding psychological reasons for embarking rapidly on another pregnancy which make it the right course of action.[152,184,191,192] The timing has to be a personal decision.

It was clear that for the majority of the parents whom we interviewed, the next pregnancy represented an important positive step in the grieving process. A new baby brings hope for the future, it offers distraction from grief, and it establishes the capacity of the parents to parent successfully. It is important to emphasise the parents' own awareness – this child is not a replacement for the earlier one, and their absorption in this new life does not mean that they have forgotten the life and death of the sibling. Rather it indicates that they are accepting their loss as part of life's experience and moving on by living with it.

However, it must be remembered that for over a quarter of these families the next pregnancy did not have a happy outcome. We have reported six pregnancies lost, and one child born with serious problems. The principal researcher also heard from three other couples after the 13-month interview who had suffered further losses of pregnancies ($n = 1$) or babies ($n = 2$). The effect of this additional pain on these families has to be balanced against the happiness of those who went on to have a positive experience.

# Other children in the family can be a source of solace

Other children in the family were identified as a major source of comfort in the parents' sorrow. They forced the parents to get up in the morning and get on with the routines of daily living, they made the parents smile, they reassured them that they could be successful parents, and they encouraged the adults to socialise. However, feelings are ambivalent, too. The parents' own relationship sometimes suffers where there are other children, and we found that a disproportionate number of families experienced this. Fathers may feel excluded, parents may have little time for each other, each parent may resent the other's approach to the siblings, regarding it as too protective or overly indulgent, and the persistent demands of the children may be irritating when tolerance levels are impaired.

Particular difficulties attach to survivors of a multiple pregnancy, and those who care for the surviving children must be sensitive to this danger. The demands of parenting and the repeated exhortations to be strong for and appreciate the existing babies may rob the parents of space to grieve.[193] Every happiness and every development with the survivor has a reverse emotion because the dead child cannot reach that point. Simultaneously celebrating and grieving is a difficult experience which requires careful management and an awareness that one baby does not compensate for another.

# Planning and working towards short-term objectives is helpful

Our findings show that for many parents, events such as holidays, moving house, redecorating the home, or special projects are helpful ploys when moving through the grieving process. They do not work for everyone and as we have seen some parents abandon any efforts to escape the pain recognising that wherever they go and whatever they do it remains with them. However, the impression was conveyed that parents welcome a staged approach to grieving. If they have a short-term goal, it helps them to view the future in a limited way, rather than facing the yawning void of the rest of life without the child. Part of this is due to the fact that they are kept occupied and their thoughts are partially distracted from their grief. By forcing themselves to be productive, they have less time to sit absorbed in melancholic thoughts, and this in turn helps them to survive the sadness. Mothers who are not yet ready to return to work or who are housewives find these bursts of activity help to structure their day and give them purpose. Almost all of the men we interviewed were in paid employment, and our findings suggest that work is a therapeutic means of coping for them, even though it may provide only temporary distraction from their sorrow.[174] It is a coping strategy not always available to their partners.

# Anniversaries and special dates may be particularly difficult for both parents

Remembering events which occurred a year previously is clearly a source of sorrow for parents. They recall detail with impressive clarity. Anniversaries of the birth and death of the baby are sad reminders of what they have lost and can never joyously celebrate. Events which are normally associated with celebration and happiness, such as Christmas and New Year, are now occasions which highlight their unhappiness.

It is significant that the women in our study were often unaware of the impact of these events on the fathers. However, many men, even those who find remembering any dates difficult, are in reality sad around the time of the anniversaries. They do not always tell their partners that they have visited the grave or wept or commemorated the event privately in some way. This seems to be a feature of their double wish not to talk about their emotions and not to upset the mother further. But listening to their own accounts of the pain they felt on seeing another pram like the one they had chosen, hearing a certain song, removing baby clothes or getting them out again, seeing another new baby in their house, watching a child in a restaurant, or weeping alone at a grave is eloquent testament to the fact that they have not forgotten.

The fathers in our study identified a significant difference in their mourning. They see the mothers as grieving for the loss of a baby, whereas they themselves are mourning the loss of a child and everyday occurrences such as another father sharing in activities with his children are poignant reminders of all that they have lost. Just because they do not share these intense emotions does not mean that their reactions should be denied. Additionally for the fathers there can be a haunting sense of powerlessness. They see it as their role to protect their family. However, they have been unable to defend this child against the greatest possible harm, a harm which has robbed him or her of life itself. This sense occurs in circumstances where no one could have prevented the tragedy, but running alongside their feeling of personal loss, it contributes to their silence about their deepest feelings.

# The parents will always have a shadow over their lives, but most progress through their grieving successfully

We found that almost all of the parents whom we interviewed at 13 months were now more sad than they had been before this loss. This is to be expected, and their belief that a shadow would always linger is understandable. The fact that they will never have an easy answer to a simple question such as, 'How many children have you got?' highlights the ongoing sorrow they must accept. However, what is heartening is the finding that by 13 months after the death, two-thirds of the parents were already more happy than they were sad. The mothers' emotions tend to be more extreme in both directions than those of the fathers, but it seems that even a year on most parents are accepting the loss and moving forward in their grieving.

# Conclusion

- Carers must be aware that bereaved parents may be grappling with other major life events as well as the death of their child.
- Grief changes people and may affect relationships, resulting in a limitation of the support that is available to parents at a time of great need.

- Men and women grieve differently, and parents may need help to understand their partner's ways of coping.
- Subsequent pregnancies and babies give parents hope for the future, but appropriate timing depends on their own circumstances.
- Existing children may be a source of solace, but may have a detrimental effect on the parents' own relationship.
- Planning for future events helps parents to move forward in the grieving process.
- Although particular dates such as anniversaries may be difficult for both parents, fathers may not voice their emotions to the mothers.
- Most parents accept their loss and begin to move forward towards a positive approach within the first year of bereavement.

# CHAPTER 12

# Support in bereavement

Grief can seem quite overwhelming following the death of a baby, and parents are shocked at the depth of sadness they experience, worrying that they will never ever feel any better.

> *Mother*: Numb. It felt as if your world had just shut.
> *Father*: I think the hurt and the anger that you feel when you lose a child, you actually have to go through it yourself to understand. You can't describe the level of it . . . I can't say it's worse than [losing someone adult you're close to] because people's perceptions of loss and human pain vary. But I lost two of my best friends in a car crash when I was living with them, and I never felt pain like that in all my life until [the baby]. The pain is so [intense] . . . I'll never feel as [terrible] as I did when we lost [the baby] – never in my life will I feel so bad and so low. And I would have quite happily stuck a tube in my exhaust and taken myself away and I've *never* been one for feeling that way . . . but I would quite happily have done it, if it hadn't been for my other daughters and [my wife]. I'm describing it as hurt, pain and all that – I'm *trying* to describe it but I can't get anywhere near it.
>
> (P 35: parents of preterm triplets)

As time goes by parents sometimes measure their progress in terms of accomplishing small steps – being able to go out and speak to people again, being able to bring the baby naturally into conversation without crying, being able to visit a new mother and baby, or feeling ready to hold a new baby. As one multiply bereaved person put it, 'If I can't see the light at the end of the tunnel, I'll string lights along the way.'[194] Aware of the difficulty people have in knowing what is the best approach to take at this time, we set out to ascertain from the parents themselves what, in their case, was or was not supportive at different stages of the grieving process.

Both their needs and the strength of support changed over time. In order to capture the sense of progression and the differences as well as the similarities, we shall report the data first for the early weeks and then for the rest of the year. Inevitably in places this will appear repetitious, but to merge the information would be to lose an important element of the process over the months following the death and beyond the first anniversary.

# Supportive people in the early weeks following the death

Only nine sets of parents (15%) felt that they had had no outside support in the period immediately following the death. The remainder cited a variety of sources of help. Lay support came from friends ($n = 35$ sets of parents, 59%), grandparents ($n = 24$, 41%), other family members ($n = 19$, 32%), other children ($n = 18$, 31%), work colleagues ($n = 15$, 25%), bereavement groups ($n = 7$, 12%), neighbours ($n = 5$, 8%) and church members ($n = 2$, 3%). Professional support was provided by healthcare professionals ($n = 24$, 41%), bereavement counsellors ($n = 7$, 12%) and ministers ($n = 2, 3\%$).

# Helpful factors in the first few months

One mother summed up the sentiments of many: 'This horror never leaves you; you learn to live alongside it.' But some things have the capacity to comfort and others have the potential to exacerbate the hurt. Needs vary from one individual to another, and the important message conveyed by these bereaved families is that other people should take their cue from the parents themselves. However, certain clear messages emerged which provide useful indicators as to how people may be sensitive to parents' needs. In order to offer some yardsticks we shall report these matters in some detail.

Everyone could identify something which they had found helpful in the early weeks following the death of the baby. It is important to remember that this was an open question, and the parents were not guided in their thinking by the interviewer, so where a clear consensus emerged the message is powerful.

# Professional support

The contribution of professional staff is different from that expected of lay people, so the support which parents value from this source will be considered separately. Of the 24 sets of parents who cited healthcare professionals as supportive in the early weeks after their loss, most identified the hospital staff, and in all cases except one (where the ward sister had visited) this was limited to the NICU team. A small number of families had surviving babies in the NICU, and they found it helpful to have an opportunity to reminisce with the staff in a meaningful way about the child who had died.

> The staff bring their names [those of the dead triplets] into the conversation. They haven't forgotten. And it's a big comfort to *know* they haven't forgotten.
>
> (P12: mother of preterm triplets)

These were people who were sensitive to the changing moods of the parents, sympathising when they were down, and comforting and cheering them as necessary. With them the parents could be natural, knowing that a laugh would not be construed as disloyalty to the dead child, and sadness would need no explanation.

> There were nurses there, they weren't just there for the [babies], they were there for us as well. It could only have been a few weeks [after the funeral], they would see what sort of a mood we were in. If we were down they'd try to pick us up. If we were up they'd try and keep us there. If it was appropriate to laugh we laughed, and to begin with at first you felt really guilty about laughing. You thought, 'It's been two weeks since [the baby] died, what have I got to laugh about?' And then we thought, 'We've still got another two girls, we *should* still be smiling and laughing' . . . They were really good and you felt a sense that they were there for us as well, and that we're really important to how the girls do as well.
>
> (P35: father of preterm triplets)

In one case the parents were comforted when the staff sent letters as from the survivors saying that the babies missed the dead sibling. However, it was hard then if contact ceased abruptly when the survivors went home, as this source of support was removed.

> As soon as [the surviving twin] came off it [the oxygen], I was on my own . . . Nobody's been in contact. And I just felt on my own. Personally, the way I was and the way I felt in having a new baby home, coping with oxygen, trying to cope with grieving, I just found it very hard . . . I coped

but there were times when I wasn't [coping] – times when I wanted to scream and break down but I couldn't because I still had [the surviving twin] and everybody kept saying – even my Mum – 'You've got [the surviving] baby to think about.' I just felt because there was twins it was so much harder than losing a [singleton] child ... [if they had come] just occasionally rather than be at a place for four months of your life – four months going through ups and downs and traumas day after day, day in, day out [and then nothing] ... but I just feel that once I got [the baby] home, nobody was as interested. You were just another notch in the day.

(P10: mother of preterm twins)

This mother's partner, however, perceived things rather differently, seeing a benefit to reduced contact. (It is important to note that, as the mother pointed out, the father was out at work all day, and she was the one left alone with the baby.)

There should be maybe somebody set aside – whose job it is ... maybe there could be somebody that gets [involved with you]. It might be somebody who's actually got an involvement with the Unit, who actually knows you as well. I don't think it would be right having somebody who doesn't know you ... but I personally think that when you come home you're left to it and sometimes you get on a lot better. Sometimes with people coming in you think maybe they're meddling a bit. That's my personal opinion. I'd just like to get on myself, and just battle on and if I am struggling then I would talk to [my wife] about it.

(P10: father of preterm twins)

Even where there were no surviving children, parents sometimes found it helpful to maintain contact with the NICU staff. In the early weeks they were uniquely placed to be supportive, as they had known the baby better than anyone.

*Father*: It's difficult for me right now to look back on her life and not get upset. But I suppose as time goes on I'll start to see the good things that have come out of it. In a way it's therapeutic for me to be able to keep in touch with some of the friends that we made at that time as well. I don't want to turn my back on it.
*Mother*: After [us] the staff up there were the people who knew [the baby] best. They knew her far better than our families did.

(P51: parents of baby with congenital anomalies)

In two cases a neonatal nurse had visited the parents after they had left the hospital, and this was seen as especially supportive because these nurses had been part of this profound experience, sharing memories and emotions with the family. Periodic socialising with selected members of the healthcare team helped two other families, easing their 'withdrawal symptoms.' However, most parents cited written contact as the means by which hospital staff offered support. They particularly appreciated cards and messages which mentioned special features about the baby.

> The cards that we got from the nurses – they'd actually write a letter and say what they remembered about her and what was special about her . . . they were far more touching and meant so much more because they actually talked about [the baby] as a real person, because they knew her – they'd got more they could say about her than [family].
>
> (P 51: father of baby with congenital anomalies)

A letter from a NICU doctor requesting that the father be given time off work had been a useful gesture for another family.

Staff working in the community were also mentioned. Nine parents cited their GP as helpful, coming to see them (in one instance several times) and listening sympathetically to their story, and in one case reassuring them about the health of a surviving baby. Some GPs were instrumental in bringing forward follow-up appointments or answering questions about the baby. One made a special point of visiting on the baby's expected date of delivery, and was perceived as very sensitive to the parents' needs, caring about how they were coping.

Three families had been supported by their health visitors (HV), with one mother specifying that the HV had gone to the NICU to obtain information on her behalf. Five others cited the community midwives. In one case the mother said that it helped just to know that someone would be coming each day and they would be able to talk about what had happened; the midwife just 'said the right things.'

The remaining factors which were identified relate to ways in which lay people were seen to be supportive.

# Opportunities for parents to talk about the baby and their experience

The single most overwhelming need that was expressed was for parents to be able to talk about the baby. Most couples initially talked together about the experience and shared their emotions. For some this meant overcoming inhibitions, but it had been worth the effort.

> Take any opportunity to share any strong feelings, frustrations with each other. Don't bottle it up. If you need to talk about it just talk about

it. Bottling it up is just not going to get you anywhere. I've learned that – because I'm a bit of a bottler. I don't speak about things – I don't find it easy. Whereas [my wife] is very much a talker. So therefore she brings that out in me. But it's true, a thought shared ... the fact that you've talked about it means that thought was then shelved, it doesn't linger on and rumble on. That's why we've got over it relatively quickly.

(P44: father of preterm quads)

However, as we have noted earlier, as time went on couples not infrequently found it difficult to talk together about this experience. When they were not emotionally available to each other it was important for them each to be free to find other listening ears.

[You should] allow the other person [your partner] to speak to who they need to speak to. I speak an awful lot to my friend but [my partner] doesn't speak to his at all, he only speaks to me. And that's fine. The only thing is that there's been a couple of hiccups with that – I am quite an open person and I do talk a lot to my friends and he was saying, because we're trying again, 'I don't want you to tell anybody until you're about three or four months pregnant or whatever. We shouldn't tell anybody.' I said, 'I *need* to tell people because I'm so excited about it, so scared about it, that I *have* to. If you don't want to tell anybody, fine,' ... but for him to expect me to bottle that up is too much. I just know that I couldn't. It would do me harm to do that, because I'd be really stressed. And if something does go wrong I would need them there anyway... and you have to be strong enough to say that because it would have been very easy for me just to say, 'Well, OK then, we won't,' and suffer on my own. But when it's something as big as this you have to be quite selfish and take what you need and do what you have to do. And if it means drifting apart a little bit, then ... if you're strong enough you'll drift back together.

(P45: mother of preterm baby)

Almost all parents acknowledged this need to talk, with only three fathers at this early stage saying that they preferred people not to mention the subject.

The difference [between us] is that [my wife] will want to talk to people about things, but I won't. My approach to these kinds of things is that I'll deal with them; I don't care about what anybody else thinks. I don't need anyone else to tell me what to think. Because I feel I have to take personal responsibility for everything to do with that [experience with the baby]) I don't get any comfort from anyone else saying, 'I understand how you're feeling,' or anything like that. That just washes over me.

I don't need it and I don't expect people to come and necessarily offer it. I know that if I want any help from anyone I can go and ask for it. Because of the way I feel, I wouldn't necessarily come across as being very sensitive to someone else's viewpoint – [My wife] would expect someone to come and offer whereas I don't. If you want any [help], you ask. If people were coming to my door and saying, 'What can I do to help?', I'd feel like saying, 'Get lost. It's a private matter for me; you're just intruding. If I want you I'll come and ask.' That's really the difference between the two of us.

(P18: father of preterm baby)

For the majority of parents it was important to go over and over their story and to have people listen attentively. They valued listeners who could cope with powerful emotion and not feel the need to change the subject, turn away or offer hollow platitudes. Where the baby had lived for some time and the parents had real memories of the child as an individual, it helped them to recall events and weep and laugh together about them. However, many of these babies had had only very short lives, and few relatives or friends had even seen them. Indeed, some of the parents commented that at times it was hard even for them to believe that this event had taken place. Consequently, those people who had shared part of the baby's life and/or death were in the special position of being able to reminisce with the parents and discuss details and perceptions, a factor which parents found especially reassuring, confirming as it did the reality of their experience. Any acknowledgement of the importance of this baby in the parents' lives and affections was welcomed. Where the child's existence or the tragedy were seen to have impinged on the lives of others as well, the sense of the baby's value was increased.

For some parents it helped, too, when other people were not afraid to introduce the subject of the baby spontaneously, naturally and appropriately.

Somebody else had a baby at the weekend. The baby arrived on the day it was due. Somebody said, 'Oh that's very rare.' And my friend said, 'Oh, that happened with your two.' And that was the first time that anybody had talked about [the baby who died] so naturally. It meant so much to me that somebody could mention that I had two children without it being a sad thing. It really did. It made me feel happy. She has no idea how much I appreciated it.

(P27: mother of baby with cardiac anomaly)

Genuine interest and concern were appreciated.

You bump into people who've never met you before and you never bring up the subject because you know how awkward they'll feel, but of course

they ask the question, 'Have you got any children?'. . . I start crying [and
they say], 'Oh, I'm so sorry. Anyway I'll shut up now.' That annoys me.
That really gets on my nerves. I hate when they say, 'Oh, I'll be quiet
about it then'. . . I can understand that they might feel awkward, but
then I want them to ask questions. When we went away [on holiday]
there was this woman who said, 'If you don't mind me asking, what
happened?'. . . It was nice for somebody to be interested . . . people think
that if they don't mention it they're not going to hurt you and to me that
hurts me even more if they don't mention it, because it feels as though
they don't care.

[P58: mother of preterm baby]

Sensitivity came from knowing the parents well enough to interpret their
cues accurately. As one father said, he could feel safe with old friends who
would let him express his thoughts about the baby; only with them could
he lose his inhibitions and talk about this deep hurt.

If friends or relatives possessed special skills they could be particularly
useful. For example, parents felt that they could talk to individuals who
held healthcare professional qualifications about the medical side of the
experience and ask questions or seek confirmation. One mother was comforted by a spiritualist friend who gave her hope that the baby's spirit lived on.

Eight parents from seven families mentioned that a bereavement counsellor had been helpful at this stage. Seven of these parents were mothers
and only one was a father. Those who were in receipt of counselling spoke
warmly of the support they derived from talking about their experience,
gaining insights into their difficulties and being helped to move on.

Many parents commented on the helpfulness of the interview in that it
provided a forum for them to talk about the baby intensively.

We needed something like this [interview] tonight. Like you're doing.
Just somebody to talk to. You've actually helped us probably more than
you know even though you're saying we're helping you. But you're helping us. We've spoken about it. We've gone right through it again which
we've never done. Somebody to do that. We've never sat and done what
we've done tonight – gone through it from day 1 – together, too. We've
never ever done it.

(P38: father of baby with congenital anomalies)

Parents were aware of the potential to 'bore' people with their repeated
story, and they welcomed the opportunity to recount the whole story to
someone who was genuinely interested. We shall return to the effect of participating in the research in more detail in a later section.

# Shared experiences

Parents who had themselves been bereaved were in a unique position to be supportive. Many respondents spoke appreciatively of the bonds which developed through sharing a common grief. Other people might *say* that they knew what the parents were going through, but the parents were irritated by such comments. Those who really *did* know could provide a depth of understanding and reassurance that no one else could. Indeed, in some cases such sharing of stories brought unexpected comfort – they could be glad that they themselves had had precious time with the baby, and that the baby had died peacefully, had not suffered, and had not survived to face a life of severe disability.

# Sensitive expressions of sympathy

Almost all parents valued sincere expressions of sympathy. Many observed that it was better to stumble over words and acknowledge inadequacy in this situation than to avoid or ignore the parents or the subject of their loss.

> I felt that people maybe don't write a letter because they just don't know what to say. They feel awkward, and they just say, 'What can I say? What can I do?' So they'd send a card, 'Thinking of you,' or whatever. But you felt that you appreciated people taking out time – it is awkward for people – and I was interested to read the letters and just to feel that it *is* difficult, but they have managed it.
>
> (P6: father of baby with congenital anomalies)

Family members provided support by being there for the parents, understanding the significance of this child in the family, and mourning the loss for themselves as well as for the parents. Grandparents were the most frequently cited family members who rallied to the support of the parents at this time. Again reactions varied, with some appreciative of the unconditional love and care of their own parents, others finding the grandparents' expressions of strong grief difficult to bear, and yet others helped by the necessity to be strong for other relatives. The grandparents provided support in practical as well as emotional ways, ensuring that the parents were fed, packing away baby things, visiting frequently and taking the parents out. One young father found his own parents helpful in explaining the behaviour of his partner, who was acting uncharacteristically in response to her loss.

Two families spoke warmly of the special help that was provided by other female relatives who had experience of counselling. However, there was a tendency in some families for the relatives to swamp the parents with attention and sympathy, and a few commented that the most supportive act had been for them to withdraw, giving the parents space to grieve in private.

Practical help which relieved parents of responsibilities and pressures was also valued as a genuine expression of sympathy. Examples included neighbours bringing meals, people taking children out, and friends accompanying the parent to potentially stressful events, walking the dog, or providing food. In two cases they listened sympathetically, and in another case they shared an experience of loss. Two mothers were invited to be involved with these neighbours' children, and they were comforted and supported by this sensitive response to their need.

Sympathetic work colleagues helped parents to integrate back into the work-force. When bosses gave time off work, paid the fathers while they were off, or arranged matters sensitively to help the parents to ease back into their jobs, the family was grateful. Concrete evidence of sensitivity to their pain and ongoing sorrow was appreciated – for example, colleagues adjusting work patterns to the moods and needs of the parents, and being flexible in response to their fluctuating emotions. If the parents had previously found colleagues awkward or unfeeling, these marks of sympathy were particularly valued. Again a number of parents had experienced a deep level of support from colleagues who had themselves lost children. Colleagues and friends could also help the parents to integrate back into their social circle as they felt ready to do so.

## Keeping busy

Hard work provided solace for many parents especially fathers, who said that they could forget their pain and sorrow for a while when they were immersed in work, although one father recognised a danger in always being busy.

> I can very easily get lost in doing things and [when relatives took over the household tasks] that certainly gave me the space not to do them and to be able to just be and feel and for us to be together without me diverting myself into being busy.
>
> (P49: father of baby with asphyxia)

The discipline of paid employment forced them to concentrate on other things, and if work was busy the days slipped by leaving little opportunity for their unhappiness to reach overwhelming proportions. Some fathers also found that it helped them if they were able to do things to protect their partners from hurt, such as ringing people to let them know what had happened, fielding questions about how they were coping, or carrying out tasks outside the home so that the mother did not have to face people.

For those women who spent most of their time at home, it was all too easy to dwell on the tragedy, and some said that initially they could not galvanise themselves into action even to perform the usual routine household chores. However, recognising this potential, some mothers deliberately took steps to try to keep things in perspective – for example, by undertaking exacting or exhausting new projects, planning for future events, disciplining themselves to go out and face the challenges of everyday life, keeping a diary, or expressing their emotions in poetry or prose.

# Other children

As we have seen, parents who had other children spoke eloquently of the enormous help they were in the recovery process. Just holding them was soothing. It was reassuring to have tangible confirmation that they could produce healthy normal children. The children themselves forced the parents to carry on the normal everyday routines. Their engaging ways made the parents smile again, distracting their attention away from the pain for a time, and their demands forced the parents to resume normal activities. Small children's artless chatter about the dead sibling helped them to integrate the baby's existence into the family's on-going lives, and older children's maturity and support comforted them. They gave the parents permission to laugh again, to play and to look forward. One mother noted a palpable difference in the support group she attended – she observed that first-time mothers took the loss much harder.

One mother added that in the early weeks she had worried that her sadness might be adversely affecting her older child. The little girl's life should have been totally happy at such a young age, she thought, and she was anxious that a significant part of it might be blanked out by the effects of this tragedy. She resolved actively to work at being happy and positive when she was with the child, and she found that the effort helped her personally to move forward.

# Drugs

A small number of parents (both mothers and fathers) took medication, such as antidepressants, to help them through the early weeks or months of their bereavement. Two mothers and one father said that they had returned to hard drugs to blot out the pain.

# Additional factors

One or two parents cited other factors which they had found helpful, and these are listed both to acknowledge their role in some cases and to raise awareness of their potential. Actively commemorating the loss helped some – for example, visiting the grave or assembling mementoes. Reading about grief and loss was beneficial for one mother, although she was then annoyed that her husband had to be forced to read books on bereavement which she had found so useful in understanding the grief process. Trying to escape the memories was a tactic attempted by some parents, by taking breaks away, but this often met with limited success.

Although no parent actually cited legal redress as a helpful factor, two sets of parents were going down this route in their search for answers. A small number of others said that they were either already talking with lawyers or contemplating doing so in order to establish whether or not they had a case.

# Unhelpful factors in the first few months

All except two sets of parents could cite events which had added to their pain and hurt soon after the death. As before, remarkably consistent messages were conveyed by the parents, even though the question was quite open. A number of factors were cited time and time again in various forms, and these are itemised before more idiosyncratic points are listed.

# Ignoring or avoiding parents or the subject of their loss

This was by far the most commonly cited hurtful experience. Professional silence hurt them, and a need for ongoing contact sometimes resurfaced many months after the death.

> I would have liked some kind of contact at the six months point, for that is the time when you definitely go off your head. I think that is the time that things begin to kick in, start to raise things. It's a time when maybe you're going back to work, having to face things, maybe starting to go out socialising, that kind of thing. That's when you're starting to filter the whole process right through . . . somebody just to say, 'Look, I realise it's six months, do you want to come for a cup of tea? Anything I can do?' Just something . . . for the first six months people expect you to be kind of

weird anyway, kind of off the wall, but after that people expect you to be better. There's, 'Well, you're six months down the line, you're back at work, you're driving a car, you're going shopping, you're on a night out.' They expect you to be better when inside you're just screaming . . . yes, I would say [it needs] somebody to make contact with you.

(P15: mother of preterm baby)

For one mother there was an additional aspect – a feeling that she was being 'ignored' by the hospital – which troubled her greatly. She had serious questions about what had happened during labour and she was unhappy about being excluded from professional meetings set up to enquire into the death. Since the subject of the enquiry was her baby, she felt that she should have been party to what was discussed. As a consequence, not only did she not have answers to her questions, but she also feared a cover-up. She felt that her only recourse was to take up the matter with a lawyer.

It was distressing, too, when lay people avoided or ignored the parents altogether. As far as one father was concerned, people should say something about what had happened at the first encounter with the parents, and if they let that opportunity go they could never make up for it with him. The avoidance had special significance for these families, because in ignoring the parents these people also denied the existence of the baby.

I hated the thought that it would just be ignored because in a way to ignore speaking to me was to ignore that she existed. And I really felt that extremely strongly.

(P46: mother of baby with brain damage)

We got [the chaplain] to say at the service, 'Don't walk by them in the street. If you see them speak to them. It's a part of their life and it's always going to be a part of their life.'

(P21: father of baby with cardiac anomaly)

However, they did recognise that it was not easy for people to approach them. In the early weeks after their loss, parents were often upset by any mention of the baby, and they frequently saw people withdrawing from them because they were embarrassed or upset. But it was their withdrawal which was hurtful, not their sympathy.

A lot of people that are close to us – and [my husband's] like that with me on a lot of occasions as well – they all show that they're walking along on eggshells because they're frightened in case they say the wrong thing and I get upset. I try to explain to them, 'If I get upset it's only part of grieving, I have to at one point get it out. If you won't let me get it out I can never come to terms with it.' Both of us know that we'll never forget [the baby] and we'll never forget what's happened and the pain'll probably never ever go away, but through time we'll learn to accept it and come to terms with it. But everybody's got to allow us to do that, in our own time, instead of forcing us to accept it or walking around on eggshells and not talking about it.

(P23: mother of preterm baby with congenital anomalies)

A small number of parents said that they resented having to be watchful or protective of others at this time. When people changed the subject or switched off and stopped listening, the parents felt that their experience was diminished.

I feel that when I'm out if I see somebody, I'm over-[bright and breezy]. But I feel I've got to be like that or they're scared to say anything to me. When I bump into people I don't want them to avoid [the subject of the baby]. They'll say to me, 'How are you doing?' And I say, 'Well, you know. I've got a bad day and a worse day at the moment.' And that gets them talking. I feel I've got to say something before they can. [You give them a cue]. But I only say that to some people, not all people.

(P 38: mother of baby with congenital anomalies)

Other parents were crushed when people were preoccupied with their own affairs and ignored the parents' tragedy, dwelling instead on their own children or their own troubles. In the initial stages of their grief the parents had little space for any one else's experiences. Still others resented people trying to push them into doing things for which they were not ready. All of these behaviours appeared to be ignoring their grief.

# False comfort or belittling comments

The second most commonly cited factor for parents was that of having their experience belittled. So many parents commented that losing a precious baby was the worst thing they could ever imagine having to face, and it was cruel when people diminished the enormity of their loss.

I know now they were just nervous, but at the time I was just so angry and I thought they'd better just keep out of my road! I know now they're just scared about what to say and then that's what they do, they say the wrong thing.

(P8: mother of preterm twins)

Examples included people telling them that they could easily have another child, or that they should be grateful for the child they already had, that it was no worse than a miscarriage, that they had not really had time to get to know the child so it could not be too bad, and that they would soon get over it.

> One thing that is horrible that some people keep saying is, 'Oh well, you're young. There's still plenty of time to have more.' And that is one of the worst things that you can say to somebody that's lost a baby, because it's not *another* baby you want, it's your *dead* baby you want back. Age is nothing to do with it. Another baby will never replace [the baby we lost].
>
> (P9: mother of baby with cardiac anomaly)

> You venture down the street and people say the stupidest things – out of kindness but ... I'm so tired of hearing, 'It wasn't meant to be,' and all these horrible clichés. You feel like screaming at people, 'Says who? Who says it wasn't meant to be?' ... and then if they don't say anything you think just as bad of them, I suppose.
>
> (P15: parents of preterm baby)

It seemed fairly common, too, for people to say that they knew what parents were going through. The parents were adamant that unless they had been through this experience themselves, others could not even begin to imagine how bad it was.

> So many people have actually said the stupidest things to us. The worst thing is, 'I know how you feel.' And I'm [thinking], 'No, no, *no*! You'll never know how I feel until you've held your baby in your arms till he takes his last breath. You'll never *ever* know how I feel.'
>
> (P 56: father of preterm baby with congenital anomalies)

# Hurtful comments

A few parents recounted specific comments which they had found particularly cruel. The first time one mother went out she was stopped by someone who asked a most hurtful question.

> I thought, 'If I stay away from [everybody], shut myself off, the gossip, the talk will all have finished by the time I venture out. They can think and they can say what they like.' But then, the very first time I went out, I was stopped and they asked me, 'How much of his brain did he have missing?' That was *my very first* experience of being out on my own ... I often felt when I went down the town I was like a fluorescent light – I would stand out in a crowd because of what had happened. That's what I had felt ... I mean I'm nobody, but at that time I was everybody.
>
> (P 20: mother of baby with asphyxia)

Another mother was told that it must be 'nice to have so much time' on her hands. One father spoke of people telling him that they were 'fed up hearing about the baby.' A mother who took active steps to get on with life and be happy for her existing child said that it was cruel and undermining to be advised by someone that it would take her years to get over her loss, and that she probably never would. Some of these experiences might seem blatantly insensitive to the reader. It is salutary, then, to listen to the mother who cited as hurtful receiving cards with messages about 'looking back on her memories.' She had none, so this was a cruel reminder for her. These parents are very vulnerable, and their heightened sensitivity must be borne in mind.

# Rocking of security

When tragedy has befallen a family, they are only too aware of the insecurity of life. It was further undermining to the parents' confidence to be reminded that other bad experiences might lie in store. Hearing of others' failure to resolve their grief, of repeated obstetric failures or losses, or of catastrophes at different stages of childbearing made them anxious about their own childbearing future. Stories of the high incidence of break-up of relationships following infant deaths also added to their burden.

# Swamping attention

It was unhelpful to be swamped with attention and to have too much probing and too many questions.

> If I needed people they'd be right there, but I don't like to bother anybody. I'll [soldier] on and I'll get through this my way. And my way of dealing with it has been on my own. I was just never being given that opportunity. I was being suffocated. They were at my door, they were shouting through the answering machine, they would not leave me alone. It was horrendous. We had 18 messages one day. I couldn't even go to the toilet, I couldn't make a cup of tea. There were people at the door shouting through the letter box – just needing a cuddle. I didn't *want* to cuddle anybody. I just wanted to be on my own ... I was given tablets from the doctor but I didn't want to take them ... If I was just given space to deal with it the way I wanted to, I would get there.
>
> (P20: mother of baby with asphyxia)

Most of the parents who cited this item referred to grandparents who did not give them enough space to grieve in private, who were often weepy themselves and who were extremely sensitive about the subject of their grandchild. But one mother said that she felt overwhelmed by relative strangers who were too curious, probing for more and more detail. Another mother commented that whilst it had been warming to have everyone caring and concerned initially, there came a point when it was not helpful for them to keep asking how she was coping. She was now trying to get on with life and did not need to be constantly reminded of her sorrow.

# Ignoring of fathers' grief

Fathers were frequently overlooked. Nine specifically mentioned their irritation or hurt when people asked about the mother but not about them.

> I found that people would ask and you'd have to tell them, 'Bad news, I'm afraid.' And then they'd say, 'How's [your wife]? How's she getting on? Is she doing all right?' More than once I felt like saying, 'Well, excuse me, there's two of us. This is hurting me as well.' People – especially women – tend to ask how she is but in fact I don't think anybody ever said to me, 'What about you? How are you coping?'
>
> (P15: father of preterm baby)

> It's like a guy's just meant to get on with it and nobody's got any feelings for [him] . . . All you ever get is, 'How's [your partner]? How's [she]?' . . . Nobody asks how am I coping. That hurts because I'm actually going through the same as what [she is], maybe in a different way, but it's still the same.
>
> (P38: father of baby with congenital anomaly)

Even one GP incensed parents by reportedly coming to the house and spending time with the mother but making no reference at all to the father's feelings.

On the other hand, some fathers were aware of inhibiting factors which precluded easy conversation on the subject. Two fathers just did not want any mention of the death. Another said that although people did ask him how he was, he felt guilty if he gave the standard reply that he was fine, but he believed that it was inappropriate to tell such enquirers this particularly intimate story. One father found that in doing all he could to spare his partner pain and protect her from the cruelty of the outside world, he himself had suffered additionally by having to recount their story so often to so many people.

> I had to go up to people and stop them coming to see [my wife] . . . to stop [her] getting hurt. It hurt. Deep down it was getting so hurtful – it was

hurting so much I started building up a barrier myself. And it's hard to knock it down. I can speak about him, but it feels like I'm getting torn up and I just build the barrier again. To knock it down is [to make myself very vulnerable again].

(P 34: father of preterm baby)

# Painful reminders

Some of these items were cited as sources of sadness in the earlier chapter, but they are included again here because they were mentioned as unhelpful things in this different context. A hurt which was difficult to avoid was seeing other pregnant women or new babies and remembering painfully what might have been. A special poignancy attached to those pregnancies which matched the dates of the mother's own pregnancy, and to observing the babies achieving milestones which would have been those reached by the dead child at that time. Even where the babies were their own – siblings of the dead baby – it was sad to compare their outcomes. Visiting the survivors was a painful experience.

If you've just got the one baby you don't have to go back into that Intensive Care room again if your baby dies. But if you've got two or three you do, you have to go back in and you see all the same machines and it's all the same people and you see the same space. And then you see another baby in that space. On the day of [the baby's] funeral we went in in the morning and there was another baby in [her] space . . . we went in and it felt empty, it just felt so empty . . . Obviously we know they can't say [to other families], 'I'm sorry, your baby'll have to go to another hospital because this is what's happened.' You can't do that. That was understandable. But it was still a bit sore . . . even just there with the [other triplets] it was back in Intensive Care again and you think, 'I don't want to be here; I hate this room.'

(P 35: mother of preterm triplets)

When other smaller sicker babies in the nursery lived, that comparison too was full of sadness.

However, being cushioned from other children was not the answer, and the parents realised that they had to face the rest of life, which included other babies. A small number of both mothers and fathers found it hurtful when friends or work colleagues refrained from telling them about pregnancies or births, tiptoed around the subject, or kept their children away. These reminders were painful, but they were a part of life and the parents wanted to be included. As some pointed out, it was better to square up to the challenge sooner, rather than be shielded from its reality only to have it assume increasing proportions. Of a different dimension was the emotion generated when pregnant women appeared to be careless of their own health and of the welfare of their unborn children. Parents spoke passionately of their sense of injustice when they saw other women abusing their bodies.

A small number of couples had watched a television programme featuring withdrawal of treatment which had been broadcast soon after their own experience of this procedure. This had been disturbing. The outcome had caused one couple in particular to question their own decision for a time.

## Contact by those who did not know of the death

Inevitably it sometimes took a while for news of the tragedy to percolate through the couple's circle of friends and acquaintances, and several families reported the horror of being contacted by people who assumed all was well, or who were agog to hear news of the delivery. In two cases a similar hurt had been generated by healthcare professionals. In the first case a midwife calling to see the mother and baby upset the grieving parents. In the other case a GP was perceived as inept.

> There was just total neglect from that doctor's [surgery]. On the morning of [the baby's] funeral, a doctor came into the house to do a baby check on him. And he had all my notes. Obviously they didn't have a file for [the baby] because there *was* no file for him. They only had *my* file. Apparently when a doctor goes out to do a check I understand they've got to have a file for yourself and for the baby. He didn't even have that. And he called in – just walked straight into the house – shouting, 'I'm here to do a baby check.' He didn't wait at the door – just walked straight in. That just shows that they never read any of the notes at all.
>
> (P23: parents of preterm baby with congenital anomalies)

For four sets of parents the pain came from mail which was designed for healthy babies and mothers, including survey forms, baby samples or a call for a hearing test.

## Inappropriate gifts

Two sets of parents experienced pain caused by the receipt of offerings which they felt were inappropriate. In one case flowers carried an association with celebration, not loss, and were not welcomed. The other mother was not comforted by gifts sent by work colleagues which she perceived as coming 'officially' as a routine duty contact.

# Things parents would have liked in the first few months

Having established what had been helpful or unhelpful in the parents' actual experience the interviewer then asked them if there was anything in addition which they would have liked at this stage, but did not get. Lest undue weight be given to certain items, comments that were the obverse of the factors which they had found unhelpful are not repeated here. However, it should be noted that the parents emphasised that they wanted the following:

- *people to be interested* in what had happened to their baby
- *everyone to avoid clichés and false reassurances or platitudes*
- *the fathers' grief to be acknowledged* and
- *space to grieve.*

More specific wishes that were cited are listed with numbers (*n*) in parentheses indicating the numbers of families who identified this as a suggested improvement, where more than one did so. The fact that only small numbers thought of any given area for improvement should not by any means lessen the weight of their contribution where such a change might be beneficial.

## More information from the hospital

This included obtaining answers to their difficult questions about what had happened, a summary of events from beginning to end, reassurance from the consultant neonatologist that the mother did not make the decision to stop treatment, and guidance on how fathers should grieve.

> Since we've been in there [the NICU], there have been kids that have died . . . You know when somebody's coming out with streaming tears and it might be that they've got bad news, it might be because their child has died. It's for a point of reference that I wish that somebody that had maybe had triplets and lost one had written a book that I could have read, that felt like that. Because at the time you lose a child, you're the

only person in the world that's done that. You're the only person in the world that has lost a triplet. But you're not. I think to have the feeling that you're not the only one and that you can read how somebody was feeling and see [that you] know exactly where you're coming from . . . I feel counselling is patronising. I don't know whether it would help or not to put my feelings down on a sheet of paper but – ? Just as a point of reference more than anything.

(P35: father of preterm triplets)

## Changes in hospital practice

Some parents looked for an apology from the hospital acknowledging that mistakes had been made, an opportunity to write to the obstetrician to say how they felt about their 'poor' management, and a facility for the hospital to register deaths and births together ($n = 3$).

## Extra support after the death

Eleven sets of parents looked for extra support. They itemised having someone to 'pick them up' immediately for support so that they did not feel forgotten, counselling being offered routinely from the outset, with the opportunity to opt out of this if they wished ($n = 3$), someone to talk to ($n = 2$), and someone like the interviewer coming to talk to them ($n = 5$).

> Instead of you having to go somewhere – *them* coming to *you* . . . having it in the safeness of your own house not in a stupid room where they've got to offer you biscuits and tea after ten minutes and there's 40 other folks sitting looking at you. And I don't want to hear anybody else's tragedy. I've got my own tragedy. And I wish there was somebody who would do what you've done and sit and listen to my tragedy. I don't want somebody to come back with *their* tragedy and say, 'I've had it worse' . . . It does help. I think that would be a better service than what everything else was . . . in your own surroundings, your own territory, makes it a lot easier to speak, I don't speak about it when I go up to the hospital.
> (P38: father of baby with congenital anomalies)

Other parents also cited a wish that information had been given from the outset about support groups – preferably by someone contacting them proactively ($n = 3$), that other fairly recently bereaved parents who had been through the same experience had contacted them ($n = 3$), that the GP had been more understanding, that grandparents had accepted what had happened without feeling a need to apportion blame, that grand-parents had not insisted that their grief was greater ($n = 2$), that friends and relatives had visited as before, and that their own church had made contact.

## Less intrusion

One couple felt that there should have been a reduction in the number of healthcare professionals attending after the death and 'swamping' the parents.

These data all refer to the early weeks after the loss. We turn now to the longer term experiences and needs.

## Supportive people in the year following the death

Most families found support in some form over the ensuing months. No mothers and only three fathers said that they had received no support from outside the family home during the year after the death. However, two families noted that whilst other people might offer their help, the real work of adjusting to their changed circumstances had to come from within. Furthermore, sometimes the parents' own behaviours could be misleading. Some reported that they gave the outward appearance of being in control or of getting on with life, reserving their tears for private moments in the house or car. They recognised that such behaviour might send a message to other people that they had 'got over' the loss. Some couples even concealed their actions and emotions from each other. It was only on the first anniversary of the death that one couple 'confessed' to each other that they had both been 'sneaking' into the cemetery to talk to the baby.

While the number of families obtaining support from lay sources was similar at both points of enquiry, there was a marked dropping off of pro-fessional support over time. Sources of lay support, in decreasing order of frequency of citation, were friends ($n = 34, 68\%$), the parents' own parents ($n = 26$, $52\%$), other family members ($n = 22$, $44\%$), existing chil-dren ($n = 17$, $34\%$), other bereaved parents ($n = 10$, $20\%$), work collea-gues ($n = 7$, $14\%$) and the church ($n = 3$, $6\%$). Professional support was provided by bereavement counsellors ($n = 8$, $16\%$), hospital staff ($n = 7$, $14\%$), ministers of religion ($n = 7$, $14\%$), GPs ($n = 6$, $12\%$), health visitors ($n = 1$, $2\%$), social workers ($n = 1$, $2\%$), psychologists ($n = 1$, $2\%$) and an alternative therapy practitioner ($n = 1$, $2\%$).

# Helpful factors in the year following the death

## People making themselves available and being able to contain the emotions

Parents greatly valued the concern and care others showed. Often it was enough just to know that such people were there for them should they need help. They appreciated those who had the sensitivity to give them space to grieve in their own way. For some this was expressed by a physical presence – someone who was able to contain the powerful emotions and sadness in whatever form it appeared. For others it was demonstrated in a willingness to drop everything to be with the parents, or a readiness to offer appropriate practical help.

> That was another thing we discovered ... the 'bowl of soup' concept, which is the best thing you can do for somebody who's been bereaved – you can make them a big bowl of soup or bake them some shortbread or do their washing for them. But it's not the big tell-me-all-your-woes thing, it's just something really basic and simple. We went that day, we went off to the funeral and when we came back, one of [our] friends had left a gallon container of soup and two big things of French bread and it was wonderful because nobody had to worry about what we were going to eat that night, and it was such a kind thing to do.
> (P25: mother of preterm baby with brain damage)

Sometimes it was unexpected people, who had formerly appeared brash and noisy, who revealed hidden depths of tenderness.

However, more than one mother found the most sensitive people to be the ones who appreciated that when she was having a bad day she just wanted to be left alone, and who did not 'suffocate' her with well-intentioned attention. The very fact that friends kept making contact was supportive in itself, since it showed that they understood that this was an ongoing sorrow. Their love and concern made the parents feel valued.

## Listening

A continuing basic need of bereaved parents was to talk. It helped them to have good listeners who did not feel that they had to have answers or offer bland reassurances. However, one mother found a psychiatrist unhelpful. This doctor listened but offered no comment, and she found this unnerving.

Friends were clearly supportive in an ongoing way during the first year after the loss, with as many as two-thirds of the parents deriving comfort and help from this source. Some indeed pointed out the value of talking to people who were less emotionally involved than close family members. The parents were free to set the tone of their conversations without anxiety about how much additional distress they were causing grandparents or uncles and aunts. When the friends had known them for a long time the parents appreciated their sensitivity, which allowed them to pace their integration into the social scene in their own way and at their own speed, without external pressure being applied.

Opportunities to share their experience with other bereaved parents who really knew what it felt like were highly valued. Additional benefits were available where these people could tell them something of what lay ahead. However, only three sets of parents cited a bereavement group as being supportive at this stage. For one of these three couples, the experience of being with other people in a bereavement group for all kinds of losses, namely Cruse, had helped to normalise the mother's own grief.

Professional listening was cited less frequently, but was nevertheless appreciated by some families. For eight sets of parents a bereavement counsellor had been invaluable during the year following the death. In one case this counsellor was also a member of the family. The mothers who had seen such counsellors on a regular basis spoke warmly of their skill and help. As one mother put it, counsellors listened well whatever the parents said, and did not make 'stupid comments.' It was also reassuring for the parents to know that whatever was said was in strict confidence.

Six families had received support from their GP. One of these mothers was greatly helped by her doctor making frequent appointments for her to come back to keep talking about her emotions. She commented that she would not have spontaneously asked to see him, but she was grateful that he was proactive, as she could go along repeatedly with a clear conscience and also be assured of a ready and sympathetic listening ear.

Another couple found their new GP much more helpful than his predecessor. After the death, this mother spent much time searching for the truth about what had gone wrong, but some staff were unhelpful and dismissive of her concerns, and she found it a lonely and isolating experience. However, this new GP proved more sympathetic: he both listened to her thoughts and facilitated access to further information and to the people she needed to see. The father did not want to have anything to do with this search, but he too found this doctor particularly helpful when he came to their house one year after the death, with time to spend listening and talking to them. This gave the father a much needed opportunity to talk about his own pain and concerns, and to obtain answers to his questions.

# Being natural with the parents

The ability to talk about the baby and what happened naturally was a skill which as many as half of the parents spontaneously mentioned appreciatively. It was difficult for them when people avoided the subject, were unable to cope with their tears or dwelt overly on the tragedy. A relaxed approach which made them feel that the other person could be comfortable with powerful emotion but was not preoccupied with the morbid detail helped them to feel at ease. Being generally treated as normal was of greatest help for a number of fathers. When work colleagues or bosses were understanding and sympathetic during the year after the death and helped them to reintegrate into the work-force and be treated as normal, this was perceived as demonstrative of sensitivity in a form which the parents found acceptable.

# Remembering the baby

Anything which showed that others were also remembering the baby was usually supportive. As before, so also in the longer term, with so few memories and so few people who had known the baby, many parents found it therapeutic to dwell on aspects of the baby or events in his or her life which consolidated the reality of his or her existence. This they could only do with individuals who had been part of the experience. Sometimes this took the form of verbal references to the characteristics of the baby in comparison to other children, or mention of the baby as a brother, sister, nephew or granddaughter. This was warming because it established the baby as a 'real person.'

For many parents, reassurance that the child was not forgotten came from cards and notes, and for a minority it came in the form of flowers on the grave or an album for photographs. What helped was knowing that others valued this short life and recalled the baby as a real little individual. Remembrances on special dates or at intervals demonstrated that the baby was still 'in their consciousness,' as one mother put it. However, as one father added, such gestures were only helpful if the person was close enough to what had happened to feel genuinely the sentiments expressed. For example, if the neonatal nurse who had cared for the child, or the chaplain who had supported the parents during the death and funeral, sent a message or anniversary card it was highly valued. In one case the chaplain had dropped in on a couple on the anniversary of the child's death, and they were both deeply moved by his care and thoughtfulness.

> The minister [hospital chaplain] came to see me. He was going away...
> for three weeks and he knew that he would be away on her birthday this
> year, so he came to see me before he went. But then I still got a card from
> him that marked when she died. It was so nice. And he's retired now.
> He's lovely.
>
> (P45: mother of preterm baby)

The fact that they still remembered a specific baby when they dealt with so
many spoke volumes to the parents about the depth of their compassion
and the value of the baby's influence on others' lives.

> People like [his nurse], I'd have thought they'd have forgotten about us,
> although I haven't forgotten about them because they are a big part of
> our life. But you feel they see that many people coming and going, how
> can they remember us? [But she does.] That makes me feel quite good.
> After over a year [she] still remembers us.
>
> (P48: mother of baby with congenital anomalies)

On the other hand, receiving a card from the NICU on which the name of
the person signing it was unfamiliar was perceived as a rather meaningless routine gesture, and hence of little real value.

> If it's a person doing 40 cards with names that mean nothing to that
> person then it's not a good thing. If it had been the midwife that was
> present [at the delivery] and it had been her own initiative, we probably
> would have been very touched. But [because we didn't know this per-
> son at all] we weren't touched at all really. We were really surprised.
> It was hand-written but she wrote that she felt *very* sad about what
> happened, and it didn't feel it was honest – it couldn't be – I mean we
> don't expect a person that doesn't know us, doesn't know [our baby],
> we don't expect *anybody* to feel strongly about this.
>
> (P17: parents of preterm baby)

It was evident that different things were expected and welcomed from different people. Their significance and acceptability varied. Some reminders
were simply too painful because they came from grieving relatives and
touched deep chords, and these required careful screening by the parents.

> I don't think it would have been [OK] from anybody else... It was really
> brief. It just said, 'Remembering [the baby]' or something. And it was fine
> because it was from [the chaplain]. But I think if it had been from my
> Mum and Dad or friends had sent it, then it wouldn't have been [OK]
> ... I think it's the distance though, he's not too close. One friend sent
> me a card on her birthday as well, which I didn't even open – I didn't

open it for about three weeks, because I just knew what it was. And it was just, 'Thinking of you at this time.' But if I'd opened *that* on her birthday it might have upset me, and I was doing well on her birthday so I just thought, 'No, I'm not going to do that.'

(P45: mother of preterm baby)

Exceptional remembrances helped a minority of parents. For one mother this involved having all of her friends put up a photograph of her dead baby in their homes. In a few other cases, friends and relatives had established a memorial in some form (such as a plaque, a seat or a shrub) to commemorate the baby's short life.

# Other children

For a third of the families it was their other children who were a major source of comfort and strength, and who helped them to face each new day as the year passed. The youngsters 'forced' them 'to be normal.' However, as we have seen, the support of children was not without complications. Many parents became conscious of changes in their behaviour towards their existing children. Some were aware of increased levels of anxiety, and some became over-protective or over-indulgent as a result.

I wish that somebody could give me a guarantee that nothing else would happen between myself, my partner and [our other child] … The unthinkable has already happened and it can happen again. Sometimes I think about it and I think: I lived in a world where I thought me and mine were untouchable – I could protect my kids. And I couldn't.

(P 38: mother of baby with congenital anomalies)

However, some mothers found that their overriding wish to protect their children had the effect of strengthening them. Not wanting to mar their children's happiness or scar them by the experience, they tried not to get upset in front of them. Answering the children's own innocent questions about the baby and dealing with ongoing references to the dead child helped to cultivate the feeling that the baby was still very much part of the family. This in turn helped the parents.

New pregnancies brought new hope for the future, as has been described earlier. Alongside the joy the pregnancy itself brought, the parents found support in the expressed pleasure of other people on their behalf, including GPs, doctors and siblings' teachers. Genuine caring and support from hospital staff during the next pregnancy were also greatly appreciated.

# Work

As before, a number of fathers commented that work had been their salvation in the year after the death. They could keep themselves busy and either temporarily forget the pain or at least keep it under control. They appreciated colleagues making allowances for their below-par activity and not putting too much pressure on them. Being given time off as necessary or being allowed a holiday was helpful, especially when such things were given readily without a lengthy explanation being required. A small number of mothers who returned to work after their maternity/compassionate leave found the same benefit in having other things to think about, although two of mothers went back too early and found that they simply could not deal with the job. Particularly thoughtful gestures warmed the parent – for example, colleagues approaching a manager to ensure that one mother had a day off on the anniversary of the baby's funeral.

# Visiting the grave

The degree to which 'visiting the baby' helped varied. Some parents spent a great deal of time at the grave, talking to the baby, thinking, remembering and tending the plot. For a number of parents keeping the grave tidy or decorated was an expression of their parental love – 'the only thing I can do for him.' However, for others the pain was too acute to bear.

> *Father*: I'm glad she's got a grave and I'm glad she's got a nice wee stone there. In the rose garden it would have just been that wee metal plate and I'm so relieved [it worked out that she was buried in the ordinary part of the cemetery] . . . that's where I want her.
> *Mother*: I don't like cemeteries. I don't like visiting cemeteries. And I find it very hard to go up there. I find it hard because I think too much goes on in my head. I can think of her all day every day without going to a cemetery. But then I start to feel guilty. 'Oh, I've not been up to the cemetery. She'll not have fresh flowers. I'll need to go up' . . . I don't like it because I don't want her to be there . . . she's always in my thoughts so a wee stone's not going to make any difference.
>
> (P10: parents of preterm twins)

However, this father had a special reason to feel good about visiting the grave. He had taken on an extra job to acquire the money for a headstone. Refusing offers of help from the family, he saw this provision as something he personally could do for his dead daughter, and he took pride in the achievement.

It has been a comfort to me that grave . . . I love going up there . . . For all I've said, 'You've got to get on with life'. . . it's definitely been a comfort to me . . . I would say, get them buried in a plot or a grave and get a proper gravestone because I think that goes a long way to the grieving process maybe – but it's something that I've not realised . . . until now.

## Realisation that worse things happen

Over the year a few parents found solace in hearing stories which seemed worse than their own. This was particularly apparent in the case of parents whose babies had lived for some time. When they heard of others whose babies were stillborn or lived only hours, they appreciated in a different way the opportunities that they had had to do things with their own baby. A number of parents even described themselves as 'lucky.'

## Opportunity to be with other babies

Being gently helped in a controlled and private way to overcome their initial reluctance to touch, hold or even see another baby was helpful to a few mothers. Other parents making their children available when they were ready helped them to stay in contact socially, and ensured that the dread of seeing babies did not impose severe limitations on their lives. On the day she left the hospital after the baby had died one mother, aware of a potential problem, deliberately went to see her sister with her children, as she felt that this would prevent any barriers rising.

## Church support

Religious affiliations were supportive to three parents. In one instance this was in the form of church members 'from around the world', who all belonged to a small close-knit sect, conveying their support and care through cards, letters and prayers which added to the love of their local community. In the other two cases, attending church services and a sense of God's presence were the sources of support.

## Relocation

The one parent who cited a social worker as having been supportive had appreciated her help in moving from a house which held such painful memories to a new location.

# Unhelpful factors in the year following the death

Support can be unpredictable. Some parents commented that they had felt very ambivalent about what would or would not be helpful, and assessment of the value of various offers or actions had only been possible retrospectively. For example, one mother was hurt when her partner did not mark the baby's anniversary in any way. Her instinctive reaction was to wish that he had given her flowers. However, on reflection she felt that flowers indicated celebration. Furthermore, she had received so many flowers when the baby died that she was unsure whether she would ever feel pleased to be given flowers again. When she tried to analyse her feelings more closely, she found that she could not identify anything which her partner might have done which would have made her feel better. As she spoke, it occurred to her that she herself had done nothing for him on that date. She now had to question why she had been angry with him for the same inaction.

Some of the elements cited bear similarities to the earlier unhelpful actions. Their repetition serves to highlight the fact that these are ongoing issues of long-term significance. Listening to the parents' hurt is a powerful reminder of the need for constant care and sensitivity. This is not a hurt which heals in a few weeks or months.

## Incompatible grieving patterns

Having shared this profound experience together, the couples assumed that they would remain close and grieve together, too. However, as has been explained in earlier chapters, both partners were hurting deeply and it could be inhibiting for either of them to speak of the child when to do so provoked distress or a withdrawal. Furthermore, they were grieving in different ways and for different things.

> *Mother*: It's different grieving because . . . He had [the baby's] life planned up until he was 16 – maybe even 18 and his first pint. Whereas I never had that – [he was just my baby].
> *Father*: [She] was just expecting a baby, I was expecting a son . . . I've lost my wee laddie but I've lost an awful lot of dreams as well.
> (P 38: parents of baby with congenital anomaly)

The experience brings you closer together but at the same time you do grieve in very different ways. You grieve for different things. [He] doesn't grieve to the same extent for him as a baby, but he does for what could have been in the future – a wee boy playing football. Whereas I just grieve for the here and now. I think you're quite separate in your grief.

(P6: mother of baby with congenital anomalies)

As before, many mothers found the fathers' silences and withdrawal incomprehensible or hurtful, while some fathers were at a loss when dealing with frequent weeping and a seemingly endless desire to talk about the baby.

I think it is a male thing about showing feelings and all the rest of it. I know myself that I try not to in front of anybody else. [My partner] is probably the only one I would cry in front of. Every guy – her father'll be the same. My Dad's the same. It's the way you're brought up. It's expected. I don't know if it's right, but that's just the way it is.

(P58: father of preterm baby)

I come from a very strong Scottish Calvinistic family where the men don't cry. I was brought up that way. So, I'm the man of the house so I *do not cry* in front of [people], so I've got to find some other way of expressing myself.

(P47: father of baby with brain damage)

These differences were difficult to analyse or tolerate when both members of the couple were equally vulnerable. A few parents commented that it had been necessary for them to take turns to be strong and comfort the other, and in that way they had staged their grieving.

# Trite expressions which belittled the experience

By far the commonest hurtful behaviour of other people over time was that of making light of what had happened or offering meaningless platitudes.

There was this period when I was not working. When I saw people they would say, 'Oh, what are you doing? Are you doing lots of painting? Are you doing lots of sailing?' And actually I couldn't [cope with] doing anything. It was all I could do to get myself out of bed. So actually everything that people said to me reinforced the feeling of complete failure. But also I felt like saying to them, 'Oh, if your two children* had just died would you be doing lots of painting and lots of sailing?' I didn't *say* that because people don't mean it – it's people just looking for something to say.

(P49: mother of baby with asphyxia)

---

* Refers to an earlier loss, too.

Some parents generously sympathised with the felt need to say something, but they emphasised how hard it was to have people saying things like 'I know how you feel' – they *could not*; 'You can just make another baby' – another child would never replace the dead one; or 'A new baby will fill the gap' – the gap could never be filled.

False reassurances or promises which were not in people's power to give were seen as empty. Making assumptions that the couple would have another baby was presumptuous, especially to those with a history of infertility. Judgemental responses to the parents' behaviours and reactions were isolating and irritating. Expecting the parents to be 'over it' or to return to their former activities was to diminish the impact of the loss and the continuing effect of this experience. Such comments demonstrated a lack of true sympathy. A GP giving sedation and false reassurances was perceived as responding inappropriately to a deep need.

## Unnatural behaviour

As the year went on, parents wanted those around them to behave as naturally as possible. Hurtful unnatural behaviours cited included suffocating attention, being mournful or morbidly preoccupied with death or the dead baby, excluding other children from the vicinity of the parents, forcing parents to talk about what had happened when they did not want to, or pressing opinions on the parents.

## Being ignored

Another frequently mentioned source of hurt was when people ignored the parents or avoided the subject of the baby. Even though the parents knew that it was fear of saying the wrong thing which prompted people to pass by as if they had not seen them, they still found this hurtful. The child had been and still was a vitally important part of the parents' lives and experience, and the tragedy of his loss was a major event which had changed them for ever, so if he was not mentioned, the parents felt the importance of this short life was diminished. In some ways even to the parents there was a strange sense of unreality, especially if the baby had never come home. They needed reassurances that he or she had been real, and if others included the baby in the conversation it helped to reinforce his or her identity.

It was particularly difficult when family members avoided the subject. Mothers were bewildered and distressed when the child's father did not or would not talk about the baby. In one case a whole family ignored the baby's existence, they were embarrassed if he was mentioned, and they spoke of another child as the first grandchild. When family members did not visit the grave or mark anniversaries this was hurtful to some parents. To them it indicated that the relatives did not care enough, they did not appreciate the loss to the parents, or they had already forgotten the child.

Work colleagues were singled out for mention by several parents in this context. One father had deliberately introduced the subject of the baby at work, but his colleagues ignored it. Another father said that even a year on he still remembered those who said nothing, and there remained a barrier between them. In general, women reported experiencing greater sympathy and understanding, but one mother remembered only one colleague ever mentioning her loss during the first 13 months of her mourning.

As has already been stated, professional support decreased over the year. However, at this second point of enquiry a number of parents actually cited hospital staff as unhelpful because they had made no further contact. When no member of the community team or a bereavement group did so either, this increased the sense that the parents were forgotten and that no one cared how they were coping.

> I think it was bad that nobody followed up – maybe [from] 2 months down the line, a phone call to the house, 'Is there anything we can do for you? I would like you to come down.' Or 'Could I come up?' – like you've done – 'Could I come up and see you for an hour? Just to see that everything's all right. Because losing a baby's a traumatic thing.' But there's no follow-up. You walk out of that hospital and they've never seen you again. If I jumped off the bridge or whatever, they would have read it in [the paper] or whatever, they'd say, 'Oh, that was [name]. That was [the baby's] Mum. She must have had a hard time.' They don't *know* if you've had a hard time or not. They've no idea. So I think their follow-up procedure really needs to be looked at. Probably personally too because I look at it a year down the line, [my husband's] got big problems ... he had nobody [to talk to].
>
> (P36: mother of preterm baby with brain damage)

It was particularly disappointing when the Unit staff who knew of the trauma of the experience and had shared in the parents' pain and sadness made no contact with them. The parents needed to know that the emotion which the staff had appeared to feel had been genuine, and their compassion for the parents did not end as they walked out of the hospital door.

> I know that they can't do this, but when it was [the baby's anniversary] I thought we might have heard something from [the] SCBU.* I don't

---

* Special Care Baby Unit.

know what I was expecting, but I think I was just expecting some sort of remembrance. But nothing came. I don't know what I was expecting – a card maybe just to say they were remembering her? Or something like that. I know that they can't because they see thousands and thousands of babies dying.

> (P7: mother of baby with cardiac anomaly)

Since my six-week check-up there's not been anything from any of the doctors at all, nothing from anybody... not once have the doctors ever mentioned, how are we getting on, or how are we coping, or anything ... I'm not a very open person when it comes to things like that ... I [wouldn't find it easy] if I was feeling down or anything [to go and] spill it all out to them, I'd rather wait until they maybe broached the subject. And then it's easier to [talk about it]. I don't like going to the doctors at the best of times now, but I just feel we've been pushed aside.

> (P23: mother of preterm baby with congenital anomalies)

## Other people putting their own emotions ahead of the parents' needs

It amazed some parents that others could rate their own needs and emotions more highly than those of the parents at this time. Different families reported the experience of a friend being upset because the mother did not confide in her, a grandmother refusing to visit the cemetery because she was too upset, and a grandfather being unable to mention the baby or deal with the death. A common experience among parents was of others concentrating on their own seemingly trivial preoccupations. To the parents their concerns appeared frivolous and insignificant, and they wondered that others should bother to talk about these matters in the face of their own real tragedy.

## Thoughtlessness/insensitivity

Although many of the parents lamented the thoughtlessness and insensitivity of certain people, some added a caveat – they recognised that their own sensibilities were heightened as a result of their experience. It was difficult for people to avoid sensitive areas because they could not know where they were.

Instances I've found hurtful have been when people have [said something] that's not even directly related [to our experience]. It's just things which to me might be significant but to them never would be, so it's the sort of thing that people couldn't plan against. So if I was to say, 'Saying *this* wouldn't help,' and ' Saying *that* wouldn't help,' it makes people awfully on edge about saying *anything*. Because to be quite honest the situations where I've felt a wee bit upset have been quite often just because I take things out of a conversation, and I know that they don't mean it – it just triggers something off in my brain and they couldn't stop themselves saying it because nobody could know it would be hurtful. It's weird.

(P29: mother of baby with asphyxia)

Parents cited a range of experiences which had upset them. These included professional errors, such as a midwife diminishing the value of time spent with the baby by saying that it would have been better if the child had been stillborn, and unsympathetic comments from hospital staff during a subsequent pregnancy. They also included insensitivity from lay sources – for example, a Christmas card sent to a mother of twin boys picturing two boys playing in heaven, friends and relatives thrusting babies at parents, 'cruel' comments about 'childbearing failure' or 'a bitter and twisted mind,' constant references to other pregnancies or babies, insensitive jokes, compassionate leave becoming annual leave, and breaches of confidentiality.

Even people who were trained in caring for bereaved families could get it quite wrong for some parents. One mother recalled someone from the SANDS organisation confidently asserting that all parents are desperate for their baby to live. The mother to whom she was speaking was not.

At one point, once I'd explained [our] situation – and I was very upset at the time – the girl said, 'Oh, I know, I know. You would just do anything for them not to die. It doesn't matter what they'll be like. It doesn't matter as long as they're still there.' And I was sitting there thinking, 'Well, actually no, that *wasn't* how it was for me.' And then of course I went away out feeling, 'That's the way I *should* have been feeling.' I was in a very fragile state by that point and I started to question my own judgement about what had happened to us. And I thought, 'No, that person has totally misunderstood how I was feeling.' And there's no point in going to something like that pretending to have a view that you don't have . . . I found it much more distressing than I expected. I found it quite *un*helpful.

(P18: mother of preterm baby)

By contrast, this mother found Cruse immensely helpful.

I think the fact that it wasn't to do with neonatal deaths made a difference. It was almost as if it was making the death of a baby more normal
or more mainstream rather than being set apart . . . But somehow Cruse
made everything very ordinary, everything I talked about. By the time I
went to Cruse I really thought I was going mad. I had lost all my confidence. I needed people to tell me what to do . . . and the relief of having
somebody who'd say, 'OK let me explain what I understand about grief
and the grieving process. And let me tell you that you're not going
mad – you're *not* mad and you're not *going* mad. And it will get better.'
Very positive stuff but without actually telling you what to do . . . she
just made everything very normal and understandable.

(P18: mother of preterm baby)

Other parents found it patronising when people assumed that grief would
follow a set pattern. These experiences were undermining and hurtful.

[The community midwife] tried to tell me what I was feeling – thank
you, but I know what I am feeling.

(P26: mother of baby with congenital anomalies)

The innocent comments of strangers occasionally hurt parents even
though they accepted at an intellectual level that these people could not
possibly have known about their circumstances. One couple found themselves angry when passers-by referred to their two surviving triplets as
twins. One mother was hurt when the undertaker referred to the fact
that there was space enough for other names on the gravestone when she
was newly pregnant again.

# Other pregnancies/babies

Bereaved parents commented that they could not escape from babies and
pregnant women – they were everywhere. They tried to school themselves
to accept this reality, and one mother even took in her baby niece soon
after losing her own baby, but she found the experience so painful that
she had to return her to her mother. Each baby highlighted their own
loss. Unsolicited samples of baby products added a painful emphasis. The
parents' sense of injustice was further increased when these other children
were maltreated.

# Being asked difficult questions

As we have seen in an earlier chapter, a recurring source of pain experienced by these parents was being asked how many children they had.

The tension between being true to the baby and sensitive to other people's feelings was not easy to resolve. However, other people who did know the circumstances could also cause further pain through their questioning. As one mother said, every time she went out people asked her how she was, and every time that question 'resurrected the pain.' When people asked difficult questions or expressed concerns about a subsequent pregnancy, a few mothers felt that perhaps they, too, should be worrying. Where there were problems of infertility, questions and comments could be particularly distressing.

A number of families experienced their own children asking questions about the baby, what had happened, and what might happen in the future. Although most parents dealt with these queries in a matter of fact way, one father found it immensely painful and admitted that he 'bit their heads off' every time. His wife took the children aside and dealt with the issues they had raised herself.

Another source of difficult questions came from within. One couple heard of a subsequent success story which left them wondering whether they themselves should have tried harder to save the baby. There were no cast-iron reassurances to convince them of the wisdom of stopping treatment.

> *Father*: [6 months after our baby died] there was something on the news that a lot of our friends picked up on. I hadn't seen it but people had spoken to us about a baby that had this terrible heart condition and it had this pioneering surgery. The hospital had told them to take the baby home to die – apparently – that's what the press said. And the parents put out a national appeal: could anyone help? And Birmingham hospital said, 'Yes, we can help.' And they did some surgery which – the way the papers put it – everything was going to be fine and dandy as if it was just one operation. And a few friends were saying, 'Oh that looks very similar to what you had.' And that was the first news of a similar thing we'd ever heard where people had gone a different way from what we had done, and immediately it made us start doubting what we did. Did we do the right thing? Should we have tried a bit harder? And we went through a bit of an awful time ... It just stirred up a lot of feelings and we wondered, could we have done something different? I think we'll always have times when we might doubt what happened, and the fact that we ultimately let him go to die as opposed to putting him through what we were told was a series of operations, all of which were particularly difficult, not very high survival rates. But you read the paper and that paper makes it sound like it's just one little operation and everything's going to be fine, and that caused quite a bit of distress at the time.

*Mother*: And we wondered if our friends were pointing their fingers and saying, 'Did you do enough?' I'm sure they weren't *now*, but that's the way we felt at the time.

(P2: parents of baby with cardiac anomaly)

# Memorial service

Before commenting on the negative perceptions, it is important to note that although no one singled it out for citation as supportive, a few parents rated the memorial service highly. It helped to know that they were not alone, and it gave them 'space to feel.'

That was wonderful, beautiful. It was the most moving service . . . a very, very worthwhile experience . . . I would highly recommend it.

(P44: mother of preterm quads)

Nevertheless, as we have seen, a considerable number of parents expressed very negative feelings about the experience. It was unhelpful to be surrounded by other grieving families, and particularly hurtful to have babies crying during the service.

It was very well organised and what not, but they had babies there – it's just ridiculous people taking babies in. They provided a crèche for people to put their babies in – nobody used the crèche and there were babies screaming in there which to me just ruined it. I was just [so upset] – all I could hear was these babies . . . really, the lack of compassion by some people! . . . I thought, people have lost their first child here, they may not go on to have other children. And I could see there were people getting very upset by that. So I was very disappointed in that. And I felt sorry for the organisers, because they had worked very hard, they'd done all they could . . . they say it on the leaflet: 'If your baby gets distressed, please take them out of the crematorium.' My Mum was sitting beside someone whose baby was in a buggy and this baby was getting quite fractious. And the girl didn't take it out, she was just going, 'Sshhh.' And my Mum was getting so upset – it was right beside her. It really was upsetting. Apart from the fact that you're upset anyway . . . I was angry afterwards, but initially I was upset.

(P6: parents of baby with congenital anomalies)

One couple, who had been remarkably positive about the care and support they had received, described the memorial service as the most dreadful event of their lives, noticeably setting them back in their grieving. Another mother had found it totally jarring. To her it held an overall message that 'It'll be OK,' but she knew that 'It won't *ever* be OK.' She felt that she was just 'being polite', not honest. The 'tea and cakes' was a 'ridiculous' farce.

# Things parents would have liked in the year following the death

There were two factors which were cited again and again as something parents would have liked but did not get: routine and regular checks to ensure that they were coping, and an opportunity to talk things over with someone sympathetic and understanding. Given that this was a completely open question with no guidance given, the frequency with which these two factors were cited is significant. None of the other items listed occurred with the same constancy.

## Checks of parental coping

During the intense period of the dying, the death and the immediate aftermath, the parents were the centre of concentrated attention. However, many felt isolated from the team who had been so closely involved with them. From their perspective it felt as if they were now forgotten and the experience was over, but for them the reality was just beginning to hit them, and as the numbness passed the depth of the hurt and loss became ever more apparent. Did anyone care whether or how they were coping? The parents gave a clear picture of their ideal support system. It would be based on the premise that this was a universally traumatic experience with ongoing powerful stresses and needs, and that everyone would need help to survive it. There would be no assumption that only those who were coping badly needed contact. It would involve periodic enquiries as to how they were faring, leaving them the option to accept support or not, depending on their circumstances and needs. Some outline of what emotions and difficulties could be expected as time went on would be provided.

It should be noted that a number of parents observed that they had been told they could contact the staff at any time, or they were given a sheet of names, addresses and telephone numbers of various organisations. However, what they wanted was for someone to contact *them*. It should never be assumed that parents would just obtain their own help, they said. It was an added burden for them to be required to be proactive in seeking such help. When they were feeling vulnerable and emotionally fragile it was difficult to pick up a telephone and speak to a complete stranger about something so intimate and painful. It took great courage to explain aloud what had happened. The ideal might be for someone who already knew the basic details of their experience to make the initial contact with them, it was suggested.

One mother commented that this contact should be ongoing for as long as parents felt a need. For her, 6 months had been a black time when the full impact of what had happened finally hit her. Others spoke of being on autopilot for weeks, or feeling as if they were in a hazy cloud at first, and the real devastation hitting them some weeks or months later. It was then that they really needed someone who understood the nature of parental grief to give them an opportunity to share their distress. So many people just could not understand this delayed reaction or continuing distress.

As part of this ongoing interest in their welfare, anniversary cards or letters would serve as indicators that neither the parents nor the babies had been forgotten. The sharing of these memories with people who had actually known the child was clearly of special significance.

## A listening ear

The importance of a listening ear was emphasised by many parents. Mothers found it therapeutic to go over and over events. Fathers found it helpful to talk to someone 'who asked the right questions' and helped them to gain insights into the experience and its effects. The therapeutic effect of the research interviews was cited in this context, and it was very evident that these represented a form of intervention in the lives of these families.

> I can see now that − you said, 'Is there anything people could have done for us that they didn't do?' − if you hadn't been here we may well have felt a need − I think I would have felt a need to have a conversation like this with someone. And I wouldn't really have cared *why* we were having the conversation. I'm glad that you're doing something with this information − that's really pleasing. But you've definitely fulfilled a specific need that *I* had.
>
> (P25: mother of preterm baby with brain damage)

Given the significance of any intervention in a research project, the effects of the study interviews are specifically described in a subsequent section.

The parents concluded that in view of their own experience, perhaps all couples would benefit from an opportunity to analyse their feeling aloud in a protected way. They looked for someone to talk to who was not emotionally involved with the child or the family, but who understood the trauma. Parents identified a number of factors to bear in mind when deciding who should perform the role of listener: he or she should be knowledgeable about the world of neonatal care, a good listener who could bear powerful emotion, someone who did not feel a need to respond with meaningless clichès and platitudes or to offer false reassurance, and someone who knew the right questions to ask and how to guide parents through the experience. The encounters should be on a one-to-one basis and definitely not in groups. Some thought that they should always be in the parents' own home. For the fathers in particular there should be no suggestion that this was a form of 'counselling', which in their perceptions involved people trying to 'sort them out' or psychoanalyse them.

Where the baby had suffered from a rare disorder there was a suggestion that it might be good to talk to other parents of such an infant. Again the forging of such a link should be initiated by someone else and should not rely on the parents making the first contact.

# Guidance for fathers

Many of these fathers were professional men in responsible senior positions. They were used to being in control and knowing what to do. However, this experience was uncharted territory, and furthermore they were expected to support their womenfolk who were behaving in ways that were difficult to understand and handle. Four of them wished that there had been something to tell them what to expect, what they might feel and what they should do. They needed a compass.

# Bereavement groups

Although a number of parents had attended bereavement groups, parents from only seven families (12%) had found them supportive in the early weeks of bereavement.

> I was very apprehensive about getting in touch with these people [at SANDS] because I had a vision of what they were – which was completely wrong ... I would say the first night it was very, very painful – even just getting there and realising all these other people had experiences ... after the initial first meeting it felt quite normal to be sitting chatting with these people and felt comfortable that the feelings you'd experienced somebody else had felt them at different times possibly, but everyone's emotions were the same and the reactions that other people had had to things were just the same. And you heard how they had dealt with it and funny situations that had come up because people couldn't handle them or stupid things people had said to them. It made you feel more that you weren't the only ones. Because there's a loneliness attached to bereavement when you're wandering around like an alien and you feel like you've got something tattooed on your forehead.
>
> (P1: mother of baby with asphyxia)

A few other parents added that it was good to know that the groups were there if they wanted them, but that they themselves had not felt this was a helpful avenue to pursue. More than one parent identified making the first contact as a major hurdle.

Those who did attend bereavement group meetings expressed mixed emotions. On the positive side, they derived comfort from shared experiences, even finding that they had much to be grateful for, as others had had worse experiences.

> The few we went to were nice. It did what I feel it should have done. It gave you [the sense] that you're not the only people that are suffering. I can remember saying to one of my friends, 'What it did for me – it made me realise there was somebody worse off than me.' And they were [saying], 'But nobody's worse off than you. You lost your baby.' But I said, 'Oh no. My baby was early. Theirs were full term. They had full-term babies and you don't expect anything at 40 weeks to go wrong.'
>
> (P 36: mother of preterm infant)

They found it reassuring, too, to see that other parents had moved on in their grieving and were happy again.

On the negative side, it was unhelpful when participants seemed to be wallowing in grief or dwelling on the past. The newly bereaved parents looked for evidence that in time they would be happy again, and seeing others who were still sad many years on was depressing.

> They dwell on the past, whereas I really wanted to go to see that there's a future, to see that there is something in front of me.
>
> (P40: mother of baby with asphyxia)

> We wouldn't want to dwell on what's happened. We want to respect what's happened but we're moving forward.
>
> (P51: father of baby with congenital anomalies)

> Maybe it's because you go to something like that that you never let go.
>
> (P50: mother of baby with congenital anomalies)

Some parents had no space to listen to others' problems because they were still too absorbed in their own grief.

> I don't think these things are [helpful]. You got the feeling that the people that went to them they were not there just for that. It was like a social club kind of atmosphere and they weren't really there to talk about the baby. They *had* all had babies that had died, that's about the only thing we had in common ... I can't – I still can't – feel anybody else's loss. My loss is worse than anybody else's. Even when I go to the cemetery and I see all these babies' graves, they're surrounding me, but my baby was

the worst. And I can't feel their loss. The only thing that helps me is that I know I'm not alone. You can think when it first happens to you that you are the only person it has ever happened to. But . . . just in the row he's in there are nine babies buried . . . you're surrounded by them. [But you can't take on board their tragedy]. That tragedy is not my tragedy and my tragedy is worse than all that put together.

(P 20: parents of baby with asphyxia)

Other parents expressed concern about the revelations of so many things which could go wrong and the undermining of their confidence in future childbearing experiences. Hearing parents speak of repeated disasters was not encouraging. Learning that things could go wrong with normal healthy babies, during labour or even after a normal birth made them fearful for their own futures.

One other mother said that while she had not wanted to go to a group meeting, she had drawn strength from a visit to the house by a member of such an organisation. The visitor was positive and happy again, which gave the newly bereaved mother hope for the future.

At the 13-month interview when parents reflected on the whole year of bereavement, a considerable number of them commented that they had not found it helpful to go to support groups. By this stage, two factors were predominantly cited as an explanation for this phenomenon. First, it was undermining of the parents' confidence to be exposed to so many stories of obstetric tragedies. They now knew of so many things which could go wrong.

We got what we needed out of the group in that it helped us to realise that we weren't the only people in the world this had happened to. But then it got to the point that you were listening to some of the people's stories and you were getting quite upset about what happened to them. And I think if you carry on going too long you hear such a range of things that happen to babies that it would put you off for life, having a child, because some horrific things have happened and it would terrify you. It did get to that point I think, of starting to frighten you at the prospect – hearing about things that we'd never even *heard* of before.

(P 2: father of baby with cardiac anomaly)

I stopped going because I felt quite scared – there were so many things that can go wrong . . . with couples, with babies, with everything. They had a book which was lovely and there were all these babies – and I didn't know that many babies died. That was what was scary. There were no two that had died of the same thing – lots of things. And you think 'Have I got to deal with [these too]?' Because something really terrible's happened, now you think something else could happen . . .

There's a test for [what our baby had] but then you're scared about still-birth, you're scared if your baby could be starved of oxygen on delivery . . . a lot of sad, sad stories. Maybe it's selfish, but you don't want to listen to anybody else's sad story – I've got mine.

(P38: mother of baby with congenital anomaly)

[My partner] used to go out scared and come back upset. So what was the point in going to the meeting?

(P38: father of baby with congenital anomaly)

Second, it was depressing to see parents years after the death re-living the pain and apparently not moving on. As several said, they felt that the parents were 'wallowing in grief' and dwelling on the past to the exclusion of the present or the future.

I thought the danger from [going to SANDS groups] was you get a lot of people who become sort of professional grievers as it were. My phrase is 'people who like to pick their scabs'. And I personally didn't think that would be helpful for [my wife] so I wasn't a supporter of that idea.

(P18: father of preterm baby)

There's folk that're going after six years. I don't want to hear that in six years they're still splitting up and going through [all that]. Six years down the line I hope we've still got loads of memories of [the baby] but we're not going to meetings or anything like that; we've handled it enough ourselves without [relying on that].

(P38: father of baby with congenital anomaly)

And one woman was there and it was *20 years ago* her son died; it was twins and one of them died, and she was crying! And it was maybe three months after [our baby] died, and I was so upset and I just thought, 'I don't want to feel this bad in twenty years time. I don't.' And it was scary . . . My initial point [in] going to SANDS was that I wanted to meet parents who'd been through the same [experience] but who were normal. Because I felt so *ab*normal, I wanted to meet someone who'd been through it and who was fine and who could laugh. But then they tell their story, you think, ['Oh no!'] . . . And I didn't want to hear that. I wanted to hear that they did move on. There *were* some who were saying that, but [the others] dominated.

(P38: mother of baby with congenital anomaly)

These parents looked for reassurance that they would eventually be happy again and that, although they would never forget the dead child, things would assume a different, more positive and hopeful perspective as they moved on in life. Some felt that the participants were too absorbed by their own grief to be available to others. One parent found that it was always the 'same people speaking, the same ground covered.' Almost all of the fathers who made a comment about the groups said that it was 'not for me,' and one other father who saw the effect on his partner concluded that the experience was 'more damaging than helpful' for the women folk, too.

> I sometimes think that they're more damaging than helpful. It's always bad news. Dying babies, this, that and the next thing. It's a vicious circle and you seem to never get out of it . . . you don't need that. It's gone. You have to think, 'What's next?'
>
> (P9: father of baby with cardiac anomaly)

# The research interview as intervention

Many parents spontaneously remarked that they had found it unexpectedly helpful to participate in this research. This inevitably means that the experience constituted a form of intervention not normally available to bereaved families. It must therefore be examined more closely.

When first approached, the parents said they had agreed to take part in order to help other families in the future who had to deal with this traumatic experience. If some good came out of their tragedy it would give extra meaning to the baby's life. However, once they had taken part they discovered that the experience had been beneficial to them personally. The benefits accrued from a number of factors, not all of which were available from discussion with friends or relatives. Knowing that others would benefit from their disclosures was indeed comforting, and confirmed their initial reactions. But more than that, the research encounter allowed them to start at the beginning and go through the whole experience. Knowing that the interviewer would not be bored by their detail, they felt empowered to take the time to reflect on the whole experience. In the process they were able to gain insights and clarify details or sequences in their minds, ironing out minor discrepancies in their perceptions and memories. No other situation offered quite the same opportunity.

> These kinds of things help me. You're obviously asking questions that [I] wouldn't think of asking [myself]. I'd be annoyed if I didn't have a realistic answer for most of your questions. It's a good thing [to have to think about them].
>
> (P50: father of baby with congenital anomalies)

> I'm quite comfortable with this [interview situation]. You're not patronising me. You're asking questions and I'm giving you straightforward answers.
>
> (P35: father of preterm triplets)

You coming to talk to us – it's given us a chance to talk because anything shared is a help. Talking about it all over again, things come to
mind, you get them off your chest. Just being able to talk about it.

(P44: father of preterm quads)

Moreover, it allowed each parent to hear the feelings of the other without
the responsibility to protect, comfort or assist – a task undertaken by the
interviewer – thereby freeing each parent to be honest and open. It was
very evident that many fathers and also a number of mothers were revealing information which they had not shared before.

. . . and just hearing him talking about how he feels – because he would
never tell *me* about any of this. I never find out how he feels about things
until he talks to other people. So to actually have somebody specifically sit down and demand an answer – well, he kind of feels obliged
[to answer *you!*] – it's not like if it was my Mum that asked the question,
he'd probably [shrug] and change the subject or whatever, but he knows
he *can* answer you. And I listen to him and I'm learning things about
what he thinks that I wouldn't have found out otherwise. And I think if
you hadn't been here doing the study I maybe wouldn't have known that
stuff. And I think I would have felt that lack of being able to go back,
revisit it, talk it through. [It's better than just talking to friends] because
you've got the knowledge and you're asking specific questions which
they wouldn't have thought of. It does put things into an order in your
mind, and you get out what you need to say and then it helps you put
a line under it.

(P25: mother of preterm baby with brain damage)

The fact that so many parents (85%) undertook a second interview seems
to reinforce further the positive dimension of the experience. A number
of them commented on the usefulness of the return visit after the first
anniversary.

*Mother*: Actually, you know you're saying, 'Has anything been useful?'
*You* have been useful – extremely useful. And this is useful, the fact
that you've come a second time – it's almost even more useful. It was
useful the first time, but now you're kind of tying it up.
*Father*: It's something you've dealt with very well. You didn't come
back and pick the bones . . . chewing it over helped the first time but
you're probably getting the message that [we now think], what has been
has been.

(P25: parents of preterm baby with brain damage)

A very important element for fathers was that the interview was not set up
as a form of therapy. They were adamant that if it had been offered as
a form of counselling they would not have agreed to participate. Since

the introductory letter expressly stated that it was designed to obtain information to help others, they had seen it as a legitimate and laudable reason
to talk about their experience. Having someone to interview them who
had both medical knowledge and a declared specific interest contributed to
this feeling.

> ... and I suppose you coming from a medical background helps people
> [express their feelings]. If you were just a lay person probably people
> might not be so inclined to be so [forthcoming] ... Actually I'm saying
> that it's helpful to have someone to talk to you, but if you knew that
> 'a counsellor' was coming to talk to you you might think, 'Oh, I don't
> know that I'm really interested in that.' But the fact that you know its
> 'a medical person,' it's different. You don't feel it's that anyone's trying to
> sort you out or anything.
>
> (P25: mother of preterm baby with brain damage)

The interview setting also had advantages over talking to staff from the
Unit. Parents could be critical without feeling disloyal or worrying about
feelings, they could re-live the whole experience in its entirety, they could
describe events without feeling that they must show appreciation or con-
formity, and time was not limited – they could take things at their own
pace and for as long as it took, and they were within the security of their
own home.

One couple, however, said that they had their own idiosyncratic motive
for taking part. They had given the consultant 'a hard time' in the hospital
and only much later came to appreciate his great skill and compassion.
They wanted to participate in the research to please him and to help to
make reparation for their own conduct at the time.

Once they had participated, no couples expressed negative reactions to
being interviewed, although some said that they had had initial reservations beforehand. The strong positive messages conveyed would seem to
support the fact that researchers can explore such sensitive ground without adverse effects on the interviewees.

# Discussion

Before we discuss the issues relating to support, it seems important to
remind ourselves of the enormity of what parents are dealing with in the
days, weeks, months and years after a child has died. A few statements
made by grieving parents capture something of the ongoing pain.

> Nothing fills the void of his absence. He's not replaceable. We can't go out
> and get another just like him ... There's a hole in the world now. In the

place where he was, there's now just nothing . . . The world is emptier. My son is gone. Only a hole remains, a void, a gap, never to be filled . . . It's the *neverness* that is so painful. *Never again* to be here with us . . . All the rest of our lives we must live without him. Only our death can stop the pain of his death.[72]

There is no adequate epitaph for the death of a child, and no sense in searching for one.[195]

Intense grief brings intense pain to those who mourn. The death of a child brings grief that comes like ocean waves in a ferocious storm. At first the pain is unbearable, and then it gets worse.[196]

And parental loss is a permanent condition. Once the rawness of early bereavement has passed, a 'shadow grief' remains which may be triggered by significant dates, specific events or a chance comment.[83] Parents think of what the child would now be doing, this 'empty historical track' being most painful at significant points in the life of a child when milestones would have been reached.[57] Dreams over time are periodically shattered and each is mourned. Every time someone asks the parents how many children they have, they again face the enormity of their loss.[57] Life is never again just as it was before. Parents must learn to live with the reality. As one father wrote 12 years on:

The wound is no longer raw. But it has not disappeared. That is as it should be. If he was worth loving, he is worth grieving over. Grief is existential testimony to the worth of the one loved. That worth abides. So I own my grief. I do not try to put it behind me, to get over it, to forget it . . . I shall remember Eric. Lament is part of my life.[72]

This was a view reinforced by our study.

The secret is not to try to forget about what happened, but to learn to live with it. It's not something to get over. But you learn to carry it.
(P27: parents of baby with cardiac anomaly)

Indeed, some parents have spoken eloquently of their wish never to get over it — by holding on to the sadness they hold on to the precious remembrances.[57] Something of the child is retained in the pain.

# Bereavement changes parents

If we are not to fall into the trap of inappropriately labelling people as pathological in their grieving, it is important to recognise that this experience changes people. Furthermore, as has already been said, there are many features inherent in the loss of a *child* that would be regarded in other circumstances of loss as predisposing a mourner to complications,[59] and additional factors which make it unique among losses.

Our findings reinforce this observation. The parents report changes in themselves which are sometimes alarming. They are frightened by the 'crazy ideas' they entertain, and fearful for their sanity, but Ironside, in her rather provocative view of bereavement, has reassured them that other people share the same sense of confusion, and that 'even in your craziest, most evil, most charmless, most miserable, most blanked off moments, you are not alone.'[197] Socially unacceptable feelings are normal. 'Hating' other successful parents, and wanting to berate or attack pregnant women or parents who are careless of their children's welfare, are understandable reactions.

Bereaved parents' values and ambitions change. Many cease to be single-minded in the pursuit of a career or the acquisition of material possessions, the value of family and friends now being more precious to them.[48,56] In the face of the enormity of their own experience, others people's priorities and trivial preoccupations seem absurd.

Feelings of anger and injustice repeatedly surfaced in our interviews. Why me? Why us? Why do unloving or inadequate parents have healthy babies who live? Parental irritation or anger can stem from many things – for example, a sense of injustice (being treated unfairly), a sense of negative entitlement (being cheated of what is deserved), loss of dreams (missing out on important events), and unrealistic social expectations (you should be over it by now).[198]

# Each family is unique

Although some of these reactions are commonly observed, the findings from our study highlight the uniqueness of each family. Reactions vary considerably, irrespective of gestational age or any other demographic factor, although a strong impression was conveyed that the shock and sorrow associated with the loss of a full-term, normally formed child are qualitatively different from that associated with the loss of an extremely preterm child. However, it is the personal significance of the loss to these parents which is important,[77] and this fact emerges in the descriptions these parents have provided. In seeking to help them through this process it is not appropriate to categorise their experience, or to compare it with the experience of others, for as has been said, 'Each parent experiences, quite simply, the loss of *their* baby.'[77]

> . . . each death has its own character, so too each grief over a death has its own character. The dynamics of each person's sorrow must be allowed to work themselves out without judgement. I may find it strange that you should be tearful today but dry-eyed yesterday when my tears were yesterday. But my sorrow is not your sorrow.[72]

Neither is it helpful to allocate specific time periods to this process without reference to the individual and their circumstances, rather than simply the calendar.[76,199] Significant psychological symptoms have been reported even years after the loss of a child.[53,87] Attempts to measure grief,[200] or to offer guidelines,[201,202] all carry their own limitations: '... describing grief as a process with different stages is fraught with difficulty. Human feelings cannot be parcelled up with neat labels and put into compartments.'[76]

Human nature and parental need are infinite in their variety. Each individual must be treated as a unique person who deserves respect and dignity.[2] As our study shows, sometimes it is important to forget the textbook answers – the 'worked examples' – and concentrate on picking up the emotions and sensitivities of a given situation, going by one's instinct, as the GP seems to do when he calls to visit a mother on her expected date of delivery. Nevertheless we believe that there are certain key elements identified or reinforced by our study which underpin any effective attempt to support bereaved parents, and we shall discuss these in the following section in the context of these preliminary comments. Many of the factors which we identified from our data reflect those already cited in the literature as helpful or unhelpful,[73,83,203,204] but their identification in terms of this population of patients who have been involved in treatment decisions is significant.

# Who can help?

## The parents themselves

It is evident from our study that although this shared experience can bring couples closer together,[69] they may not always be available to each other as time goes on. Mothers and fathers invest different hopes and ambitions in their children. The loss of dreams at different stages of life will impinge on them in different ways and with varying intensity, losses which may periodically resurface throughout the parents' lives, triggered by incidents, dates or memories which may hold more meaning for one parent than for the other.[90] Furthermore, it is well established that mothers and fathers grieve differently.[90,198,205,206] Our data confirm the general picture of women weeping and talking, and men working and keeping quiet. Each is so absorbed in their own grief that there may be no room for comforting the other.[196] For those who do make space, there are other perils. Sometimes one partner may comfort the other at the cost of not fulfilling their own needs. Evidence exists of fathers avoiding dealing with their own grief by this strategy.[90] We also had parents 'cracking' at different times, each trying to be strong for the other at different points in the process, attributing later problems such as a 'complete mental breakdown' to earlier suppression of their own needs.

As a result of these differences and tensions, the parents may feel out of synchrony with each other.[89] In our study, almost half of the couples had struggled to maintain their relationship, a phenomenon that is well documented in the literature.[90,198] And even those relationships which did survive were often substantially changed by the experience.[59] It is clear then that although to some extent the parents themselves are uniquely placed to help each other, for a variety of reasons they may need to look outside the dyadic relationship for support in their grieving.

### Lay people

We found that almost all parents obtained some support from outside their relationship. In both stages of grieving our finding was that friends play a significant role. Relatives may be too close emotionally. They too are grieving – but for a different person. So whilst the mother is mourning the baby she cannot cradle in her arms or feed at her breast, and the father is grieving the son he will never take to the zoo, the grandparents are mourning not only the loss of their grandchild and the sense of continuity, but the painful loss their own children are enduring. Each is having to come to terms with their own personal sorrow. Inasmuch as their unique closeness and emotional bond bind them to the parents and make them sensitive to their needs and wishes, close relatives can be extremely supportive. However, where they fail to recognise the devastating pain that the parents are feeling, or they are egocentric or competing for attention, or impose unrealistic expectations on the parents, they can be a source of additional stress and secondary losses.[59,174,198] In addition, intentions may be misunderstood. We found that grandparents are sometimes perceived as too upset to listen to the parents, to hear their story, or to visit the grave. On experiencing this withdrawal but not hearing its explanation at the time, it is not uncommon for parents initially to interpret the grandparents' unavailability as evidence of their not really caring. For other parents there is a barrier to sharing grief because they themselves do not want to inflict deeper hurt on their own parents who carry burdens of their own (for example, unresolved grief for their own lost children). In their sadness each generation can be unavailable to the other at a time when both need sensitive support. Sometimes it is only from outside this network of criss-crossing pains that healing peace can be found.[197] Trusted friends who can tolerate the parents' strong emotions and who are not emotionally linked to the baby may be more available.

## Other children

The parents in our study who already had living children reported that, for the most part, they were a great source of comfort and support. Not only did they offer tangible evidence of their capacity to parent successfully, but by their very normality they helped the family to return to its usual routines and adjust to everyday living again. Although a small number of parents reported looking with sadness at the other children and mourning the fact that the dead child would never reach the milestones or have the experiences which they enjoyed with the other siblings, we found little suggestion of their grief being complicated by the fact that they were simultaneously trying to relinquish their role as parent to the dead child and maintain the same role in relation to the living child,[59] except for one group of parents. The exceptions were those parents who had had multiple births in which one or more of the babies had survived.

Our study highlights the special problems faced by families where one or more of the babies survives. There appears to be some uncertainty in the literature about the effect of survivors on parental mourning. Although grief reactions are not thought to differ between such parents and those of singleton deaths in the short or long term,[207] other researchers have found that depressive symptoms may interfere with the mourning process,[208] and some have even identified the presence of a surviving twin as a predictor of a morbid grief reaction.[209] There is, however, some evidence that healthcare staff as well as family and friends may downplay the loss, assuming the parents to be suffering less because one or more of the babies still lives,[207,208] and this was the experience of our respondents in these circumstances. For example, one mother was extremely distressed by events not of her own making or choosing. After a year of being told by 'everyone' to be strong for her surviving child, she was caught in an untenable situation. Her own mother insisted on holding a party to celebrate the surviving twin's first birthday, and simultaneously this respondent's husband sat alone on the grave of the dead twin. It is clear that all those who seek to support such families, both professional and lay helpers, need to be alert to this danger.

## Next pregnancies

Our finding of a 52% rate of new pregnancy reflects other reported rates.[190] In our sample, this new pregnancy was cited as a major source of happiness and support to the parents. However, the literature is divided on the wisdom of a rapid return to pregnancy following the death of a child,[43,44,145,190,210] and mothers themselves have maintained that the decision is a personal one, influenced by many factors.[192] This was our finding – that it is personal to each couple. A certain amount of ambivalence seems to be inevitable as the parents feel that their present happiness in a new pregnancy is disloyal to the dead child.[81] However, both throughout the literature and in our study grieving parents have emphasised the fact that having another child does not replace the one who was lost.[51] By providing a focus for their nurturing instincts, a sense of continuity and a hope for the future, new pregnancies and babies help the parents to move on in their adjustment to their changed circumstances, but another child can never fill the 'specific void left by the child who died.'[51] No child is replaceable, and thoughtless comments which deny this reality are a source of pain to parents in these circumstances.

## Healthcare professionals

Our findings show that healthcare professionals have the potential to offer a specific form of support which families find valuable. We shall detail just how this may be provided in a subsequent section but, in general, if they have not known the child, they have the experience of other families and their own medical knowledge to provide accurate information and reassurance. If they have known the baby, they can also reminisce and speak knowledgeably about the specifics in their case. Either way, an ongoing interest in the welfare of the family is greatly appreciated. Our study demonstrates that it is critically important that families do not feel 'deserted as well as devastated'[53] after the death of their child.

Although only eight families in our study were involved with a professional counsellor, we found a strong positive reaction to their involvement. The capacity of the counsellor to facilitate the effective expression of pain, bear their distress, make appropriate responses and maintain an ongoing interest made her assistance both welcomed and helpful. Other studies have also demonstrated a positive effect of such an intervention following perinatal loss,[87,174] although some caution in interpreting these results is necessary because the control group in one such study[174] received minimal attention by today's standards, including no opportunity to see their baby in some cases. In our own research many fathers specifically raised the subject of counselling. It was clear that they had an inbuilt resistance to such a concept, regarding it as an admission of weakness and inability to cope. However, inasmuch as they clearly derived great benefit from talking during the interviews, it appears that the principles of counselling do work for them, and the way in which the therapy is promoted may be germane to the uptake of any support along these lines.

## Ministers of religion

Ministers of religion are another professional group whom parents singled out for mention in the context of support. Those parents who find them helpful are warm in their praise. However, we found that more people feel supported by them as time goes by, rather than in the early weeks of bereavement. This might suggest that parents' needs for comfort and help with the difficult existential questions may not surface until the acute phase of grieving has subsided, or it might be a feature of a reduction in other avenues of support as the months pass.

## Bereavement groups

Other bereaved parents are reported to be important sources of support for bereaved parents.[43,52,196,203] They bear the mark of pain.[211] They are united by a 'common bond of suffering that joins bodies in their shared vulnerability.'[1] They provide an opportunity to share feelings in an atmosphere of understanding and acceptance, which allows parents to see that they are not alone in experiencing such painful grief, and that recovery is possible.

Some parents do derive comfort from this source, even though in our sample they were a small minority. They can feel a real sense of identification, understanding and acceptance with other parents whose lives have been similarly shattered, who will think nothing of them suddenly breaking down in tears or talking again and again about their dead child.[57] For those parents who do derive support from such a group it is salutary to hear that making the initial contact is an extremely difficult thing to do, a fact borne out by the literature.[57,73]

However, attending groups is not for everyone.[57,212] As we have found, some parents are simply not 'joiners' of groups, while others shy away from a situation which identifies people by their bereavement, or which seems to encourage preoccupation with death, or exposes parents to even more anxiety. Parents find it deeply troubling to hear so many sad stories, or to discover how often things go wrong, or to learn that parents can and do suffer repeated losses. They look for reassurance that people move on in their grieving and become happy again in time. To hear women still crying and profoundly upset 6, 10, 20 years on undermines their confidence and depresses them.

# What types of help do parents find supportive?

Our findings in general support those already identified – that the key elements are caring, sharing and remembering.[57] However, bearing in mind the circumstances (treatment decisions having been made) it is important to look at some of these features in more depth.

## Caring

Many people make well-intentioned efforts to provide support, but the parents in our study identified two main factors which represented for them genuine caring and compassion, namely a valuing of the life of the baby, and a recognition of their own enormous loss. Nothing should be done or said to diminish the importance of either of these. No matter how short the life or how right the decision to withdraw treatment, dismissive comments are extremely painful for parents.[213] Meaningless platitudes, or appeals to the parents to consider themselves fortunate, are an understandable reaction in situations such as this where security in a happy outcome from pregnancy has been shaken, but they are misguided. 'Lightning never strikes twice' (we, the parents, know that it sometimes does). 'You didn't really know him' (but we *did* know the baby he was). 'It's nature's way of sorting things out' (so are earthquakes and flu epidemics, but it doesn't make them any more palatable). 'You can always have another' (but another child won't replace this one). 'I know how you feel' (you cannot possibly know). Only the parents may justifiably 'count their blessings', and it ill behoves others to do so for them. As bereaved parents themselves have advised:

> If what you are about to say to someone in grief offers an easy or simple answer, don't say it. There are no easy answers – there is only accompaniment . . . offer love, not advice or opinions.[196]

It is not just what is said that matters, but how and when parents are approached, too, if support is to be sensitive and caring. There is a time to be with parents and a time to leave them alone. The families whom we studied illustrate how often people gauge wrongly what is needed. Those who suffer so many intrusive calls that they have to escape from the house may be as unsupported as those who see other people crossing the street to avoid them. Bereaved people have a need to find their own meaning in bitter experiences, and they sometimes need space and privacy to do so. No one can shield them from the hurt – it has to be lived through. Richard Selzer, recovering from a coma caused by Legionnaires' disease, summed up his own interpretation of privacy. He was asked by his physician why he was anxious to be discharged from hospital. He replied that he wanted not just privacy – he was in a private room – but also 'solitude. A condition that does not include people like you coming in here whenever they feel like it and asking me what else I want.'[214] As from professionals, so from family and friends: 'Even the most benevolent interruption remains an intrusion when it is uninvited.'[1]

It is so difficult to find the right words, and parents speak eloquently of the messages conveyed without words. The spontaneous embrace, and the tears that can convey a pain understood and shared.

But please: Don't say it's not really so bad. Because it is. Death is awful, demonic. If you think your task as comforter is to tell me that really, all things considered, it's not so bad, you do not sit with me in my grief but place yourself off in the distance away from me. Over there, you are of no help. What I need to hear from you is that you recognize how painful it is. I need to hear from you that you are with me in my desperation. To comfort me, you have to come close. Come sit with me on my mourning bench. . . . Your tears are salve on our wounds.[72]

True compassion recognises that there are many triggers to a parent's sorrow, even long after the death. These parents remind us again of the traumas resurrected by other pregnant women (especially those who do not take care of themselves during pregnancy)[81] and by anniversaries – the conception, the expected date of delivery, the birth, the death or the funeral[173] – or the cards which mark them,[215] by special celebratory days such as Christmas or New Year or Mother's Day and Father's Day.[57,72,81]

In the context of never diminishing the loss parents experience, special mention must be made of the fathers. It is clear from our findings that it is fairly common for fathers to be marginalised and excluded.[93,216,217] They themselves may add to the belief that it is women's work to weep by hiding their emotions and 'being strong,' and appearing to recover from the loss more quickly.[205,218,219] However, as one grieving father commented:

Our culture says that men must be strong and that the strength of a man in sorrow is to be seen in his tearless face . . . why is it so important to act strong? . . . I have been assaulted, and in the assault wounded, grievously wounded. Am I to pretend otherwise? Wounds are ugly, I know. They repel. But must they always be swathed? I shall look at the world through tears. Perhaps I shall see things that dry-eyed I could not see.[72]

It is important to remember that fathers are grieving, too. They just have different ways of showing their reactions and different ways of dealing with the loss, as we have seen from the families whom we studied. Not only do fathers need to be remembered in any support services,[69] but mothers may need help in understanding that their menfolk may have gone back to work quickly, and they may still be attending sports fixtures or drinking in the pub with friends as if nothing had happened, but they are also weeping as they drive along the road past the cemetery, and spending time sitting on the grave or looking at photographs of the baby when they think no one is watching. They too are grieving,[206] and their grief is not so much for the baby they cannot push in the pram today, as it is for the child they cannot play with on the beach, the son they will never take to the football match, or the daughter they cannot escort up the aisle on her wedding day.

## *Sharing*

Our findings provide evidence that sharing their experience is a vital part of mourning for these parents. The bereaved commonly have an immense need to talk, and to tell their story many times over.[1,80] Parents of newborns are no exception – they welcome an opportunity to discuss what happened to their baby.[57,67,83,174,209] Doing so helps them to adjust to their new reality.[48] Not to be able to talk in this way has been associated with unresolved grief.[83,220] The difficulty seems to be in finding sensitive and willing listeners. It may be important to the parents to remember, but other people appear to expect and want them to forget. Friends and family weary of the endless repetition. Consequently, the parents become reluctant to trigger powerful emotional upset, and they have even been found to perform elaborate charades, pretending that they are over the death in order to protect others – even partners – from being exposed to their grief.[83]

The importance of talking is highlighted by our study. By talking, parents begin to assimilate and understand what is happening in their world, and to adjust to a different situation. Their narratives may well have a painful and challenging quality which is uncomfortable to hear, but this 'uncomfortable quality is all the more reason they have to be told.'[1] Sharing their story, and sorting it out, is part of the remembering.

> We need to tell someone else a story that describes our experience, because the process of creating a story also creates the memory structure that will contain the gist of the story for the rest of our lives. Talking is remembering.[221]

Listening to the parents' story is an essential function of effective support. This listening may include providing a verbal, sharing presence (a willingness to talk with parents about their experience and to share one's own similar experiences) and a listening presence (being with them and not avoiding them – a non-verbal communication of sympathy and understanding).[222] Being willing to listen and to keep listening, with a genuine sense of sincerity and without giving advice, or responding with clichés, and being able to remain with them while they express their emotions and re-live their memories, can be immensely therapeutic.[45,223] However, our results show that parents rarely find such a capacity in one person. Instead, they rehearse their story with different people. Newcomers to this role have some advantages, as people who knew the parents before the tragedy occurred are to some extent working at trying to rediscover their old selves. The 'stranger', on the other hand, has no such expectation and is intent on discovering the new selves of the parents.[1] Carers who come on the scene after the event may therefore have an advantage over old friends and close family in this respect.

Being a listening presence requires empathy. Empathy is a rather over-worked word nowadays, and is often taken to mean 'walking in another's shoes.' Our study would seem to support the preferable notion of 'walking alongside' – of entering the private perceptual world of the parent suffi-ciently to understand what it is like from their point of view, feeling what they are feeling without actually being involved in the emotion person-ally.[80] The centre of attention is *their* pain, not that of the listener.

Being with someone in their grief can be a frightening and draining experience. The 'crossing the street' phenomenon is well recognised and can be understood. It is all too easy for an angry or deeply hurt bereaved person to take offence at even the most kindly meant words or actions. To the 'vulnerable bereaved, most people can appear to be clodhopperingly insensitive.'[197] Knowing this, and aware of their own sense of inadequacy, people are embarrassed and unsure about what to say. Avoiding having to speak to the bereaved parent protects them from saying the wrong thing. However, our findings show that although these parents understand the motives which drive people to avoid them, they none the less find it deeply painful to experience. Feeling their withdrawal further isolates the parent, as one mother found:

> I live in silent sadness now because people cannot talk about it with me – perhaps they don't want to or think I don't want to. But I don't want Sian to be forgotten. When programmes crop up on TV about child loss, the people in the room grow silent and can't bear for their eyes to meet mine. Everyone's heart goes out to me, but no words are spoken.[93]

It is perhaps salutary to hear the words of another mother of a two-year-old child who died of leukaemia. She wrote that she did not look for answers from people, 'just the silent expression of empathy, and perhaps the comfort of a hug.'[129]

We found that it is especially hard for these vulnerable parents to feel that the onus is on *them* to make all the running in order to set other people at ease.

> What did I find hard? People who couldn't look me in the eye and I there-fore had to go out of my way to accommodate and reassure them in order for us to be able to resume a normal relationship. Those who told me that 'these things happen for a reason and if I can't see it now I will in years to come.' I know these folk are well-meaning and, believe me, I am the eternal optimist and I *can* find *some* good out of all this tragedy but tell me, what possible true reason or consolation can there be in such a tiny, beautiful, innocent little boy being plunged half-cooked into the world, and then plucked away so rapidly?[93]

Sharing may also involve providing information. In seeking to complete their story, parents need to have all the pieces of the jigsaw in place. The mother who tramps from professional to clinic to hospital for many months searching for answers, the parents who seek redress through the courts, the couple who are still angrily waiting for an explanatory letter 13 months after the death, all bear testament to the powerful need for a cohesive and complete story. Lawsuits are expensive and immensely draining. The costs to the NHS are high and rising, and cases currently take an average of five years to settle.[224] Some vulnerable parents felt that they could not face such a painful experience even though there might have been a case to answer. A new fast-track scheme is being developed in England to cut the costs of litigation for medical negligence. A system of 'pre-action protocols' launched in April 1999 aims to facilitate resolution within 12 months.[224] The system involves healthcare professionals being encouraged to be open and honest with patients, lawyers and each other, to hand over all relevant records within 40 days or face financial penalties, and to admit mistakes within three months. The consultants in our study who openly shared their knowledge of events are operating within the spirit of this system, and the parents who have experienced this openness speak warmly of its value. On the other hand, those who feel doors or ranks close are left dispirited, mistrustful, and fearful of future encounters with the NHS.

## *Remembering*

Mourning requires memories,[67] but when a baby dies there may be few of them. It has been suggested that in any assessment of who is helping parents to grieve there are two elements to consider – first, who helps them 'to create the experience of their baby's existence,' and second, who helps them 'to understand this experience and to mourn and accept their loss.'[173] We found that tangible reminders of their baby are clearly important things to preserve. Parents told us how they clung to the bloody sheet, the unwashed bonnet which still retained the baby's smell, or the splint which had rested next to his arm. These are the objects which will always carry direct associations.[225] They do not want to forget the child, but sometimes they fear that they will forget details of his or her short life,[56] so things which keep those memories fresh are welcomed.

Less concrete memories also needed to be cultivated and facilitated. Our findings support the value of mutual reminiscing. In most cases, for parents of neonates there are few people who have shared those memories. The staff who have known the child most intimately have a crucial role to play, not just in helping the parents to accumulate memories during the dying process, but also in preserving those memories through reminiscences and shared stories, by completing the picture with those additional snippets of information that bring understanding and acceptance. Parents appreciate some continuity in the maintenance of contact.[203] When such contact is inexplicably broken off, there is a void which represents for the parents a loss of interest and a forgetting. A clear message emerges from our study – that parents regret the abrupt severing of the relationships which they have built up during the life of the child. The loss of contact cuts off a crucial source of memories. The nurse who rings the parents to find out how they are coping and whether they would like her to join them for a coffee and a chat, or the consultant who meets with the parents three times over many months, do more than offer emotional support – they help to keep the memories of these babies alive and fresh.

# Are these families different from other grieving parents?

By weaving the literature through our findings we have tried to demonstrate that most of these observations about support have already been identified over the years in various different contexts and with varying degrees of authority. We have added the personal accounts of parents to the more quantifiable research studies, and the psychological underpinnings to the more clinical implications. Bringing these facets together in this way is perhaps more novel.

Our findings show that parents change through this experience, and that their support needs fluctuate as well. Most feel that they mature through the process, but it is important to remember that 'the growth that comes from parental bereavement is always a consolation prize'.[57] Most parents would give up all the maturity to have the child back. One difference between our respondents and those studied elsewhere is that the babies of all of the parents we included had been the subject of discussions about treatment limitation. Alongside their yearning for the child, these mothers and fathers are dealing with the burdens and benefits of continuing existence. As we have seen, some fear continued existence in a severely impaired state more than they fear death. Some harbour doubts about the decision, the speed of treatment withdrawal or the accuracy of the prognosis. However, as with all other parents, they need to express these feelings and to be helped to make sense of what has been done. It could be argued that their need for empathic listening is perhaps even greater than that of other bereaved parents, and the number of people who could contain and be responsive to those fears and doubts without offering platitudes is probably smaller. We found that some parents do not share with close relatives the fact that a decision had been made to stop treatment, thereby cutting off one avenue of support. Other parents feel that since no one else they know has ever had such an experience, no one in their circle of friends and relatives can possibly understand their pain. They, too, have limits set around their social support network.

It is perhaps because of this, and because they have shared such a profound experience with the staff in the NICU, that these parents regret the loss of contact with those who share their memories and have accompanied them through the decision making and the death. There is much to reflect on and much to make sense of, but few memories to preserve. These families clearly require all the help they can get from the few people who are best placed to support them.

# Conclusion

- The pain of parental bereavement is ongoing, but it changes in intensity over time. Reminders of the permanence of the loss are painful.
- Parents want routine checks by healthcare professionals to ensure that they are coping. Periodic contact demonstrates that they have not been abandoned.
- Parents benefit from opportunities to talk to a knowledgeable, empathic listener who is capable of bearing their powerful emotions, especially where there are barriers to open communication between the parents.
- In general, parents look for support which facilitates their grieving and in time integrates them back into their social circle. Their usual avenues of support may not be available to them at this time. They should be encouraged to give clear cues to other people as to what they find helpful or unhelpful at different stages of the bereavement process.
- Some warning of the emotions the parents might expect to experience may be helpful, particularly for fathers.
- Shared memories are important, and NICU teams should ensure that cards and contacts come from those who actually knew the baby.
- If unanswered questions remain, every effort should be made to supply information which enables the parents to complete their understanding of what happened.
- Other children help parents to return to their normal routines, but those families with surviving babies born at the same time as the dead child are especially vulnerable. Not only are they simultaneously grieving and celebrating, but they have constant painful reminders of what they have lost. Other people, including healthcare professionals, must be on their guard against being too demanding and not giving such parents space or permission to grieve.

- A subsequent pregnancy may help parents to face the future with renewed hope, but the appropriate timing of such an event depends on personal circumstances.
- A minority of parents find a bereavement group helpful. A specific difficulty arises with regard to making contact with such a group, and parents may prefer someone else to initiate this contact.
- There are three key elements to effective support, namely caring, sharing and remembering.

  *Caring* involves valuing the life of the baby and acknowledging the parents' loss. It allows family members to grieve in their own way and at their own pace, recognising the particularly vulnerable position of fathers, who are inclined to be overlooked.

  *Sharing* involves responsive, empathic listening and the supply of information, where necessary, to enable parents to understand what has happened.

  *Remembering* involves facilitating the sharing of memories with those who knew the baby, and the collection and preservation of mementoes which keep his or her memory alive.
- Mothers may need help in accepting that their male partners are still grieving once they have returned to their usual routines.
- For families who have been involved in a decision to withdraw treatment, there are potentially additional doubts and fears which may require sensitive awareness and careful handling over and above that required by other grieving parents.

# CHAPTER 13

# Parents' opinions

The men and women in our study had been forced to address difficult questions about treatment limitation. Theirs were not theoretical opinions but those acquired through bitter experience: they should be heard. It was only after they had detailed their own experience that the parents were asked if they had any opinions in general about stopping treatment. Since no attempt was made to guide their thinking, it is all the more remarkable that clear categories emerged.

## Limitation of treatment: opinions held shortly after the death of the baby

Although many parents expressed their amazement at the capabilities of modern medicine, one father felt that things might be simpler and better if the technology did not exist for such heroic measures in some instances. The capacity to treat such critically ill children raised difficult questions to which there were no easy answers.

## Individual decision

A strong feeling was conveyed that the decision had to be an individual one for each baby, with a third of the parents (20 of 59, 34%) citing this as an important factor in relation to when treatment should be limited. Parents frequently qualified their opinions by saying that they spoke for themselves and would not want to impose their own views on other families. What was right for one family might not be so for another, and what was in the best interests of one baby might not be for another. Furthermore, they recognised even at this stage that if they themselves were ever faced with the same decision again, they might choose differently. They were

acutely aware of the many feelings and facts which could influence choices
at such a time.

# When to withdraw or withhold treatment

In response to a specific question about when treatment should be withdrawn or withheld, 14 sets of parents (24%) replied that if there was any
hope of survival the child should be treated: they deserved a chance. Three
couples specifically mentioned preterm infants in this context. On the
other hand, one mother was definite in her view that no baby under 28
weeks should be treated.

Three main reasons were given for withholding treatment – if the child
was severely damaged, if death was inevitable, or if the baby was suffering
(*see* Figure 13.1).

When it came to making a decision about where to draw the line, a clear
message was conveyed by the parents – the baby's interests were paramount.

> I think looking back now I would feel guilty if we just kept him on the
> machine. And maybe 3, 4 in the morning when we had slept – but for
> two days we had gone down to the room [to be with the baby – and on
> this night we had] gone to bed and maybe been woken up at 5 to be told
> he'd died. I think I probably would feel guilty to this day if that had been
> the scenario. I think I probably would have felt I didn't agree to take him
> off the life support to ease my own conscience rather than to give him a
> comfortable passage into death. I would have thought that would have

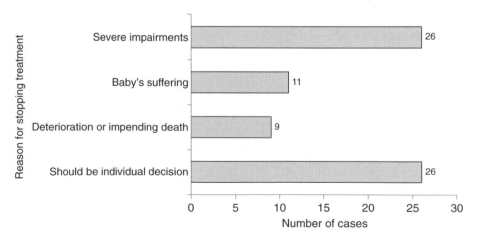

**Figure 13.1:**   Parents' opinions about when treatment should be withheld ($n = 59$).

been a decision for *me* rather than for *him*. I'm happy in my own mind that we did it for him rather than for ourselves.

(P27: father of baby with cardiac anomaly)

Much as they might wish the baby to live, the parents had to consider his interests, or as a few expressed it, they must not be 'selfish.' Perhaps the most obvious situation where death seemed preferable to continuing life was where the child was clearly deteriorating and death was inevitable, a reason cited by a fifth of the parents ($n = 11$, 19%). In such circumstances they believed that it was both futile and cruel to prolong the dying process.

Where there was no direct evidence of impending death, the burdens of pain, distress and indignity had to be weighed against the benefits of possible survival. These all carried a cost to the baby which parents worried about. Indeed, suffering was a major preoccupation of these parents throughout the interviews.

> I wonder if they try too hard; if they maybe put [the baby] through more than she [should have had to suffer]. I don't know if maybe there comes a point where it's not your baby anymore because there's no blood in there that's hers, etc. So I wonder. But then again, when do you stop trying? I started to think when she turned bad. Up until then I'd been really praying for her to live and then it was: 'Well, she's just going through too much now. She just doesn't seem like my baby any more. Her body's full of drugs, and there've got to be long term effects of that.' In fact her whole body was full of drugs and other people's blood … [At the time, when it was my own baby who] was ill, I would have tried to do anything – they could have cut off one of my arms if it makes her right … But afterwards I've now sat and thought how bad her life would have been if she had lived … Is it really right for me to make the decision to keep her alive when it's going to involve her in so much pain and distress? … Up until [the day she started to deteriorate] I was being really selfish and I just wanted her and that was it, and I didn't care what she was going to be like, I just wanted her. And then I started to think, 'Well, what about her?' Because she just looked so ill … It got to the point where you thought, 'Well, if that was me lying there with all these strange people looking down, all these bright lights,' you would just wonder, would you want to carry on?

(P45: mother of preterm baby)

I think that the process that we went through [limiting treatment] allowed our son a little dignity which I don't think we would otherwise have had. And I am very relieved that the process worked the way it did … I found it unbearable when I thought that a legal or medical opinion would mean that I would be living for the rest of my life with a child who would have pain and suffering. We were spared that. And he was spared that. It was appalling to think that you were going to have a child who wasn't going to have the kind of life that we could give him, that we would want him to have.

(P18: parents of preterm baby)

Although only nine families (15%) specifically cited suffering as a reason to stop treatment, many more expressed their anxieties about the effect on babies of aggressive treatment and prolonged damaged lives. Clearly the family suffered, too, but this was always a secondary consideration.

The question of the quality of the child's life was raised by the majority of parents in some form.

I don't think it's a question of the condition [– for example, Downs or a particular heart defect]. It's a question of whether you can pre-dict whether that person is going to have a sufficient quality of life – whether it's going to be walking, smiling, appreciating, taking things in.

(P51: father of baby with congenital anomalies)

Only two families (3%) specifically said that future disability should not be brought into the equation when deciding whether or not to treat. For them, if there was a chance of life, the child should be treated. It is important to note that in one of these cases both the parents had worked extensively with disabled people.

However, 26 sets of parents (44%) spontaneously cited severe impair-ments as a reason for allowing a child to die.

I don't think you should sustain life which isn't a life. These babies – they're not just an object on a machine.

(P16: father of preterm baby)

Given the sensitivity of the subject for these grieving parents just a few weeks after their own baby had died, it was necessary to tread lightly in this area. But, for some, gentle probing seemed appropriate and they were asked to expand on what a severe impairment might entail. No one felt able to define their limits precisely, although as one mother commented it might be difficult to identify parameters in the abstract, but a parent knew instinctively whether the damage was too severe when faced with a given scenario. This woman and her husband had themselves held the view before having children that they would not want an 'imperfect child.' When their first child was born with an obvious but medically minor defect, she had been 'shocked' and 'hysterical.' However, as a picture emerged over many weeks of problems of increasing severity their opinions changed. By the time the baby died they knew the strength of parental love which could overcome obstacles, and the depth of parental grief. Perfection was not now an absolute requirement. It was clearly difficult to draw lines which would hold in reality as well as in theory, as many parents found. There were few absolutes. Indeed, parents who had themselves made a decision based on the quality of future life said that they could not predict even what *they* would choose if such a situation presented a second time. Furthermore, one couple who had had several impaired fetuses had in fact come to different conclusions on different occasions.

Although rigid boundaries could not be set, the clearest concept to emerge was that of dependence. If the child could not lead an independent life – either from medical intervention or from other people – then that life was better not extended.

## Active measures to end life

Although the subject was never introduced by the interviewer, five families spontaneously raised the issue of 'euthanasia' (by which they meant active termination of a life). They all believed that there was a place for it in hopeless or 'no purpose' situations. Perceptions of what was permissible clearly varied. Two of these sets of parents believed that euthanasia was permissible for babies and was practised. In both cases they reported that morphine was given to their infants, and in their perceptions this had been a contributory factor in the death of the child. They saw this as a form of euthanasia. Two families expressed their surprise that active measures to end life seemed to be permissible for babies but not for adults. However, another family believed that such active measures were not permitted. They personally wished that doctors had given their own baby a dose of morphine sufficient to end his life soon after a bleak prognosis was given, but they reported being told that this was illegal. Such a measure would have spared them all the agony of a prolonged and distressing death, they felt.

## Limitation of treatment: opinions held 13 months after the death of the baby

When the parents were asked 13 months after the death the same question about the limits they would set, a similar picture emerged. As before, the question was an open one and no attempt was made to guide thinking, so these similarities are striking. One couple declined to state a view, the father adding that they feared philosophising at all about these issues lest they become unhappy with the conclusions they reached.

Parents conveyed a belief that in general the public are ill-informed about these issues. As a consequence, theoretical views tend to be inherently different from opinions that arise from lived experience.

> I've had people actually ask me – just in general conversation – saying, 'Do you not think it's freakish [treating these babies]?' ... I don't see it like that, but obviously other people do ... A lot of these babies are probably the only babies these mothers and fathers can have, and I think it's good that they can do that. It might not be nature's way of doing it, but it makes a lot of people happy at the end of it. It might be their one and only child. All the people that tend to criticise, you feel are people that can have the 'norm baby' – it's not people that have been in situations like all these mothers that *can't* have the norm baby. And *that's* the people that say, 'Oh, I think they're tampering with nature; that's ridiculous.' But when I look at [my baby] I think, 'Well, that's my girl. If they didn't do what they did for her, I wouldn't have her.'
>
> (P10: parents of preterm twins)

Their own experience had forced parents to address these issues and in many cases altered their opinions. They were now attracted to articles, books or programmes on these topics, and this encouraged them to reflect further on the questions and solutions they offered. Two couples drew attention to the different policies which they now knew obtained in different centres. One couple considered this unacceptable.

> From hospital to hospital the protocols are all different. That's, I think, what you find unacceptable. If somebody could say, 'Oh well, if you'd have been at that hospital down in London that would have been dealt with in a completely different way,' I think that's wrong.
>
> (P1: mother of baby with asphyxia)

The other couple had concluded that there should be a universal moral principle guiding decision making, but that doctors and parents should have the latitude to decide within that broad framework on the basis of the circumstances in each case. One other couple was disturbed by the revelation that the management of a child might hinge on which consultant happened to be on duty within a given Unit.

> Everything hung in the balance according to which paediatrician you have as to what was going to happen. We might well have been landed with something we didn't want to do if it had been one of the other doctors on that team. And my impression was that [our neonatologist] could have been the only person on that team who had the same opinion as we did [that it's best not to treat a baby who's born on the edge of viability]. So it's a lottery. It was just luck that we had him. And my

impression is that younger doctors who are coming through are much more inclined towards technical intervention . . . and it worries me that perhaps as time goes by and more technical intervention is possible the pressure's going to get much much worse on parents, and there will be no guidelines saying, 'Have you stopped to think? Have you really thought about the implications of what you're doing?'.

(P25: mother of preterm baby with brain damage)

# Individual decision

Opinions about decision-making itself have been discussed in detail earlier in this volume. Overall, a strong belief was conveyed that the decision has to be made for each individual case, and that the parents should be involved in making it to the extent to which they feel able.

*Father*: In a strange way I suppose we thought [making that decision to stop] was a parental act. We didn't get a chance to make many parental acts, but making that decision on behalf of [our baby] was a kind of parental duty.
*Mother*: I just think about it in relation to [our baby] and I feel it was right it was our decision because it's our child and you're still living with it a year later. At the time I didn't feel so strongly that this is my son and I must make the decision, because I hadn't had time to get to know him . . . Now over a year later I feel very strongly that this was my son and it's my responsibility.

(P27: parents of baby with cardiac anomaly)

Most parents limited their comments to the effect on their own family, but one father set his opinions within a broader context. There had to be limits to parental freedom, since the wider society would be affected by decisions to save the lives of children who went on to have severe disabilities.

My feeling are quite mixed up . . . I suppose ultimately it has to be a person's family who make that decision . . . it seems to be a decision about whether you take on that commitment to care [but] in many cases probably it isn't [*you* who takes on the real burden], it's going to be somebody else that finishes up providing the care. So I am quite mixed as to whether it [should be] parents or whether it [should be] somebody making that decision on behalf of the society that's going to care for people if it looks as though they're going to be very severely disabled. And I feel wide open, vulnerable, thinking about it at all because I could criticise myself severely for anything I've said.

(P49: father of baby with asphyxia)

Although the majority believed that parents should have a major role in decision making, a minority thought that it was too burdensome a decision for parents. Their voice must also be heard.

> When that was just put to us – [perhaps we should let her die] – we said, 'No,' because it's a horrific thing to think of. That was without thinking it through though, and the consequences of saying, 'No,' and what that was going to lead us on to and how we'd have to change our lives. And it's also like you're denying that child every right to life. It's like you're killing them, you're murdering them.
>
> (P9: parents of baby with cardiac anomaly)

It is important to draw attention to the strength of feeling parents showed after more than a year of reflection on these serious issues. The majority expressed themselves forcefully – parents should have a say in whether treatment should be stopped in these tragic circumstances. Even some of those who felt that it should be a predominantly medical decision commented on the fact that the parents were best placed to decide when it became a question of the family's tolerances and values. They were the ones who had to live with the consequences.

> I do recall [the consultant obstetrician] in particular throughout the pregnancy making us make decisions about things I didn't *want* to make decisions about. I just wanted it to happen and not to have to think about it. But actually he was absolutely right because when it came to the crunch, it happened in a way that we could both cope with ... So whilst I think that for a lot of people the onus being put on them might be very uncomfortable – it *is* uncomfortable! – but it's the longer-term [feelings] that are important in the end ... it's not until you're faced with it that you get a feeling for what you *do* think is right.
>
> (P50: mother of baby with congenital anomalies)

One father took this thinking a stage further. In his judgement the doctors were the only people who could determine whether treatment withdrawal was a legitimate option, but it was the parents who had the information to enable them to determine the area of discretion appropriate in their case. There was a prevailing belief that a screening process was in operation which was protective; parents would not be asked to consider withdrawal if there was any real hope for a child.

Again and again parents made reference to their desperate wish to have the baby survive, and some added that this desire posed a real danger, as it might cloud their judgement and make them 'selfish.' The longer treatment was prolonged, the more attached they became and the more difficult it was to let the baby go. This was consistent with the stories of a few fathers who had remained resolutely detached from the child initially in order to be strong when they had to make the hard decisions.

# When to withdraw or withhold treatment

No parents could set fixed parameters around circumstances where limitations should be applied. In general terms, as many as 11 sets of parents (22%) specifically said that babies should be given every chance if there was some hope of survival with a reasonable quality of life. One father raised a doubt which added a different dimension to the issue: medical advances were so swift that there was always a chance of a cure for various conditions being just around the corner, so this possibility should be borne in mind before treatment was withdrawn too hastily.

As before, there was an overwhelming focus on the best interests of the baby. Sometimes the cost to the child was too high and in these circumstances, as one father put it, better to have emotional or mental agony for the parents than for the child to suffer physically. Since this was again an open question, it is all the more remarkable that the categories identified by the parents were so similar to the previous set of responses (*see* Figure 13.2). The biggest difference was in the emphasis now placed on the suffering involved. This became the most frequently cited reason to stop ($n = 20$ sets of parents, 40%). Also at this stage the issue of dependence emerged spontaneously ($n = 7$, 14%): if the child could never live an independent life, it would be better that he or she die in infancy.

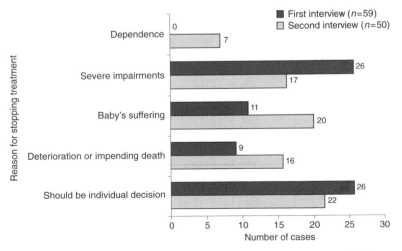

**Figure 13.2:** Parents' opinions about when treatment should be withheld: comparisons over time.

## Active measures to end life

By 13 months after the death, just three sets of parents spontaneously raised the matter of euthanasia. All three felt that there was definitely a place for actively ending babies' lives in certain circumstances, dying in comfort and with dignity being far preferable to painful, lingering or distressing deaths.

> If you've exhausted every possibility medically, you've got to have them as comfortable as possible. If that involves pumping drugs into them to stop the pain and if there's nothing else you can do to stop the pain, and if they've only got a couple of hours left, then there's no point in having that couple of hours in pain.
>
> (P7: father of baby with cardiac anomaly)

Only one of these three families was among the five who had raised the issue at the first interview. This was the family who felt that morphine should have been given early in the life of their own child, to end his life and prevent a lingering dying process and much distress.

> You've got all these people telling you that you can't have this [euthanasia]. But they're not going through, what you've just gone through so why should they run your life for you? The way I think it should happen is, if you don't want it to go any further, that child's having problems, is in pain or whatever – and he must have been in pain because he was on morphine – why didn't they just say to us, 'Well, let's stop it now; let's finish it now'? And it would have been three weeks less pain. Because the more time you spent there – you were up every night, every day – you got closer and closer to the boy. Because he was yours, you had that bond. But I think you should have the choice.
>
> (P39: father of baby with brain damage)

In both of the other cases the observation related to what the parents felt should obtain in general, and not to their own specific circumstances.

## Religious beliefs

At the first interview, soon after the death of the baby, the influence of religious beliefs which might relate to the issue of stopping treatment was explored. This was not designed to tap into associations with a particular religious organisation, but rather to understand those personal convictions which might have impinged on the parents' decisions, opinions or ways of coping.

Twenty-six sets of parents (44%) had no religious beliefs about the subject at all. One father who had had no religious beliefs before said that this experience simply reinforced his atheism. In a further six couples (10%) one parent had a faith which influenced their thinking, but their partner had none. Having no belief at all was seen by some parents as particularly disadvantageous. It eliminated the parents from a source of comfort in their loss. One atheist father commented that he believed that religion was created for just such a purpose, so comforting were its ideas. He himself promoted the concept of heaven and perfection after death to his older children, even though he was personally sceptical. In seeking such comfort, some parents attended church services who did not normally do so, while others called on the chaplain to provide compassion and ceremony in their time of need.

> All the time I'm praying for [my baby] and then when they said there was nothing they could do, I thought, 'Phht, there's no God.' But it was really strange how on the night [he died] how much I needed this minister there. And [my husband] felt the same and he's not religious. But he felt the same. He thought, 'I can't just let him go; who's going to look after him?' We needed him there. So he came but even he didn't try to say that God works in mysterious ways. Even he said to us, 'I don't know why God does these sorts of things.' And a man at my work was saying only the other day, 'I thought what's this minister going to say? What can he *possibly* say? But,' he said, 'he was really good.'
>
> (P9: mother of preterm twins)

Two mothers had actively sought a meaningful faith since the death of their child – one concluding that the ideas simply were not believable, and the other still engaging in deep discussion with the minister. One father who had rejected his Catholic upbringing found that guilt which he associated with his childhood teaching resurfaced at this time.

Parents from 32 families (54%) could identify some religious belief which related to limiting treatment in general or the death of their own child in particular. For some this concerned the actual life and death decisions. Two parents, both of whom were staunch Roman Catholics, believed that babies should always be treated until their time came to die. One indeed referred to switching off the life-sustaining machines as 'murder'. Several other parents (from six families) observed that, in their view, religious scruples should never be allowed to interfere with what was best for the baby. Parents from three families specifically cited the example of switching off the ventilator in this context.

For others it was more a matter of the solace which beliefs could offer.

> We do believe that he's in a better place. He's not going to have any pain. And there is a reason that he got taken. We do believe that now. I've

never really thought about it before. Because we're not really into the Bible or Jesus or anything like that. We don't go to church but we've always believed in God. And see when you're in that situation, you do pray – for a miracle – which is something we've never ever done. But we did pray for a miracle. And it's funny how you do get a belief. If we thought [our baby] was just lying down in a graveyard, I think we would go insane, that he isn't anywhere else. So it's comforting to think that it was God's will.

(P40: mother of baby with brain damage)

Several parents described having what they perceived to be religious or spiritual experiences which had comforted them – for example, seeing the baby's soul leave, seeing images in the sky, or feeling the child's presence. A more general belief in an afterlife was cited by 10 families (17%). It was a great comfort to them to believe that they would see their babies again, or that the child was now perfect, free from pain, with loved ones, being well cared for, or now able to do everything. Parents from three other families (5%) expressed a belief in God but uncertainty about an afterlife (although they all hoped that there was such a thing), or about the need for babies to suffer. Comfort for parents in 11 families (19%) came from a belief that God was working to a divine plan, and that there was therefore a reason why this terrible thing had happened. One other parent observed that aggressive medical treatment was part of that divine plan.

For many parents this experience of losing a baby had shocked them into re-examining their own opinions and beliefs. When things had been going smoothly for them, they had felt no real necessity to address the deep issues of life and religion. The results of such reflection could be positive or negative. For some parents, the fact that their convictions had been worked out through bitter experience made their faith more personal. Three parents now had a stronger belief in either a spiritual dimension to life or the hope of an afterlife. A religious experience had strengthened one mother's conviction. Two parents, both brought up as Roman Catholics, had now modified their ideas because what they had been taught did not match with their own real life experience. Another couple had started to go to church since they lost the baby and drew strength and comfort from doing so.

However, seven (12%) now seriously questioned their faith, wondering why God could allow such a tragedy to happen and where babies' suffering fitted into a loving God's plans.

No matter how much Jesus wanted him, we wanted him more. Everything I read in the Bible, I said, 'Well no, I don't agree with that.'

(P34: mother of preterm baby)

Two had tried going to church to seek comfort, but just could not equate their own experience with the picture of God the church promoted.

> You want to believe there is a God so He's looking after her. You just don't know. But I'd like to believe that there is a God and she is being looked after. But it is hard . . . You always believe but it's when something devastating happens that's when it tries your faith. If anybody had asked me before I'd have said, 'Yes, [I believe in God],' but now if anybody asked me I'd have to say, 'I don't know.'
>
> (P7: mother of baby with cardiac anomaly)

One mother had lost the little faith she had, and another was still very angry with God and had not been back to church since the tragedy. Two fathers and one mother temporarily lost their faith but had now had it restored. One of these fathers confessed that it had shocked him how easily he had abandoned a lifetime of belief in the face of one catastrophe.

Some parents had looked elsewhere for comfort. Three mothers had taken up spiritualism. Two parents specified that they had derived comfort from believing that something of the child continued on – one mother felt her child's presence in certain places in the house, and one father believed that his baby had been reincarnated. One mother drew solace from the belief that her baby girl, who had lived for several weeks and had 'a near-death experience' earlier on, had developed special gifts as a result of this which singled her out as exceptional.

# Changed views

Few parents had had any idea of what intensive care involved. Although most expressed gratitude for what could be done, a small number reflected sadly on the dilemmas that modern capabilities had created. Even one mother who was herself a healthcare professional said that she had not been aware of how neonatal care had advanced, and had she known, she would not have elected to have her own babies treated so aggressively.

> Before I had the [babies] I [thought] why would anyone want to torture their children that way? Why would anybody want to risk having a mentally handicapped child? Now I understand why people do it . . . So I don't *agree with* the treatment of extremely premature children, but I can *understand* parents wanting to have it and I would never ever now make a judgement on them. I mean, I think it would be wrong, but if I knew that someone had a 26-week baby and they wanted all the treatment for it, I still think it's cruel – I think what I did to my own children was cruel – but [I can understand them]. And what can you do? As a

doctor you can't say, 'No, it's not going to work.' For one thing it gives you more time with your children ... I still think it's the wrong thing to do, thinking medically and because I think it's cruel to children – but if I heard that that's what parents wanted to do I wouldn't think they were stupid or selfish or whatever, because I've been there and I can understand it.

(P 33: mother of preterm twins)

Only a small number of parents reported changes in their views about treatment for babies as a consequence of this experience. One couple was now firmly against aggressive treatment for babies with severe impairments. Four sets of parents, having had preterm infants themselves, were now in favour of treating such babies when previously they had thought it to be unnatural and cruel.

When I read stories before about babies being born that size I thought, 'That's not right. It's just not nature. It shouldn't be allowed.' And then it happened to me. And I told [the consultant and the consultant asked me did I still feel like that] and I said, 'Oh no.' I had to give [my baby] every chance that we could, but it was always in the back of my mind, are you tampering with nature in doing this? And [my husband] even asked her, 'Are there any of them that escape unscathed? Have they all maybe got a small price to pay in later life?' But at the time we just thought we have to do everything possible for him. But I still can't answer whether it's right or wrong ... I was always one of these people who would say, 'Och, I wouldn't do that. Nobody would get to do that. I'd do this.' And now when I hear people saying that, I say to them, 'You don't know how you would do.'

(P9: mother of preterm twins)

One of these mothers still felt that it was cruel, but she now thought it was justified provided that the infants were 28 weeks or more, with a good chance of a normal life.

Two sets of parents were now supporters of euthanasia. One couple had previously thought it was a bad thing, but circumstances had made them change their minds. Their own experience had shown them that prolonging certain lives carried too high a price in terms of suffering.

Two fathers and one mother had had their views on abortion challenged. They described themselves as strongly against abortion in the past, one father indeed having been militant in his opposition. Personal experience of their child's struggle had made them reflect anew on the issues, and they were all now less sure that there was a 'black and white' answer to such a matter. Even though their own inclination was still to be against abortion for themselves, they were less confident that it was right in all cases, and they were less judgemental of others who reached a different conclusion. One other mother who did not identify a change of view on this matter earlier spoke movingly of her own crisis of conscience when severe impairments were diagnosed during her pregnancy which helped her to see the complex interplay of emotions, beliefs and hard choices. If she, with her strong convictions against abortion, had been torn, it was easy to see why others who were less confident in their beliefs could make different choices.

Two sets of parents were now against having amniocentesis to detect abnormalities. Both had done so for this pregnancy, believing that they were not made of 'the stuff of saints' and would not have the resources to cope with children with real difficulties. They now realised that their views on disability for their own children had changed, and their tolerance was higher than they had thought it to be. They were now not so sure that they only wanted a perfect baby. Having experienced parental love, they had come to realise that they would rather have had the child live with some problems than have him die.

The strength of parental love had surprised many parents. This in itself, they felt, provided a form of safeguard, as parents could not do anything which was not in the child's interests. The baby definitely came first, and they would endure anything themselves to do what was best for him or her.

> Before [the baby] I probably would never have even thought of the child inasmuch as [I'd have thought about how] it would have affected *our* lives. If somebody had said to me, 'Why are you having this amniocentesis?,' I think it would have been more like, 'Oh well, I don't know if *I* could cope with a Down syndrome baby, or this type of baby, or that type of baby,' whereas now I *know* I could cope with it. I just don't know if I would want the *baby* to have to cope with it ... I would definitely be thinking of it more from the child's [point of view] because I would just get on with it and I would have to cope with it. Before I'd have probably been more selfish and said, 'I don't know if *we* could cope.'
>
> (P45: father of preterm baby)

Four parents had had their confidence in medical skill challenged. For one there had been a total loss of faith in hospitals, doctors and scans after the screening system had failed to detect a lethal congenital anomaly antenatally. Another was disenchanted with the 'conveyor-belt' approach, and felt that staff should listen to mothers more and tailor management to the mother's own requests, experience and needs. One father now worried that resources might be constraining the use of technology in certain hospitals. He felt that care for his partner had been less than optimal, and that their social circumstances had led to their being discriminated against. The fourth parent, a mother, had earlier anxieties about the doctors' prognosis which made her question their judgement and the whole matter of treatment limitation in that Unit. Her confidence was challenged by a report of a baby in similar circumstances to her own who had been treated and who lived. Some weeks later that baby died, and she then changed her mind: perhaps the doctors had been right after all, because she was spared the additional pain of losing a child whom she had grown to know and love even more deeply over time.

# Advice that parents themselves would give to other parents

As the respondents pointed out, this was the most devastating experience: 'Imagine the worst situation, multiply it by 10 and you get somewhere near' how bad it is, as one father put it. A recurring message was given that these newly bereaved parents had learned many things in the process. In order for us to learn from their personal growth, parents were encouraged to say what advice they would give to other parents in similar circumstances. However, they were often hesitant about giving advice, and anxious not to impose a standard or expectation on others. Every experience and each family was different. There was no recipe for parents to help them survive the experience, but each must find their own way through it. They also pointed out that needs and wants varied at different times, and it was important to take the experience one step at a time. Because of this, five of them declined to offer any advice, and a number of others felt that the best thing they could do would be to 'be there' for these families, not to advise them.

However, the parents were encouraged to offer suggestions, and their advice related to three main areas, namely the decision making, the dying process and the bereavement process. The precise numbers of citations are unimportant although, where appropriate, indications are given of the weight of opinion. In reality, individual parents not infrequently provided illuminating insights.

# During decision making

## *Seek information*

Parents' main recommendation for this part of the experience was to communicate with doctors and obtain as much information and advice as possible – questioning, challenging and complaining if necessary. They strongly reinforced the importance of accurate and comprehensive information in the decision-making process.

### Request the things which you personally want

Parents emphasised the value to them of having things done in the right way for the family; not ensuring this left them vulnerable to long-term regrets. Having hesitated to ask for things themselves, they encouraged others to have more courage. As they pointed out, these are extraordinary circumstances and no parent should worry about their ideas being too bizarre to request.

### Ensure that the timing is right

Sensitive timing was identified as important to the parents in both the short and the longer term. They advised that others should not be pressured into making premature choices, as they might be left with recurring doubts. These are crucial decisions with which the parents will have to live for the rest of their days, and they should be based on deep beliefs, not spur-of-the-moment choices.

> What's important is that you can live with your decision, at the end of the day, in the longer term. And that's the really difficult bit . . . Much as it's sad for the baby who dies, it's the people who are left who have to come to terms with that. So their wishes and views have to be important.
>
> (P 50: mother of baby with congenital anomalies)

### Decide together

A joint decision was regarded as preferable to a unilateral one. Parents advised couples to talk together and to keep talking to make sure that they are of the same mind about the final decision. However, once the decision has been made they should live with it and not endlessly question its rightness.

# Dealing with the dying process

### Do what feels right

A strong recommendation was made for parents to do all they could to make this a special time, taking advantage of the guidance which staff could offer through this uncharted territory. However, the parents cautioned other families to take account of their own tolerances and wishes. This was their baby, not the hospital's, and they should not be reticent about asking for what was right for them. Several parents who had felt that certain things were expected of them advised other parents not to succumb to that type of pressure, no matter how benign it might appear to be.

### Build up memories

Spending time with the baby, gathering mementoes and building memories
were cited as essential if the parents were to be able to remember the child
as an individual and as part of their family. Parents recommended that
others should concentrate their efforts on accumulating these memories
and mementoes while they could.

### Be aware of the options available

Being aware of what is possible is a first step in making informed choices,
and parents advised other families to seek this information. They should
know, for example, that they can take the baby home after death, but they
should also know that it can be devastating to relinquish his or her body
from home.

## Coping with the loss

Most of the advice that parents offered related to coping after the death.
They recommended that others should make use of any resources available to them which would help them through this traumatic experience.

### Talk

The most commonly cited recommendation, identified by almost all of the
parents, was to talk and to keep talking. Some parents specified a particular person to talk to, such as the partner, other bereaved parents, or a
professional person with good listening skills.

### Do not suppress emotions

Many parents advised strongly that feelings should be expressed and not
bottled up. This included many fathers who had themselves found it difficult to release their grief, but who now knew that this had been counter-
productive for them personally as well as for their partners. Other parents
recommended openly expressing their emotions, not being afraid to shout
and cry if that felt right, going with their emotions on bad days, and not
struggling to put on a brave face. They believed that suppressing sorrow
as deep and painful as this only led to trouble or illness. Some wanted to
reassure other parents that it was natural and normal to harbour strange
thoughts and ideas. As one mother put it, 'There's probably nothing
you can think that's so outrageous but that no one else has thought.'
One devoted father, who recommended openly acknowledging troubling

thoughts, spoke with feeling. He had stayed off work for nine weeks to spend every minute with the baby, but he admitted that he had harboured ideas of rejecting her at one stage – a thought which appalled him later.

> After we'd been told about the brain damage and whatever, trying to come to terms with having a baby with severe brain damage – it's going to ruin our lives. I couldn't get over that. And I got a bit selfish and I thought well, perhaps it would be the best thing to let her die. I felt terrible. I kept that to myself but that's how I felt. I got to the point where I couldn't go in and look at her – I wasn't going in as regularly. And when I did go in if the saturations did come down, instead of going, 'Oh, they're down,' and getting someone there and then, I felt as if I could have turned my back and walked away. I just can't explain how bad I feel about that now. But I didn't do that. But because I *thought* about it, that was bad enough. I just felt terrible that I had even contemplated that. Things were getting worse and worse and that was the kick in the teeth. I didn't think things could get any worse.
>
> (P9: father of baby with cardiac anomaly)

### Grieve naturally

In many different ways respondents advised that parents should grieve naturally in the way that was right for them. There is no one way which is correct, and whatever felt right for them *was* right for them. If they were having a bad day they should not try to put a good gloss on it. If they were angry or weepy they should express those emotions. The pain had to be felt fully before they could think of moving on. Accepting the reality of what had happened was a necessary part of learning to live with it. Parents also cautioned others about being railroaded by people with set expectations – rather they should try to take control of their own lives, going with their own instincts and inclinations. Support came from a shared feeling, not an imposed solution. Some parents noted the importance of working through the grief naturally, and this was not something to suppress artificially with drugs if it could be avoided. Timing is important, and a number of parents emphasised the value of taking things one day at a time, and not trying to rush the grieving process.

### Help each other

Parents advised other couples to beware of the stress that this experience exerts on their own relationship. Many spoke strongly of the need for couples to work at helping each other through this difficult time, recognising the potential for a breakdown in communication. They need to be tolerant of the other partner's emotional unavailability at times, and their very different reactions and requirements. Making time for each other was recommended, as well as talking about any problems and working at solutions. The men were advised to be patient with their womenfolk, who tended to be emotional for a long time. Women were advised to recognise a male reluctance to talk or weep, and not to interpret it as a sign of lack of grief or love.

### Seek support from others

Newly bereaved parents were recommended to seek out others who could listen sympathetically and appropriately. Talking repeatedly about their experience is essential, and they should not suppress their feelings simply in order to protect others. They were advised to give other people cues to facilitate appropriate responses and support.

### Try to move on

Some parents gave advice relating to accepting what had happened and making a concerted effort to move on. Too much retrospection could lead to a form of 'wallowing' which some of these parents had seen in others and from which they recoiled. There is no danger that they will ever forget; the memories are to be savoured and lived with, not buried. However, in the remembering it is important to maintain a balance between the positive and the negative, and to look forward as well. This includes, for example, not giving up hope, establishing a routine or keeping busy in order to get through each day or week or month, having short-term goals, and hanging on to whatever anchors the parent could find, in the knowledge that the storm would eventually abate. They conveyed a strong sense that although this is a profoundly painful experience, the parents will survive it and find a measure of happiness again. They might even identify positive outcomes such as inner strength, different priorities and greater sensitivity.

# Discussion

These parents have highlighted the fact that experience changes theoretical views. More than three-quarters of them were conscious of now thinking differently about important issues. Since theirs is the voice of experience, it carries a special weight.

Our study shows that the experience of bereavement changes parents as people as well as changing their views. Priorities change, sensitivities are heightened, and life and family are valued at a deeper level. Their sense of security is shaken by the tragedy. If the unthinkable has already happened, what else might not overtake them? Such an experience seems particularly to undermine confidence in their capacity to reproduce safely. As has been said, another pregnancy becomes for some 'one more chance for a speeding truck to ruin' their lives.[226] Caught up in these profound thoughts, it is small wonder that the normal everyday trivia which preoccupy most people seem absurd and irritating. Against this overall change in their approach to life we shall examine some of their opinions which add to the debate on what ought to be done in these cases.

# The decision should be an individual one

Our data demonstrate the uniqueness of each family's own beliefs, values and tolerances. The parental recommendation that each decision should be made on an individual basis, making reference to their specific circumstances, is a powerful one. Blanket rules are clearly inappropriate.

It is evident that experience itself changes perspectives. Although it is relatively easy for people who have had no exposure to these procedures to assert what should or should not be done, our findings show that it is a very different thing to be weighing up the consequences of different choices for one's own child. Parents are clearly amazed at what is medically possible, but they are also sobered by the implications of aggressive and invasive modern intensive care. If these measures contribute to saving a life they can be seen as a necessary part of treatment, but when the baby's life may not be saved, or it will be of questionable quality, other issues have to be considered. The balance of burdens and benefits for all concerned must be carefully weighed. The parents' conclusion that each case must be decided on its own merits echoes that reached by staff in NICUs.[12]

# Quality of life is a major factor in parents' deliberations

Our findings demonstrate that the quality of life a child might expect is a crucial consideration in the minds of parents. Severe impairments which limit their independence, or the suffering resulting from such impairments or from continuing treatment, weigh heavily with them. It is very clear that the child's interests are of paramount importance, and that the parents' opinions concur with professional recommendations.[10] As the British Medical Association has noted, the law has confirmed that there are two essential and key factors which must be considered when deliberating whether or not to treat, namely the patient's best interests and an assessment of the benefits and burdens of the treatment. Assessing best interests in the case of a baby is not an easy matter, and they believe that it should include additional criteria: whether or not the child 'has the potential to develop awareness, the ability to interact and the capacity for self-directed action, and whether the child will suffer severe unavoidable pain and distress.'[10] These are the factors which parents spontaneously identify. It should be noted that, compared to the opinions of doctors and nurses working with such families,[12] proportionally more of the parents specifically cite suffering and dependence as reasons to withdraw treatment, drawing attention to their sustained view that the long-term consequences of decisions made in the NICU must be considered in the first hours and days of a child's life. Indeed, as our data show, one year after death, suffering is the reason most commonly cited by parents for stopping treatment. The agony of parental grief is more tolerable to them than the thought that the child will suffer.

## The majority believe that parents should be actively involved in decision making

As we have seen in an earlier chapter, the majority of parents regard decision making about treatment withdrawal on behalf of the child as part of parental responsibility. They have few enough opportunities to act as parents, and yet they have unique insights into family values and circumstances. Moreover, they have an overwhelming love for the child and want what is best for him or her. They believe that the power of such love, coupled with the medical contribution to the decision-making process, will provide all of the safeguards necessary to protect such babies from any potential abuse of parental rights. The fact that in our study their opinions about the right decision were sustained over time, most parents were satisfied with the management of the decision in their case both at the time and a year later, and we found no evidence of guilt associated with their taking responsibility for the decision, would suggest that fears about the consequences to parents are ill-founded.[12,17,27] However, an important point which emerges is that parents do not feel that they are bearing this responsibility alone. They believe that doctors would not give them the choice of stopping treatment unless they themselves believed that continuing intensive care was not in the child's best interests. They are also very aware that they are reliant on the medical team to give them the information they need to guide their choices, the facts often being accompanied by guidance or even recommendations as to the preferred option.

# Some parents advocate the active ending of life where death is the expected outcome of treatment limitation

It is evident from the way in which they describe and react to a number of issues that parents perceive medical practice differently from doctors and nurses. This may be a contributory factor in their expressed views about what they refer to as 'euthanasia.' The clinical co-researchers are confident that usual practice in their own study Unit lies within the current RCPCH guidelines,[9] but in the perceptions of a few parents at least, the use of morphine equates to a form of euthanasia. Although the number of individuals who specifically discussed this factor is too small to be significant, the strength of the feelings and arguments expressed demands attention. Irrespective of how the parents interpreted what was actually practised in the Units, some families clearly want it to be legally possible to speed up death in certain circumstances. Many more have stated that in their judgement there is no value but there is certainly great harm in prolonging the dying process, adding to suffering and distress and compromising dignity. If the child is going to die anyway who benefits from extending that distressing process?

Professional bodies are strongly opposed to any change in the law to make active ending of life legal.[9,10,153,154] Doctors are understandably cautious about this. As has been pointed out:

> There is one important difference between the two acts [passive and active euthanasia]. Active intervention with lethal substances removes all possibility for the patient to continue living. Failing to administer an antibiotic or turning off a respirator still permits the patient to live ... Passive euthanasia in this way is more tolerant of error.'[36]

However, the distress of parents faced with hours or days of watching their baby dying slowly and unpleasantly must be heard, and our findings suggest that the debate should be reopened to examine what ought to be done in these profoundly difficult circumstances.

# Parents may derive comfort from religious beliefs

It appears that an experience as traumatic as this makes parents ask deep questions about life and death and an afterlife. We found that very few parents believe that religious scruples should influence decision making.

Rather, the principal effect of religion identified by our study was its capacity to offer comfort. Solace comes from a belief in a divine masterplan, and hope of an afterlife with a future better than the present.[2,57] It is clear from our data that parents are deeply troubled by their powerlessness to protect their child from harm – they have been unable to stop death from claiming him, and they cannot help him now.

> It was the opposite way round to what it should be. It should have been him standing looking down at me [in that grave]. That's the one recurring thought that I have . . . there was nobody there [in the afterlife] to protect him and show him the way. These are hard things to live with. Especially I think it's even worse when it's a boy, for the father. There's a kinship there, isn't there, between men? There is a definite bond there.
>
> (P 20: father of baby with asphyxia)

Parents look for reassurance that the child is now in a better place, being taken care of, and free from pain. Some actively seek such reassurance from within religious or spirit realms, but not all find it. In cases where previous convictions are undermined, important anchors may be removed at a time of great need.

# Parents' advice to others hinges around being actively involved and expressing their emotions

In giving advice to other bereaved parents based on their own experience, our respondents identified priority issues. The recommendation to be actively involved and to acquire memories is a powerful one. Time with the baby is short, but the parents will have to live with the consequences of what is done for the rest of their lives. Because the territory is uncharted and their emotions are so turbulent, parents who have lived through this experience know that there is a tendency not to be assertive. They now recognise that this is not the time for reticence, but rather parents should hold out for what they need or want, whether it be obtaining information, choosing to do or not do specific things during the dying process, or timing events in line with their own preferences or tolerances. In this way they will be left with minimal long-term regrets.

Coping with this experience strains personal resources. Our data indicate how much parents are in need of help and support. Nowhere is this more powerfully felt than in the necessity to talk. The loss of a child is so devastating, and the emotions so profound, that they cannot and should not be suppressed. However, finding people to listen is clearly not always easy. As we have seen, the parents may well need listeners from outside their immediate family. The strong advice from those who have been in this position is to seek out someone who can bear their pain and help them to make sense of their experience and work through their grief. Only in this way will they come to accept what has happened and move forward with hope in the future.

# Conclusion

- The loss of a child changes parents' priorities and attitudes and undermines their security.
- Parents believe that the decision should be individually tailored to the circumstances of each case.
- Quality of life, dependence and suffering are important factors in the reasoning of parents in deciding when to stop treatment.
- Parents think that they themselves should have the opportunity to be actively involved in decision making and the dying process, in line with their own tolerances and preferences.
- The debate on the management of babies in difficult cases where death does not swiftly follow treatment withdrawal should be reopened.
- Religious conviction may bring solace, but it rarely influences decision making.
- Opportunities to talk about their experiences are crucial to the parents' healthy progress through the grieving process.

# CHAPTER 14

# Some concluding thoughts

Our empirical research set out to identify and describe important ethical and clinical issues surrounding the withholding and withdrawing of invasive intensive treatment, to see how they are resolved in real life, and to assess the consequences of current management. In order to illuminate understanding of these sensitive issues it was essential that the study met certain criteria. It must address the real moral issues, conceptualise those issues appropriately, arrive at justifiable conclusions and address all of the significant components of the issue.[113,227] The ethics underpinning this research are sometimes more implicit than explicit, but in this concluding chapter we shall look at them more expressly as we gather together some of the loose threads that remain after detailed discussion of each part of the decision-making process.

## Parents' opinions on the boundaries

Having lived through the experience of their child dying, the parents whom we studied give a clear message: limits should be set to what is attempted in our efforts to save the lives of imperilled infants. Their considered view is in line with those of others on this matter. In general, they want everything done to cure their child's problems and they are supportive of technological interventions which may save the lives of their children,[158,228] but they fear severe impairments,[229] and they regret the imposition of prolonged pain and suffering in cases where the prognosis is bleak.[21,34] They do not view as a kindness an aggressive fight which results in children surviving with devastating impairments, enduring protracted dying processes, or suffering without any prospect of future benefit. When we analysed the reasons that parents gave for withdrawing or withholding treatment, it was clear that suffering and the prospect of a poor quality of life are the two main factors which influence their choices. Doctors tend to look first at more technical and prognostic medical factors to determine the chances of survival and the factual consequences of treatment, and then weigh up the implications in terms of pain and future impairment.

Although a tiny minority of the parents we studied concluded that they would always want everything done for their own child, almost all believed that careful choices should be made on the merits of each case. They do not want decisions to be made by default. A balance has to be struck between the ethical and the technologically medical, and technology must not be permitted to assume control until there is no choice left. Cases such as the notorious American ones (Linares and Messenger), where fathers took it upon themselves to ensure that their children died,[114,230] highlight the strength of parental feeling on this matter. They support the view that authority must not be assumed without responsibility.[231] Moral choices, even though they may on occasion be fallible, are preferable to a pursuit of medical treatment without true compassion and practical wisdom. It does not seem compassionate to them to stand by and watch a child slowly deteriorate. As one father put it, doing so betrays a lack of maturity:

> It was the maturity [of his opinion that we liked]. He was cognisant of the fact that the doctors who were technophiles about the machinery will keep the kids going. His view was that they haven't lived [long enough in] their lives to see the problems that that child would go through, beyond the fact that they've managed to keep them going. But he thought that their [the child's] challenges later on in life were greater than [those facing the staff at that point]: do they resuscitate?
>
> (P25: father of preterm baby with brain damage)

As has been said, 'the virtue of compassion is integrally linked to the ethical use of power in the physician–patient relationship.'[232]

However, the limits and tolerance of parents may be at variance with those of doctors and nurses. We shall deal with their different perspectives in a later section, but it is important to recognise at this point that although all may agree that limits are desirable, exactly where those boundaries lie may be more open to dispute. For example, tolerance of impairment appears to differ. Although parents and healthcare professionals view mild to moderately disabled health states similarly, parents have been found to be more accepting of severely disabled health states than the healthcare professionals.[120] Doctors and nurses working in NICUs tend to have a more pessimistic view about the outcomes for sick preterm infants than do parents, and it has been suggested that they underestimate the capacity of parents to cope with babies with disabilities.[233] In addition, the parents' perceptions of health states more closely match those of the surviving children reaching adolescence than do the perceptions of the healthcare professionals, with both adolescents and their parents tending to be more tolerant of disability than the staff.[120] Does this make the parents the more appropriate agents to make decisions on behalf of their infants? Or does the experience and medical knowledge of the doctor carry greater weight?

# The decision-making process

When any decisions on this matter are made there is a process to be undergone. In essence there are two main aspects to the decision to stop aggressive treatment. The first relates to the actual determination – whether or not to treat. Facts form the foundation of any good moral decision. What do we know? What could we know? The implications of these facts must then be considered. A minority of consultants act alone, but most discuss the options with colleagues and attempt to establish a consensus, which may or may not be a unanimous view, and which is then taken to the parents. Sometimes it includes advice or a recommendation from the medical team. There is a persuasive argument for doctors allowing a measure of value judgement to temper their presentation of the medical facts, since 'good advice, which we should expect from our friends and doctors, consists in more than information.'[234] As the parents have indicated, the experience and authority of the consultant at this time represent a vital factor in the process. They not only look to him to convey the facts and the arguments to inform choices, but they also look for evidence that he is to be trusted and that the case he presents is well reasoned, logical and fits with what they see and know. The extent of involvement of parents in the actual decision varies, but if they are to take any responsibility for the choices, it is at this point that their opinions are sought. The exact timing of their involvement will vary with the changing fortunes of the baby, the urgency of the need to decide, the consultant's perceptions and preferences, and the family's tolerances and resources.

Once that decision has been made, the second task is to guide the parents through the withdrawal and dying process. Here the experience of the medical team plays a different part. Their exposure to many other such situations gives them the confidence to be able to predict the sequence of events to some extent although, as we have seen, predictions of the time it will take have been found to be worryingly inaccurate. Experienced staff can reassure the parents, help them to accept the inevitability of the death, and facilitate optimal involvement in the dying process. There can be no blanket policies, but it is evident that efforts are made to ensure that each event is orchestrated in a way that is responsive to the individual family's needs and wishes.

Two other functions accompany this process. One is that of facilitating a healthy grieving process with minimal regrets. The parents will never forget this child, but in time most can move on to lead happy and positively orientated lives. Confidence that the right decisions were made, that they did all that they could for the baby, and that they have a logical and full explanation for what happened aids this process. So, too, does reassurance from the medical team, provided that it is based on facts and accurate knowledge as well as experience. On the other hand, confidence is undermined if gaps are left in the parents' knowledge, or if there appears to have been medical collusion to protect them from the truth or to cover up negligence.

The other important function is to preserve the integrity of the medical team. There is often little space for debriefing and recuperation, attention soon being diverted to the needs of the next family. These cases drain personal, collective and administrative resources, and what is possible may of necessity be constrained as a result.

# Who should decide

Whilst a number of people are involved in the decision-making process, we found that the ultimate responsibility is borne by one or both of two groups of people, namely the medical team and the parents. Doctors usually seek the opinions of colleagues or specialists. Parents occasionally discuss the issues with family, friends or ministers of religion, but these other people rarely take any responsibility for the actual decision.

It is clear from our own earlier work,[12] as well as from many other studies and official guidelines, that it is generally accepted that the parents should be involved. The parents themselves strongly uphold their right to be so included, not only in the UK but also in the USA[21,233,235] where it is considered essential to involve them because it is the families who 'bear the emotional and financial consequences' of aggressive treatment for infants.[236] However, in practice although staff working in NICUs agree that they should be involved, they consider that it would be too weighty a burden for parents to take responsibility for the ultimate decision. We found that only 3% of doctors and 6% of nurses thought parents should do so.[12] In the current study we find the parents calling into question this notion that they will find it too onerous. As we have seen, the majority believe that they *should* accept this responsibility; it is part of being a parent. In their own perceptions the majority considered that the ultimate decision had indeed been theirs, and others who did not make the decision themselves subsequently wished that they had done so.

Serious concerns have been raised about the consequences to the parents in terms of guilt or doubt, but we found no evidence of resultant guilt associated with their own decision making. Many parents certainly do dwell on the decision and the events surrounding it, but this is hardly to be wondered at. These are momentous happenings with tragic outcomes. As one father put it, 'This is not a decision I ever want to be fully at peace with.'[27] However, the parents whom we studied show a high level of satisfaction with both the process and the final decision. It is quite evident that they are able to separate out the process from the outcome; dissatisfaction is not an inevitable concomitant to the giving of bad news.[104] Neither are guilt, regret or doubts about the wisdom of the decision inevitable.[237] There is, of course, always the possibility of error, but no more so when deciding to stop than in continuing. Indeed, it has been argued that there is less risk of regret or guilt if the parents have had time to think through the questions and implications and are 'convinced, intellectually and emotionally, that they are doing the right thing for their child.'[237] This seems to be the critical issue – the parents need to be *personally persuaded* that this course of action is the best for their child. It is abundantly clear that the baby's interests are of paramount importance to them – his or her suffering and quality of life are high-priority considerations. We found lingering doubts only when the parents had been unconvinced of the wisdom of stopping treatment. If they have not been given and seen for themselves concrete evidence of a poor prognosis, they have no yardstick by which to measure and confirm the rightness of the decision to withdraw or withhold treatment. If the child appears to be fighting to live, doubts may arise about the accuracy of the medical assessment.

There is a persuasive argument to be made for sharing decision making.[131,234] Both doctors and parents bring different knowledge bases and perspectives to the decision-making process, and each is reliant on the other to some degree in forming a wise opinion about the best way forward. The parent relies on the doctor for certain medical information, and the doctor relies on the parent for facts about their values, preferences and circumstances. Only by sharing their perspectives can they work towards a common understanding and conviction that this is the appropriate decision, in these circumstances, for this child.

In the real world with its less than ideal situations, however, things are not so simple. The contributions, roles and experiences that the two groups – the medical team and the family – bring to this exchange are not only very different but may not be equally powerful, and may be limited by certain constraints. For example, the medical staff – who have seen

these conditions many times and repeatedly assessed the wisdom of continuing to treat – bring a level of expertise to this decision which is beyond
dispute. They can say with some authority what is probable and what is
possible.

> [The neonatologist's] view was much more mature [than ours] because
> he had seen the variation and the different elements that are so difficult
> to put down. But the maturity of his 30 years on a case-by case-basis,
> with the knowledge that he's seen the babies that have been successful,
> the babies that he's seen that haven't been successful, who've struggled.
> I would respect his view far more because our view is from our circum-
> stances, and that's just one slice of the whole pie that he's seen.
>
> (P25: father of preterm baby with brain damage)

But they are fallible and they do sometimes get things wrong. Various constraints, demands and limits may influence what they can or do actually
do. For instance, perceptions of the law may force them to act in ways
which run counter to their intuitive sense of compassion or benevolence.
A cultural imperative to strive to avoid death may make them reluctant to
admit defeat, parental expectation or the fear of recrimination may influence their practice, and their own sense of personal weakness or preferences may make them guarded in their recommendations.

The experience and authority of the parents are of a very different nature.
Their relationship to the child gives them special privileges, responsibilities
and duties that are recognised throughout Europe.[238] However, they too are
subject to constraints and limits. For example, their own powerful emotions may incline them in a certain direction, they may find it difficult to
tease out the interests of the child from those of the family, and their own
limited understanding of medical matters may colour their perceptions of
the facts and arguments which are germane to good decision making.


# Differences in perception

It is apparent both from our research and from anecdotal evidence that in
any given case the doctors and the parents may perceive the identity of
the decision makers differently. There are a number of possible reasons for
this. The first has to do with the interpretation of cues that each gives to the
other in this intense interaction, which may materially influence how each
responds. For almost two-thirds of the families whom we studied, discussion about withdrawing treatment took place within the first week of life,
and for more than a fifth of families it took place within the first 24 hours
after delivery. Not only are emotions turbulent at this stage, but also there

has been little opportunity to forge relationships or discover basic philo-
sophies of life or expectations. Some things must be taken on trust, but
ideas about responsibilities and roles may be misplaced, and cues may be
misinterpreted.

The second reason relates to the complexities that surround giving the
parents the information they need to make an informed choice. For
the majority of these parents there was no warning of the problems to
come. They had simultaneously to cope with news of a tragic development
and the possibility of impending death. The necessity to make considered
assessments with critical consequences at such a time is a daunting task.
In these sensitive and immediate situations, doctors are not looking for
gut feelings or beliefs that are not thought through. They want parents
to go through a careful deliberation on the basis of accurate information,
to understand the likely consequences, and to balance the burdens and
benefits. In order to facilitate this process, the medical team itself needs to
establish clearly what the facts are, and what the arguments are for each
possible course of action. However, by going to the family with the full
authority of a confident professional consensus, they may be powerfully
influencing the parents' decision. Some parents are more conscious of this
potential influence than others.

The third reason is related to the second, but it represents a factor of
which both medical staff and parents are very well aware. There exists an
imbalance of power, knowledge and experience between the two parties.
Even in families where at least one partner was him- or herself a healthcare professional, the parents were conscious of this divide. They are therefore reliant upon medical information to form a considered opinion. The
extent of their acknowledgement of this element might have coloured
their perception of just who ultimately took responsibility.

Fourth, parents make certain assumptions about the role of the medical
team. It is taken for granted that doctors diagnose disease, order treatments,
assess benefits and burdens and likely outcomes, and determine management. The parents whom we studied based their decision on the information
and advice provided by the medical team. It could be that in saying that they
personally decided, they were assuming medical involvement.

A possible fifth explanation arises from the nature of the decision
making process. A number of consultants have emphasised the fact that
they would never mention possible withdrawal of treatment unless they
were themselves convinced of its medical appropriateness in this case. It is
the medical team who are deciding the initial boundary lines. The parents
may subsequently help to refine the limits in this case, but they do not set
the markers which define medical futility or 'no purpose.'[9] Moreover, when
the doctors come to the parents to discuss the options, they have usually
already obtained some idea of the preference of the medical team. This is

weighty. Nevertheless, if they are truly consulting the parents, the decision is still an open one at this point – they have an opportunity to take a different line. The parents, not having been part of the earlier debate, may perceive themselves as having the deciding voice until closure comes with the final decision. The medical team, on the other hand, may feel that they themselves have already decided and the parents are simply concurring with their choice. This may account for the apparent discrepancy in perceptions.

# Is parental autonomy an illusion?

Given the imbalance of power, experience and authority, are parents in reality deciding, or is this an illusion created by the practices that NICU teams have adopted? To what extent is putting forward persuasive arguments a form of respect for parental autonomy, and to what extent is it an attempt (albeit benign) to overcome parental autonomy? In order to give parents the scope to make their own unaided decision, it would be necessary for teams to present all of the available information in an impartial way, providing both the facts and the arguments to back up the case for and against each available course of action. In the perception of both the medical team and the parents, these facts are commonly presented with guidance as to the preferred medical option, or a recommendation as to the best decision in this case. Not only so, but these additional pieces of information are often couched in terms of consensus recommendations. Although this may be a form of manipulation of parents to bring them to a medical decision, it is not necessarily a negative construction to put on what happens. The majority of the parents in our research were satisfied with both the decision and the process. They may not recognise these influences but even were they to do so, the result may not be unwelcome to them. They are after all very aware of their own limited understanding, and they clearly trust the medical team to have the best interests of the child at heart.

Furthermore, far from frustrating parental autonomy, in presenting a carefully reasoned argument and convincing parents of the practical, medical and ethical wisdom of that choice, doctors may indeed be enabling the parents to choose more rather than less autonomously. There are at least three ways in which this may be true.[234] First, by thinking about the facts and their significance to the family in a different way from that in which their unaided thinking might go, the parents' choice will be more active and a truer reflection of their considered choice. Second, for a choice to be autonomous it should be informed not only by the facts but also by what is of value. Doctors can represent what others think to be of value, allowing the parents to set their own ideas into a broader context. Third, by having to think and then rethink their own choices in the light of the medical team's arguments, and give reasons for rejecting alternative choices, the parents will reach a conclusion which they can more rationally defend. Overall, the parents' own conclusion is then based upon a rationally argued foundation which takes account of all the elements involved in making wise judgements.

# Communication

Bearing in mind all of these influencing factors and potential difficulties, it is not surprising that good communication emerges as a key element in effective decision making. This is nothing new. Consecutive Confidential Enquiries into Stillbirths and Deaths in Infancy, in examining risks which might be attributable to suboptimal care, have highlighted the need for good communication and for listening to what mothers themselves have to say.[239–242] Communication is regarded as a critical factor in both process and outcome, a two-way process which involves an 'ability to talk and write in terms which the other party, whether parents or professionals, can understand; willingness to hear and understand another's point of view; and mutual understanding about the outcome at the end of the discussion.'[240]

When it comes to decisions about withdrawing treatment, it is evident that considerable efforts are made to communicate effectively, but a number of elements may present obstacles to clear understanding. The parents whom we studied have helped to raise awareness of those factors which require vigilance. Doctors and parents are often divided by factors as varied as class, culture, knowledge, personality and language. At the time when these crucial decisions are under review, families are emotionally traumatised and physically exhausted by the experience of having a critically ill newborn. A stream of detailed information with recommendations to stop treatment may be perceived as arrogance by a vulnerable teenager. A statement of a 10% chance of survival may seem to have been false hope to a grieving mother, a 90% probability of death being closer to her acknowledged truth. Averting the eyes or an unscheduled meeting without witnesses may be construed as attempts at cover-up, or as personal discomfort with what has happened.

Our research found that with no warning of coming disaster, when the subject of treatment limitation was broached parents were taken by surprise. Yet doctors believe that they share information with the parents honestly. This raises questions of perception, protection and communication. Recognising the potentially devastating effect of a 'death sentence', no matter how humanely and sympathetically it is given, some clinicians worry that 'warmth and humanity are becoming submerged in figures.'[243] As part of this desire to soften the blow, some neonatologists do what they can to preserve some hope, believing it to be cruel to remove a crutch which might support parents through a difficult and often protracted experience. However, the parents in our research have clearly stated that being given the facts fairly and squarely is preferable to being given false hope. A number of factors may be coexisting here.

The first has to do with the wisdom that comes with hindsight. When they reflected on their decision-making experience, these parents all knew that their baby had died. If a doctor had said, 'There is a 10% chance your baby will pull through' to parents whose baby *did* survive, there would not have been the same sense of let-down, even though the information was equally true in both instances.

The second factor relates to the difference between giving and receiving bad news. At the time when things are going wrong for a baby, parents vary in their capacity to accept and deal with news of a poor prognosis. Some mothers confessed to being hysterical, and some fathers recalled being angry and 'difficult' with the doctors. Such reactions might make doctors back off and give parents more time to absorb the reality of a bad prognosis. The parents reviewing the experience months later might well perceive this as the doctors protecting them from the truth. To take the case of the couple who were given information by five different consultants as an example, the mother admitted to being 'hysterical.' All of the consultants, she felt, had softened the news and encouraged her to hope. To the mother they had all handled it badly, being unduly protective and offering false reassurances. On the other hand, clinicians describing this incident might well have reasoned that this woman was just not receptive to the full truth at that point – perhaps someone else putting it in a different way would get through to her, and this second, third or fourth time might reinforce the strength of the opinion. In the end a junior doctor, thinking that the parents already knew, stated baldly that the baby was going to die. The reality penetrated and the mother was immensely grateful for this blunt truth. She could now do what she wanted to with this baby while she had the chance. It could be argued that the previous five senior doctors and time had all prepared the mother to assimilate this truth.

The way in which news is conveyed is a third element which also potentially influences perceptions. Although there may be nothing falsely hopeful about a doctor saying in a level tone, '10% of these babies survive intact,' to a parent it may be qualitatively different from a doctor saying in grave tones, '90% of these babies do not survive,' or to a third doctor saying cheerily, 'Well, one in every 10 of these babies goes on to do just fine.' The optimistic parent may cling to the hope that hers is that one baby in 10 and believe that she has had encouragement to think so. Objectively the information is the same, but perceptively and emotionally it is not. Many other features of an exchange may also colour a parent's understanding of what has been said, including tone of voice, eye contact, non-verbal cues, previous experience, personality and mood.

Given the need of the medical team to offer support to parents through this traumatic experience, but also the need of parents for honesty, it would appear that a compromise may be called for. To meet parental wishes, the prognosis should be as pessimistic as it is in truth. However, hope and encouragement may be offered with promises of as satisfactory a dying process as possible. To know that death itself is inevitable is a hard blow, but its impact may be softened if parents know that the staff will do all in their power to give the baby a pain-free and dignified dying process and the parents an experience which is as good as it can be.

Not only is communication important during the decision-making process and the dying process, but also the need continues beyond that – beyond the family's time in the Unit, beyond the death and the funeral. Parents feel a strong need to talk, and to talk repeatedly, with people who can help to reinforce the reality and value of their experience and facilitate their gaining understanding of what has happened. Being listened to is an essential component of their grieving. If the family are to have an opportunity to talk at length to those who have the necessary finely honed skills to bear their pain and help them in their grieving, who will finance such a service and how will these listeners be trained and supported themselves? The needs are clearly spelled out by the parents. The implementation of change needs wider consideration and debate.

# Meeting parental wishes

Important as it clearly is to pay due heed to what parents have identified as helpful in this process, it is also necessary to acknowledge the constraints which may limit what is possible or desirable. Resources are finite. Furthermore, the parents' voice is one of many, and others must be heard, too. Some of the issues which emerge will require further careful deliberation, weighing up the consequences of change and the competing interests of different people. This point is probably best made through a number of illustrations.

For example, parents strongly recommend having one consultant assigned to a given family, to convey the information consistently, listen to their reactions and preferences, and liaise with the rest of the team. Fragmented management appears to be more likely to engender misunderstanding. Having too many people involved detracts from their need for privacy and alters the dynamics of communication. A first response might be to exclude everyone else and concentrate on the family's needs alone. However, the consultant may not always be available, and he will have other sometimes competing demands on his time and resources. The nurses spend long periods of time with the parents, and the family will put demands on them which are not best met if they have not been included in discussions. Specialists may be particularly well equipped to convey certain forms of information, but the named consultant may be less well able to do so. Junior doctors have to learn how such situations should be handled. Given that there are no set rules of practice, and each case is different, much relies on an intuitive sense of what will be right for this family – a sense which is largely acquired through practice and experience. It could be potentially damaging to families to have inexperienced staff learning the hard way on them. It would be better that they learn through watching the master at work. It may then be necessary to look into ways of including others sensitively without detracting from the rapport that is established between consultant and parent.

A second example relates to the sensitive handling of requests for autopsy. This is quite evidently an extremely delicate issue. Parents speak of their shock when asked for permission, and their abhorrence of the idea of the child being cut. However, given the definite advantages of obtaining post-mortem information, it would be an inappropriate response to say that we should not mention this subject lest we add to the parents' pain. Instead we must look again at just how and when families are asked, who asks them, what is said and what arguments are brought to bear. Do they fully understand the genetic implications? Have they addressed all of the relevant issues? It is only by identifying the causes of refusals, and restoring confidence in the post-mortem system, that we shall halt the current decline in autopsy consent rates and potentially spare parents long-term regrets.

Follow-up care provides a third illustration where the parents' voice must be set alongside the needs of others. It emerges as an area where change is needed. Parents must not feel abandoned as well as devastated. They give a powerful message about their wish for ongoing contact which helps to keep memories alive, to make sense of what has happened and to support them in their bereavement. However, resources are finite and further demands cannot be added to staff's existing burdens without careful appraisal of the implications. If the parents are to be given routine early appointments to be seen after the death by the consultant who cared for their child in life, what about his other responsibilities? What boundaries will be set to maintaining contact, and who will decide when visits should cease?

The matter of protracted deaths is a fourth example where families clearly call for changes to be made, but competing claims may be heard.

Parents are deeply concerned about the suffering their child endures. Where death is inevitable they see no value in extending the pain – either that of the child or theirs. Some call for a legalising of active measures designed to induce the death of the baby. We have suggested that the debate on this issue be reopened in the light of what parents have told us. Active ending of life might indeed be one topic for consideration, but so too might be the better preparation of parents for what could happen, or improved support for the family at this time. It is relatively easy for anyone after the event to say that this or that would have been better. However, prospectively much is uncertain, and the unexpected does occur. Moreover, even if active termination of life emerges as the key issue here, the consequences and implications of any changes to the law or to policies must be carefully weighed. The interests of the baby and the parents are indeed important, but so too are the interests of families yet to come, and those of the staff, of the community and the wider society.

The autonomy of any given parent is inextricably woven into the fabric of the whole community. It may not be possible to provide the ideal for a given individual. As Warnock puts it, 'As far as public morality goes, the concept of the acceptable is necessary, in that it may set the best goal possible in the circumstances.'[244]

> The ethical, then, arises when someone begins to see that he must postpone his immediate wishes for the sake of the good. And 'the good' here embraces both his own goodness, and the goodness of the society of which he is a member. It arises, to lapse into metaphor, when people begin to see that first their own society, then human beings at large, are all in the same boat, and it is a precarious boat that will sink if there is no co-operation among those on board. Thus arises a willingness to be generous, to share, to restrain one's natural wishes when their fulfilment would damage the rest of the boat-load. In a precarious situation, people must assert and share certain values, or perish. It is this realisation, it seems to me, which lies at the root of the ethical. This is what opens up the possibility of altruism, as each person thinks for himself about his own relation to the rest.[244]

Individual decisions may be made within the privacy of the family or the NICU and be dictated by personal conscience, but the wider debate belongs in the public domain.[245]

McLean has explored the issue of the moral and ethical as applied at the individual and global level: 'What is moral has an ethical constituent and what is ethical has a moral component.'[246] At an individual moral level, people's ideas of right and wrong are shaped by many factors uniquely personal to them, producing an infinite variety of shades of opinion. Subjective and inter-subjective judgements and practical wisdom are needed to work out what ought to be done in particular cases. Absolute consensus at this level is unlikely. On the other hand, ethics can be seen 'rather as an intellectual framework against which actions and opinions can be tested and which gives to us the principles from which we can seek to achieve a resolution of complex and sensitive issues which is adequate to provide public standards.' Although it may be impossible to reach moral agreement on the topics under consideration, it is more likely that ethical commitment will be shared. 'Ethics consists in part of making such commitments explicit and seeking to apply them consistently.' It is this development of the more general from the particular which is the next step in the process of extrapolating wider principles from our data.

# The value of empirical research in this sensitive area

Not only are volumes written on the philosophical constructs which underpin decision making, but a limited number of empirical studies have been attempted to illuminate the clinical reality – for example, the process of moral reasoning required of decision makers.[41,247,248] We believe that our own programme of empirical research fulfils a number of functions. At times the data simply generate questions, but in ethical debate the questions often matter more than the answers.

## It challenges authority and experience

There is a danger that with years of experience clinicians may become familiar with certain ways of practising and have little to challenge their ideas. Our research allows clinicians to see how practice varies, so that they can assess what they themselves do against various outcome measures. The voice of these parents may well challenge their thinking and policies. For example, it exposes differences in the extent to which teams involve the parents, in the administration of opiates, and in the timing of recalling bereaved parents for follow-up appointments.

## It illuminates understanding of the reality of ethical decision making

Most clinicians have not themselves been through the experience of losing an infant. In providing a distilled view from parents who have done so, these results provide a form of surrogate experience. The differences in their perceptions compared to those of the staff make salutary reading and help clinicians to look afresh at customs and practices which have developed without adequate review or assessment. For example, these parents reveal how doubts may arise if they are given no concrete evidence of a poor prognosis, of if deaths are lingering and unpleasant. They also give insights into the effects of false reassurances or inconsistent information.

## It highlights important philosophical questions

In unpacking the real-life experience, our research helps to raise awareness of the underlying important questions and the ethical implications of various practices. For example, it enables us to reflect in a meaningful way on a number of questions, such as just who should take responsibility for the decision? What is the relationship between parents and professionals in making these decisions? Would it be right in reality to make the decision professionally, but to deceive the parents (however benignly) into thinking that they had taken responsibility when in fact they had been manipulated into choosing a certain course of action?

## It explores the limits of tolerance and acceptance

Both medical/nursing staff and parents have spelled out to us their own beliefs about where limits lie. These are considered opinions based on real-life experiences. Their conclusions and explanatory arguments help to set the boundaries around accepted practice, and define grey areas which need further discussion and clarification. For example, serious questions emerge about what should be done with severely asphyxiated babies who no longer require aggressive treatment, about the legality and wisdom of administering drugs in certain doses or combinations, or about the acceptability of withholding hydration and nutrition.

## It gives insights into what constitutes good process

In its analysis of rich qualitative data from representative samples of respondents, our research provides a framework of factors which are universally applicable without losing sight of the uniqueness of each individual experience. It has the capacity to raise awareness of those things which are potentially damaging. It makes no effort to produce prescriptive guidelines, but rather provides a forum within which clinicians can be helped to develop sensitive, individually tailored care. For example, it exposes the special vulnerability of very young parents and of parents who are themselves healthcare professionals. It spells out the range of opinion about the setting for bad news or deaths, about who and what parents find supportive at each stage, and whether they do in fact benefit from seeing or bathing a dead child.

# It provides a yardstick for what other parents think

Knowledge to inform decision making comes from many sources. Our research findings offer a measure of what many parents in similar circumstances felt was right in their case, which may then be set alongside other evidence. The parents' cumulative view carries a certain kind of authority because they have not only lived through the experience, but they are also living with its consequences. Their voice should be heard and heeded. For example, they are uniquely placed to identify those factors which they found persuasive in deciding to stop treatment, and their reasons for consenting to or rejecting autopsy.

# It offers a comprehensive picture

There is a real danger of distortion in the presentation of a small part of a large study. Where the issue is a contentious or sensitive one, there is a temptation to sensationalise one finding or statement and exaggerate its importance. In its comprehensive reporting, our research provides an authoritative and unbiased account of the perceptions and views of both the parents and the staff, and the many factors which impinge on and influence practice and opinion. For example, it sets an overall context of compassionate care which helps to prevent data on the inadequacy of current follow-up practices or of registering deaths from assuming intolerable proportions.

# What ought to be done

Both in law and in ethics it is well recognised that in most cases parents have the authority to decide on their children's welfare. It is evident from our results that at an individual level the majority see decision making about treatment limitation as part of that authority and responsibility, and they appear to have the capacity to take on the role of final arbiters without adverse sequelae. Our findings provide a powerful argument for shared dynamic decision making. Furthermore, we may confidently conclude that parents ought to be given the *opportunity* to accept responsibility for decision making, although the fact that a significant number declined to do so indicates that they should not be *obliged* to make the ultimate decision themselves.

By analysing in detail aspects of the management of these cases which parents find helpful or unhelpful, the research helps to delineate those factors which constitute good process. In doing so it provides a framework for what ought to be available. For example, it is highly relevant to know that parents find a protracted death particularly distressing and worrying, and that they are preoccupied with the suffering involved for their babies. However, by also identifying idiosyncratic preferences, the research cautions against check-lists and rigid guidelines. The couple who left before the baby had died because in their culture blue ears signify the end of meaningful life, and the father who was incensed by a nurse cuddling his dead preterm child as if he were alive, both remind us that death and involvement mean different things to different people. The fact that a number of parents felt they had had insufficient evidence of a poor prognosis alerts staff to the need to establish the level of confidence that parents have in the information they receive, and the importance of showing them convincing signs. The sum of these individual accounts therefore tells us that a flexible package of care tailored to individual need ought to be provided.

However, at a more global moral level there is no simple answer to the question of whether this research answers the fundamental issues relating to limitation of treatment. What ought we to do in these types of situations? Within what moral framework ought we to be operating? The voice of experience which comes from people who have lived through the reality does take us part of the way in that it illuminates the issues. It tells us what these people with considered views and knowledge, who are representative of the populations to be found in our NICUs, think we ought to do. However, a moral judgment has still to be made. There can be no one authoritative voice; no one exercises autonomy in isolation. How ought we to balance these voices and claims against those of others? The parents' distress or despair must be set against the possibility of saving the child's life. The view of the majority that aggressive treatment should be withdrawn sooner than it currently is must be set within the context of the time it takes to be sure that the outcome is almost certainly bleak. Furthermore, what is relevant and appropriate today may not be so in ten years time, as medical knowledge and advances will influence received wisdom. The social consequences of limiting treatment or of actively hastening deaths must be considered. Against the wish of a parent not to have a baby's life prolonged must be set the consequences to a doctor of providing the means to enable that death, the effect of such practices on the integrity of the team and the wider profession, and the consequences for the rights, duties and liberties of others if changes are made to existing laws.

Knowledge acquired from this research thus brings us closer to what we ought to do because it sheds light on the important issues and aids ethical reflection, even if it cannot of itself provide an absolute resolution of the issues. Facts are available which hitherto were not. However, knowing what ought to be done is always an ideal, and we can only approximate towards it. There are many factors to be taken into account. The voice of experience and of authority is one factor among many. It weighs more heavily now that it has been heard, and it brings us closer to that ideal.

# Conclusion

We believe that these results will help clinicians to understand better what it feels like to be faced with this momentous choice on behalf of one's baby, and to appreciate the consequences of their own actions. One father in our study provided a useful analogy.

> It's the old golf bag scenario. You have a golf bag but you have to use the right club at the end of the day. [But you know what clubs you've got in the bag.] You need to know which one to use and you need to know how hard to drive.
>
> (P 50: father of baby with congenital anomalies)

This study has described the clubs which are in the clinicians' bag and the range and scope of each of them. There are no fixed rules for their use, but there is little value in rigid parameters in situations of infinite variety. Good clinical judgements are about knowing which rules (both formal ones and the rules of thumb) to apply when, and in what circumstances. As Warnock has said:

> Ethics is a complicated matter. It is partly a matter of general principles, or even rules ... but largely a matter of judgement and decision, of reasoning and sentiment, of having the right feeling at the right time, and every time is different.[244]

The judgements which must be made are partly subjective assessments based on and influenced by many factors, but they are partly inter-subjective inasmuch as the fittingness of judgements can be confirmed or questioned through critical openness to other people's responses. In deciding whether or not to withhold life-saving treatment from neonates, fallible human beings are approaching parents with facts or with opinions or recommendations which may be wrong – wrong for the child or wrong for the parents. Parents are considering these decisions in the setting of their own beliefs and preconceived ideas and misperceptions which may not be conducive to a good moral decision on behalf of their baby. Communication in these circumstances, too, is subject to misunderstanding and distortion. The fact that such a high proportion of these couples were satisfied with the management of their cases speaks of a model of care which is in tune with most parents' needs, although it does not necessarily follow that as a result each decision was ethically right.

These decisions are among the most difficult of any which have to be made in NICUs. Our research provides rich insights into the lived experience of treatment withdrawal from the point of view of parents who have faced the dilemmas of choice, experienced the dying of their child and who are still living with the consequences of these decisions. Exploring what they say requires the discussion to be firmly grounded in real-life experience, and to incorporate a blend of both art and science. For as one mother of two boys with a rare congenital anomaly said:

> ... the values and objectivity of science are of little use to me in facing the ethical issues raised by the diagnosis of my sons and the implications for family relationships ... My sons are special people, beyond their genetic flaw, and it is love not science that puts meaning in our lives.[249]

The conclusions have to make sense and ring true for the families themselves. We have tried to retain a balance in reporting our findings, and not to obscure the pain and difficulty by dealing too explicitly with theoretical frameworks and complex philosophical or ethical constructs. By addressing issues of autonomy and paternalism, of ethical reasoning and of responsibility, as they are in real life, we have tried both to enrich the subject of philosophical medical ethics[250] and to assist medical teams to provide yet more sensitive care for families in the future who must tread this profoundly distressing path. The parents we have met have made it possible.

> It is the province of knowledge to speak and it is the privilege of wisdom to listen.
>
> (O W Holmes (1872) *The Poet at the Breakfast Table*)

# CHAPTER 15

# Recommendations

Attention is drawn to the detailed conclusions which are reached at the end of the individual chapters, and which present specific information relating to each stage of the experience parents go through. This chapter outlines the general conclusions which may be drawn from the whole.

## For practice

- Mothers' concerns during pregnancy and labour should be listened to sympathetically.
- Parents should be given full, frank information at each stage, sufficient to allow them to make informed choices.
- When things go wrong or problems are anticipated, the paediatric team should be involved as early as possible to avoid fragmentation of care.
- Information should be consistent, delivered in a compassionate way, and as far as possible provided by one senior doctor.
- False reassurances should be avoided.
- Parents should be offered the opportunity to be actively involved in decision making about possible treatment limitation.
- Wherever possible they should be shown concrete evidence of a poor prognosis.
- Parents should have opportunities to be involved in the dying process as much as they wish to be, with the options presented but not pressed on them.
- Respect, dignity, privacy and compassionate support should always be provided.
- Parents should be adequately prepared for what might happen during the dying process.
- The debate on how to manage protracted deaths should be reopened in order to determine a compassionate solution to a distressing problem.

- The rationale for having an autopsy should be clearly explained to the parents so that they can make an informed choice about giving or with-holding consent.
- The important role of staff who were closely involved in the life and death of the child should be recognised in the following areas: attending the funeral, remaining in contact with the family, and seeing them at follow-up bereavement visits. Resources should be made available for them to perform this function effectively.
- Particular care is needed in ensuring that all families receive appropriate follow-up care from the staff who were closely involved in the life of their child. The service provided should be responsive to the need for emotional support as well as for information, it should begin soon after the death, and it should take place in a setting and style which respects the parents' vulnerability.
- Periodic checks should be made to ensure that the family has adequate support and opportunities to talk about their experience to enable them to move forward in their grieving, taking account of the particular difficulties which the couple may experience in mourning simultaneously but in different ways.

# For education

- The importance of taking into account the parents' own needs and wishes should be emphasised to all clinicians entering neonatal practice, using information such as that offered in this report to alert them to the range of tolerances and preferences.
- Junior staff need to be prepared to deal with these difficult situations, but their education should never jeopardise the welfare of individual families.

# For management

- The importance of consistency and continuity should be recognised by managers, and resources made available to ensure that seamless care is provided wherever possible.
- Provision should be made to continue to support the families after discharge from hospital, to ensure that they are helped in their subsequent grieving and do not feel abandoned as well as devastated by their loss.
- The simultaneous registration of births and deaths should be re-examined with a view to exploring sensitive alternatives for the family facing this task soon after the loss of their child.

- Viable alternatives should be sought to the lack of official recognition of stillbirths below 24 weeks' gestation in cases of multiple births.
- The implementation of changes recommended in this report should be carefully monitored.

# For research

- The reasons why parents do not consent to autopsy should be investigated in order to halt the decline in the number who give permission.
- The experience of families from ethnic minority groups should be explored in order to find out the extent to which their needs and wishes differ, and what factors are important to bear in mind in their management when treatment limitation is an option.
- The experience of other families in different specialty areas in relation to treatment limitation should be studied in order to determine which factors can or cannot be generalised across all groups.

# References

1 Frank AW (1995) *The Wounded Storyteller. Body, Illness and Ethics.* University of Chicago Press, Chicago.

2 Wyatt J (1998) *Matters of Life and Death. Today's Healthcare Dilemmas in the Light of Christian Faith.* Inter-Varsity Press, Leicester.

3 Miller P (1987) Death with dignity and the right to die: sometimes doctors have a duty to hasten death. *J Med Ethics.* **13**: 81–5.

4 Van der Maas PJ (1997) End of life decisions in mentally disabled people. *BMJ.* **315**: 73.

5 Amundsen DW (1987) Medicine and the birth of defective children: approaches of the ancient world. In: RC McMillan, HT Engelhardt and SF Spicker (eds) *Euthanasia and the Newborn: Conflicts Regarding Saving Lives.* Reidel, Dordrecht, 3–22.

6 Ferngren GB (1987) The *imago dei* and the sanctity of life: the origins of an idea. In: RC McMillan, HT Engelhardt and SF Spicker (eds) *Euthanasia and the Newborn: Conflicts Regarding Saving Lives.* Reidel, Dordrecht, 23–45.

7 Vaux KL (1987) Danville's Siamese twins: religio-moral perspectives on the care of defective newborns. In: RC McMillan, HT Engelhardt and SF Spicker (eds) *Euthanasia and the Newborn: Conflicts Regarding Saving Lives.* Reidel, Dordrecht, 65–80.

8 Kuhse H and Singer P (1994) *Should the Baby Live? The Problem of Handicapped Infants.* Gregg Revivals, Aldershot. Reprint.

9 Royal College of Paediatrics and Child Health (1997) *Withholding and Withdrawing Life-Saving Treatment in Children: A Framework for Practice.* Royal College of Paediatrics and Child Health, London.

10 British Medical Association (1999) *Withholding and Withdrawing Life-Prolonging Medical Treatment: Guidance for Decision Making.* BMJ Books, London.

11 Levetown M, Pollack MM, Cuerdon TT, Ruttimann UE and Glover JJ (1994) Limitations and withdrawals of medical intervention in pediatric critical care. *JAMA.* **272**(16): 1271–5.

12 McHaffie HE and Fowlie PW (1996) *Life, Death and Decisions: Doctors and Nurses Reflect on Neonatal Practice.* Hochland and Hochland, Cheshire.

13 Wall SN and Partridge JC (1997) Death in the Intensive Care Nursery: physician practice of withdrawing and withholding life support. *Pediatrics.* **99**: 64–70.

14 Dracup K and Raffin T (1989) Withholding and withdrawing ventilation: assessing quality of life. *Am Rev Resp Dis.* **140**: S44–6

15 Dutch Paediatric Association (1992) *Doen of laten?* Dutch Paediatric Association, Utrecht.

16 American Academy of Pediatrics (1994) Guidelines on forgoing life-sustaining medical treatment (RE9406). *Pediatrics.* **93**(3): 532–6.

17 Anspach RR (1993) *Deciding Who Lives: Fateful Choices in the Intensive-Care Nursery.* University of California Press, Berkeley, CA.

18   Norup M (1998) Treatment of extremely premature newborns: a survey of attitudes among Danish physicians. *Acta Paediatr.* **87**: 896–902.

19   Duff RS and Campbell AGM (1987) Moral communities and tragic choices. In: RC McMillan, HT Engelhardt and SF Spicker (eds) *Euthanasia and the Newborn: Conflicts Regarding Saving Lives.* Reidel, Dordrecht, 273–89.

20   Goldstein J, Freud A and Solnit A (1979) *Before the Best Interests of the Child.* Free Press, New York.

21   Stinson R and Stinson P (1983) *The Long Dying of Baby Andrew.* Little-Brown, Boston, MA.

22   Veatch RM (1984) Limits of guardian treatment refusal: a reasonableness standard. *Am J Law Med.* **9**(3): 427–68.

23   Anderson B and Hall B (1995) Parents' perception of decision making for children. *J Law Med Ethics.* **23**: 15–19.

24   Penticuff JH (1988) Neonatal Intensive Care: parental prerogatives. *J Perinatal Neonat Nurs.* **1**(3): 77–86.

25   Maroney DI (1995) Realities of a premature infant's first year: helping parents cope. *J Perinatol.* **15**: 418–22.

26   Ross LF (1998) *Children, Families and Health Care Decision-Making.* Oxford University Press, New York.

27   Rue VM (1985) Death by design of handicapped newborns: the family's role and response. *Issues Law Med.* **1**(3): 201–25.

28   Alderson P (1990) *Choosing for Children. Parents' Consent to Surgery.* Oxford University Press, Oxford.

29   Hegedus KS and Madden JE (1994) Caring in a Neonatal Intensive Care Unit: perspectives of providers and consumers. *J Paediatr Neonatal Nurs.* **8**(2): 67–75.

30   Fulbrook P (1992) Assessing quality of life: the basis for withdrawal of life-supporting treatment? *J Adv Nurs.* **17**: 1440–6.

31   Levinsky NG (1984) The doctor's master. *NEJM.* **311**: 1573–5.

32   Paris JJ (1996) Manslaughter or a legitimate parental decision? The Messenger case. *J Perinatol.* **16**(1): 60–4.

33   Bogdan R, Brown MA and Foster SB (1982) Be honest but not cruel: staff/parent communication on a Neonatal Unit. *Hum Organiz.* **41**(1): 6–16.

34   Harrison H (1986) Neonatal Intensive Care: parents' role in ethical decision making. *Birth.* **13**(3): 165–75.

35   Guillemin JH and Holmstrom LL (1986) *Mixed Blessings: Intensive Care for Newborns.* Oxford University Press, New York.

36   Frohock FM (1986) *Special Care: Medical Decisions at the Beginning of Life.* University of Chicago Press, Chicago.

37   Hill S (1989) *Family.* Michael Joseph, London.

38   Kay R (2000) *Between Two Eternities: Saul's Story.* Hodder Headline, London.

39   Pinch WJ and Spielman ML (1990) The parents' perspective: ethical decision-making in neonatal intensive care. *J Adv Nurs.* **15**: 712–19.

40   Strauss RP, Sharp MC, Lorch SC and Kachalia B (1995) Physicians and the communication of 'bad news': parent experiences of being informed of their child's cleft lip and/or palate. *Pediatrics.* **96**(1): 82–9.

41   Holm S (1997) *Ethical Problems in Clinical Practice: The Ethical Reasoning of Health Care Professionals.* Manchester University Press, Manchester.

42  Cecil R (ed.) (1996) *The Anthropology of Pregnancy Loss.* Berg, Oxford.

43  Oglethorpe R (1989) Parenting after perinatal bereavement – a review of the literature. *J Reprod Infant Psychol.* **7**: 227–44.

44  Zeanah CH (1989) Adaptation following perinatal loss: a critical review. *J Am Acad Child Adolesc Psychiatry.* **28**(3): 467–80.

45  Neidig JR and Dalgas-Pelish P (1991) Parental grieving and perceptions of health care professionals' interventions. *Issues Compr Pediatr Nurs.* **14**: 179–91.

46  MacGregor P (1994) Grief: the unrecognized parental response to mental illness in a child. *Soc Work.* **39**(2): 160–6.

47  Hazzard A, Weston J and Gutterres C (1992) After a child's death: factors related to parental bereavement. *J Dev Behav Pediatr.* **13**(1): 24–30.

48  Braun MJ and Berg DH (1994) Meaning reconstruction in the experience of parental bereavement. *Death Studies.* **18**(2): 105–29.

49  Brabant S, Forsyth CJ and McFarlain G (1994) Defining the family after the death of a child. *Death Studies.* **18**(2): 197–206.

50  Rando TA (1986) *Parental Loss of a Child.* Research Press, Champaign, IL.

51  Simonds W and Katz Rothman B (1992) *Centuries of Solace: Expressions of Maternal Grief in Popular Literature.* Temple University Press, Philadelphia, PA.

52  Mooney B (1988) Preface. In: O Cox (ed.) *Sunday's Child. When Loving Means Letting Go.* Ashgrove Press, Bath, 5–7.

53  Judd D (1995) *Give Sorrow Words.* Free Association Press, London.

54  Buckman R (1996) *I Don't Know What to Say: How to Help and Support Someone Who is Dying.* Pan Books, London.

55  Moreland L (1995) Ruth: death by murder. In: D Dickenson and M Johnson (eds) *Death, Dying and Bereavement.* Open University and Sage, London, 305–7.

56  Knapp P (1986) *Beyond Endurance: When a Child Dies.* Schoken, New York.

57  Klass D (1988) *Parental Grief: Solace and Resolution.* Springer, New York.

58  Morrison B (1997) *As If.* Granta, London.

59  Rando TA (1991) Parental adjustment to the loss of a child. In: D Papadotou and C Papadotos (eds) *Children and Death.* Hemisphere, London, 233–53.

60  Bourne S and Lewis E (1991) Perinatal bereavement: a milestone and some new dangers. *BMJ.* **302**: 1167–8.

61  Stroebe M and Schut H (1999) The dual process model of coping with bereavement: rationale and description. *Death Studies.* **23**: 197–224.

62  Walwork E and Ellison PH (1985) Follow-up of families of neonates in whom life support was withdrawn. *Clin Pediatrics.* **24**(1): 14–20.

63  Theut SK, Pederson FA, Zaslow MJ, Cain RL, Rabinovich BA and Morihisa JM (1989) Perinatal loss and perinatal bereavement. *Am J Psychiatry.* **146**(5): 635–9.

64  Vance JC, Najman JM, Thearle MJ, Embelton G, Foster WJ and Boyle FM (1995) Psychological changes in parents eight months after the loss of an infant from stillbirth, neonatal death or sudden infant death syndrome – a longitudinal study. *Pediatrics.* **96**(5): 933–8.

65  Kimble DL (1991) Neonatal death: a descriptive study of fathers' experiences. *Neonatal Network.* **9**(8): 45–50.

66  Lang A and Gottlieb A (1993) Parental grief reactions and marital intimacy following infant death. *Death Studies.* **17**(3): 233–55.

67  Mander R (1994) *Loss and Bereavement in Childbearing.* Blackwell, Oxford.

68  Kowalski KM (1987) Perinatal loss and bereavement. In: L Sonstegard, KM Kowalski and B Jennings (eds) *Women's Health: Crisis and Illness in Childbearing.* Grune and Stratton, Orlando, FL.

69  Dyregrov A and Mattheisen S (1987) Similiarities and differences in mothers' and fathers' grief following the death of an infant. *Scand J Psychol.* **28**: 1–15.

70  Foster DJ, O'Malley JE and Koocher GP (1981) The parent interviews. In: JE O'Malley and GP Koocher (eds) *The Damocles Syndrome: Psychosocial Consequences of Surviving Childhood Cancer.* McGraw Hill, New York.

71  Schwab R (1992) Effects of a child's death on the marital relationship: a preliminary study. *Death Studies.* **16**(2): 141–54.

72  Wolterstorff N (1997) *Lament for a Son.* SPCK, London.

73  Penson J (1990) *Bereavement – A Guide for Nurses.* Harper and Row, London.

74  Henley A and Kohner N (1991) *Miscarriage, Stillbirth and Neonatal Death: Guidelines for Professionals.* Stillbirth and Neonatal Death Society, London.

75  Fisher M and Warman J (1993) *Bereavement and Loss: A Skills Companion.* National Extension College, Cambridge.

76  Hindmarch C (2000) *On the Death of a Child* (2e). Radcliffe Medical Press, Oxford.

77  Kohner N and Leftwich A (1995) *Pregnancy Loss and the Death of a Baby: A Training Pack for Professionals.* National Extension College, Cambridge.

78  Kohner N and Henley A (1995) *When A Baby Dies. The Experience of Late Miscarriage, Stillbirth and Neonatal Death.* Pandora Press, London.

79  Dickenson D and Johnson M (1995) *Death, Dying and Bereavement.* Open University and Sage, London.

80  Tschudin V (1997) *Counselling for Loss and Bereavement.* Bailliere Tindall, London.

81  Brost L and Kenney JW (1992) Pregnancy and perinatal loss: parental reactions and nursing interventions. *J Obstet Gynecol Neonatal Nurs.* **21**(6): 457–63.

82  Benfield DG, Leib SA and Vollman JH (1978) Grief response of parents to neonatal death and parent participation in deciding care. *Pediatrics.* **62**(2): 171–7.

83  Peppers LG and Knapp RJ (1980) *Motherhood and Mourning.* Praeger, New York.

84  McHaffie HE (1988) The artistry of interviewing. *Senior Nurse.* **8**(1): 34.

85  McHaffie HE (1996) Researching sensitive issues. In: L Frith (ed.) *Ethics and Midwifery: Issues in Contemporary Practice.* Butterworth-Heinemann, Oxford.

86  Chochinov HM, Wilson KG, Enns M and Lander S (1997) 'Are you depressed?' Screening for depression in the terminally ill. *Am J Psychiatry.* **154**(5): 674–6.

87  Boyle FM, Vance JC and Najman JM (1996) The mental health impact of stillbirth, neonatal death or SIDS: prevalance and patterns of distress among mothers. *Soc Sci Med.* **43**(8): 1273–82.

88  Videka-Sherman L (1982) Coping with the death of a child: a study over time. *Am J Orthopsychiatry.* **52**: 688–98.

89  Dyregrov A and Matthiesen SB (1991) Parental grief following the death of an infant – a follow-up over one year. *Scand J Psychol.* **32**(3): 193–207.

90  Riches G and Dawson P (1996) Making stories and taking stories. Methodological reflections on researching grief and marital tension following the death of a child. *Br J Guidance Counsel.* **24**(3): 357–65.

91  Tournier P (1978) Foreword. In: J Powell *Why Am I Afraid to Tell You Who I Am?* Fount/Harper Collins, London.

92  Lovell H, Bokoula C, Misra S and Speight N (1986) Mothers' reactions to perinatal death. *Nurs Times.* **82**(46): 40–2.

93  Benson J and Robinson-Walsh D (1996) *Love, Labour and Loss: Stillbirth and Neonatal Death*. Scarlet Press, London.

94  Martinson IM (1991) Grief is an individual journey: follow-up of families post death of a child with cancer. In: D Papadotou and C Papadotos (eds) *Children and Death*. Hemisphere, London, 255–65.

95  Burgess R (1984) *In the Field – An Introduction to Field Research*. Allen and Unwin, London.

96  Cotterrill P and Letherby G (1993) Weaving stories: personal autobiographies in feminist research. *Sociology*. **27**(1): 67–79.

97  Cowles KV (1988) Issues in qualitative research on sensitive topics. *West J Nurs Res*. **10**: 163–79.

98  Grafanaki S (1996) How research can change the researcher. *Br J Guidance Counsel*. **24**(3): 329–38.

99  Polkinghorne DE (1991) Qualitative procedures for counseling research. In: CE Watkins Jr and L Sneider (eds) *Research in Counseling*. Erlbaum, Hillsdale, NJ, 163–204.

100 Zussman R (1992) *Intensive Care: Medical Ethics and the Medical Profession*. University of Chicago Press, Chicago.

101 Draper ES, Kurinczuk JJ, Abrams KR and Clarke M (1999) Assessment of separate contributions to perinatal mortality of infertility history and treatment: a case–control analysis. *Lancet*. **353**: 1746–9.

102 Baird DD, Wilcox AJ and Kramer MS (1999) Why might infertile couples have problem pregnancies? *Lancet*. **353**: 1724–5.

103 Lazarus RS and Folkman S (1984) *Stress, Appraisal and Coping*. Springer, New York.

104 Krahn GL, Hallum A and Kime C (1993) Are there good ways to give 'bad news'? *Pediatrics*. **91**(3): 578–82.

105 Buckman R (1995) Breaking bad news: why is it still so difficult? In: D Dickenson and M Johnson (eds) *Death, Dying and Bereavement*. Open University and Sage, London, 172–9.

106 Green JM and Murton FE (1996) Diagnosis of Duchenne Muscular Dystrophy: parents' experiences and satisfaction. *Child: Care, Health Dev*. **22**(2): 113–28.

107 Nash R (1995) Breaking it gently. *New Generation*. **14**(4): 9.

108 Blackburn S (1999) Enhancing parenting in the high risk nursery. In: *Neonatal Nurses Association Yearbook*. CMA Medical Data, Cambridge, 2/30–35.

109 Crowther ME (1995) Communication following a stillbirth or neonatal death: room for improvement. *Br J Obstet Gynaecol*. **102**(12): 952–6.

110 Finlay I and Dallimore D (1991) Your child is dead. *BMJ*. **302**: 1524–5.

111 Gorovitz S (1993) *Drawing The Line. Life, Death and Ethical Choices in an American Hospital*. Temple University Press, Philadelphia, PA.

112 McHaffie HE (1992) Social support in the neonatal intensive care unit. *J Adv Nurs*. **17**: 279–87.

113 Pearlman RA, Miles SH and Arnold RM (1993) Contributions of empirical research to medical ethics. *Theor Med*. **14**: 197–210.

114 Paris JJ and Schreiber MD (1996) Parental discretion in refusal of treatment for newborns. A real but limited right. *Clin Perinatol*. **23**(3): 573–81.

115 Shelp EE (1987) Choosing among evils. In: RC McMillan, HT Engelhardt and SE Spicker (eds) *Euthanasia and the Newborn: Conflicts Regarding Saving Lives*. Reidel, Dordrecht, 211–31.

116 King NMP (1992) Transparency in Neonatal Intensive Care. *Hastings Center Rep.* **May–June**: 18–25.

117 Rhoden N (1986) Treating Baby Doe: the ethics of uncertainty. *Hastings Center Rep.* **16**(4): 3–42.

118 Schneiderman LJ, Kaplan RM, Pearlman RA and Teetzel H (1993) Do physicians' own preferences for life-sustaining treatment influence their perceptions of patients' prefences? *J Clin Ethics.* **4**(1): 28–33.

119 Catlin AJ (1998) *Physicians' Perceptions of the Dilemma of Neonatal Resuscitation for Extremely Low Birthweight Preterm Infants.* Unpublished Doctor of Nursing Science Dissertation, Rush University, Chicago.

120 Saigal S, Stoskopf BL, Feeny D *et al.* (1999) Differences in preferences for neonatal outcomes among health care professionals, parents and adolescents. *JAMA.* **281**(21): 1991–7.

121 Jennett B (1984) *High-Technology Medicine – Benefits and Burdens.* Nuffield Provincial Hospitals Trust, London.

122 American Medical Association (1984) *Current Opinions of the Judicial Council of the American Medical Association – 1984.* American Medical Association, Chicago.

123 O'Callahan JG, Fink C, Pitts LH and Luce JM (1995) Withholding and withdrawing life support from patients with severe head injury. *Crit Care Med.* **23**(9): 1567–75.

124 Kent G (1996) Shared understandings for informed consent: the relevance of psychological research on the provision of information. *Soc Sci Med.* **43**(10): 1517–23.

125 Van der Heide A, van der Maas PJ, van der Wal G *et al.* (1998) The role of parents in end-of-life decisions in neonatology: physicians views and practices. *Pediatrics.* **101**(3): 413–8.

126 May WF (1991) *The Patient's Ordeal.* Indiana University Press, Bloomington, IN.

127 Dimond B (1998) Genetic screening: who decides? *RCM Midwives J.* **1**(4): 117–19.

128 Fallowfield L (1997) Truth sometimes hurts, but deceit hurts more. *Ann NY Acad Sci.* **809**: 525–36.

129 Cox O (1988) *Sunday's Child. When Loving Means Letting Go.* Ashgrove Press, Bath.

130 Truog RD (1999) 'Doctor, if this were your child, what would you do?' *Pediatrics.* **103**(1): 153–4.

131 Lantos JD, Tyson JE, Allen A *et al.* (1994) Withholding and withdrawing life-sustaining treatment in neonatal intensive care: issues for the 1990s. *Arch Dis Child.* **71**: F218–23.

132 Brody H (1989) Transparency: informed consent in primary care. *Hastings Center Rep.* **19**(5): 5–9.

133 Carr J (1988) Six weeks to twenty-one years old: a longitudinal study of children with Down's syndrome and their families. *J Child Psychol Psychiatry.* **29**(4): 407–31.

134 Marck BA, Field PA and Bergum V (1994) A search for understanding. In: PA Field and BA Marck (eds) *Uncertain Motherhood.* Sage, Thousand Oaks, CA.

135 Kerr SM and McIntosh JB (1998) Disclosure of disability: exploring the perspective of parents. *Midwifery.* **14**: 225–32.

136 Tannen D (1993) *You Just Don't Understand. Women and Men in Conversation.* Virago, London.

137 Allende I (1995) *Paula.* Flamingo, London.

138 Jellinek MS, Catlin EA, Todres ID and Cassem EH (1992) Facing tragic decisions with parents in the neonatal intensive care unit: clinical perspectives. *Pediatrics.* **89**(1): 119–22.

139  Stark J and Thape J (1993) Decision making in neonatal intensive care: a collaboration of parents, physicians and nurses. *Assoc Women's Health, Obstet Neo Nurs Clin Issues.* **4**(4): 589–95.

140  Woolley H, Stein A, Forrest GC and Baum JD (1989) Imparting the diagnosis of life-threatening illness in children. *BMJ.* **298**: 1623–6.

141  Harrison H (1993) The principles of family-centred neonatal care. *Pediatrics.* **92**(5): 643–50.

142  Fallowfield L (1993) Giving sad and bad news. *Lancet.* **341**: 476–8.

143  Association for Medical Education in Europe (1997) *Teaching and Learning How to Break Bad News.* Association for Medical Education in Europe, Dundee.

144  Awoonor-Renner S (1991) I desperately needed to see my son. *BMJ.* **302**: 356.

145  Forrest G (1989) Care of the bereaved. In: M Enkin, MJNC Keirse and I Chalmers (eds) *A Guide to Effective Care in Pregnancy and Childbirth.* Oxford University Press, Oxford, 161–70.

146  Stroebe M and Schut HAW (1998) Culture and grief. *Bereavement Care.* **17**: 7–10.

147  Stroebe M and Stroebe W (1987) *Bereavement and Health. The Psychological and Physical Consequences of Partner Loss.* Cambridge University Press, Cambridge, 119–22.

148  Rand CS, Kellner KR, Revak-Lutz R and Massey JK (1998) Parental behavior after perinatal death: 12 years of observation. *J Psychosom Obstet Gynaecol.* **19**(1): 44–8.

149  Buckley M (1998) Death rights. *Nurs Times.* **94**(25): 26–32.

150  Carr D and Knupp S (1985) Grief and perinatal loss: a community hospital approach to support. *J Obstet Gynecol Neonatal Nurs.* **14**: 130–9.

151  Hutti M (1988) A quick reference table of interventions to assist families to cope with pregnancy loss or neonatal death. *Birth.* **15**: 33–5.

152  Leon IG (1992) Perinatal loss. A critique of current hospital practices. *Clin Paediatrics.* **June**: 366–74.

153  House of Lords Select Committee on Medical Ethics (1994) *Volume 1. Report.* HMSO, London.

154  (1994) *Government Response to the Report of the Select Committee on Medical Ethics.* HMSO, London.

155  Campbell AGM and McHaffie HE (1995) Prolonging life and allowing death: infants. *J Med Ethics.* **21**: 339–44.

156  Joint Working Party of the Royal College of Pathologists, the Royal College of Physicians of London and the Royal College of Surgeons of England (1991) *The Autopsy and Audit.* Royal College of Pathologists, London.

157  Rushton DI (1991) West Midlands perinatal mortality survey, 1987. An audit of 300 perinatal autopsies. *Br J Obstet Gynaecol.* **98**(7): 624–7.

158  Rushton DI (1994) Prognostic role of the perinatal postmortem. *Br J Hosp Med.* **52**(9): 450–4.

159  Sirkia K, Saarinen-Pihkala UM, Hovi L and Sariola H (1998) Autopsy in children with cancer who die while in terminal care. *Med Pediatr Oncol.* **30**(5): 284–9.

160  Kumar P, Angst DB, Taxy J and Mangurten HH (2000) Neonatal autopsies: a 10-year experience. *Arch Pediatr Adolesc Med.* **154**: 38–42.

161  Maniscalco WM and Clarke TA (1982) Factors influencing neonatal autopsy rate. *Am J Dis Child.* **136**: 781–4.

162  Craft H and Brazy JE (1986) Autopsy – high yield in neonatal population. *Am J Dis Child.* **140**: 1260–2.

163 VanMarter LJ, Taylor F and Epstein MF (1987) Parental and physician-related determinants of consent for neonatal autopsy. *Am J Dis Child.* **141**: 149–53.

164 Saller DN, Lesser KB, Harrel U, Rogers BB and Oyer CE (1995) The clinical utility of the perinatal autopsy. *JAMA.* **273**: 663–5.

165 Khong TY, Mansor FAW and Staples AJ (1995) Are perinatal autopsy rates satisfactory? *Med J Austr.* **162**: 469–70.

166 Dhar V, Perlman M, Vilela MI, Haque KN, Kirpalani H and Cutz E (1998) Autopsy in a Neonatal Intensive Care Unit: utilization patterns and associations of clinico-pathologic discordances. *J Pediatrics.* **132**: 75–9.

167 Khong TY (1997) Improving perinatal autopsy rates: who is counselling bereaved parents for autopsy consent? *Birth.* **24**(1): 55–7.

168 Landers S, Kurby R, Harvey B and Langston C (1994) Characteristics of infants who undergo neonatal autopsy. *J Perinatal.* **14**(3): 204–7.

169 Rushton CH (1994) Ethical decision making: the role of parents. *Capsules Comments Pediatr Nurs.* **1**: 103–12.

170 Riggs D and Weibley RE (1994) Autopsies and the Pediatric Intensive Care Unit. *Pediatr Crit Care.* **41**(6): 1383–93.

171 Khong TY (1996) The contribution of the pathologist after a perinatal loss: what should we be telling parents? *Austr NZ J Obstet Gynaecol.* **36**(1): 15–17.

172 Laurent C (1993) A sad necessity. *Nurs Times.* **89**(13): 22.

173 Mallinson G (1989) Life crises: when a baby dies. *Nurs Times.* **85**(9): 31–4.

174 Forrest GC, Standish E and Baum JD (1982) Support after perinatal death: a study of support and counselling after perinatal bereavement. *BMJ.* **285**: 1475–9.

175 McPhee SJ, Bottles K, Lo B, Saika G and Crommie D (1986) To redeem them from death. Reactions of family members to autopsy. *Am J Med.* **80**: 665–71.

176 Abdul RH and Khong TY (1995) Perinatal infant postmortem examination. Survey of women's reactions to perinatal necropsy. *BMJ.* **310**: 870–1.

177 Martin J (1995) Doctors' mask on pain. In: D Dickenson and M Johnson (eds) *Death, Dying and Bereavement.* Open University and Sage, London, 83–4.

178 Adshead G and Dickenson D (1995) Why do doctors and nurses disagree? In: D Dickenson and M Johnson (eds) *Death, Dying and Bereavement.* Open University and Sage, London, 161–8.

179 Kubler-Ross E (1974) *Questions and Answers on Death and Dying.* Macmillan, London.

180 Harmon RJ, Glicken AD and Siegel RE (1984) Neonatal loss in the Intensive Care Nursery: effects on maternal grieving and program for intervention. *J Am Acad Child Adolesc Psychiatry.* **23**: 68–71.

181 Fox R, Pillai M, Porter H and Gill G (1997) The management of late fetal death: a guide to comprehensive care. *Br J Obstet Gynaecol.* **104**: 4–10.

182 Laing IA and Halley GC (1995) Enough is enough – when to stop neonatal care. *Curr Paediatrics.* **5**: 53–8.

183 Chitty LS, Barnes CA and Berry C (1996) Continuing with pregnancy after a diagnosis of lethal abnormality: experience of five couples and recommendations for management. *BMJ.* **313**: 478–80.

184 Theut SK, Zaslow MJ, Rabinovich BA, Bartko JJ and Morihisa JM (1990) Resolution of parental bereavement after a perinatal loss. *J Am Acad Child Adolesc Psychiatry.* **29**(4): 521–25.

185 Hunfeld JA, Mourik MM, Passchier J and Tibboel D (1996) Do couples grieve differently following infant loss? *Psychol Rep.* **79**(2): 407–10.

186 Wallerstedt C and Higgins P (1996) Facilitating perinatal grieving between the mother and the father. *J Obstet Gynecol Neonatal Nurs.* **25**(5): 389–94.

187 Gray J (1992) *Men are From Mars, Women are From Venus. A Practical Guide for Improving Communication and Getting What You Want in Your Relationships.* Thorson, New York.

188 Gentry J, Kennedy P, Paul C and Hill R (1995) Family transition during grief: discontinuities in household consumption patterns. *J Bus Res.* **34**: 67–79.

189 Cook AS and Oltjenbruns KA (eds) (1998) *Dying and Grieving: Life Span and Family Perspectives.* Harcourt Brace, Fort Worth, TX.

190 Hughes PM, Turton P and Evans CDH (1999) Stillbirth as risk factor for depression and anxiety in the subseqent pregnancy: cohort study. *BMJ.* **318**: 1721–4.

191 Murray J and Calnan V (1988) Predicting adjustment to perinatal death. *Br J Med Psychol.* **61**: 237–44.

192 Davis DL, Stewart M and Harmon RJ (1989) Postponing pregnancy after perinatal death: perspectives on doctor advice. *J Am Acad Child Adolesc Psychiatry.* **28**(3): 481–7.

193 Bryan E (1995) The death of a twin. *Palliative Med.* **9**: 187–92.

194 Bigelow G and Hollinger J (1997) Grief and AIDS: surviving catastrophic mutiple loss. In: DL Infeld and NR Penner (eds) *Bereavement: Client Adaptation and Hospice Services.* Haworth Press, New York, 83–96.

195 Luard E (1996) *Family Life: Birth, Death and the Whole Damn Thing.* Bantam Press, London.

196 Munday J and Wohlenhaus-Munday F (1995) *Surviving the Death of a Child.* Darton, Longman and Todd, London.

197 Ironside V (1997) *You'll Get Over It. The Rage of Bereavement.* Penguin, Harmondsworth.

198 Moriarty HJ, Carroll R and Cotroneo M (1996) Differences in bereavement reactions within couples following death of a child. *Res Nurs Health.* **19**: 461–9.

199 Lewis E and Bourne S (1989) Perinatal death. In: M Oates (ed.) *Psychological Aspects of Obstetrics and Gynaecology.* Balliere Tindall, London.

200 Harrigan R, Naber MM, Jensen KA, Tse A and Perez D (1993) Perinatal grief: response to the loss of an infant. *Neonatal Network.* **12**(5): 25–31.

201 Welch ID (1991) Miscarriage, stillbirth or neonatal death: starting a healthy grieving process. *Neonatal Network.* **9**(8): 53–7.

202 Ward B and Associates (1996) *Good Grief: Exploring Feelings, Loss and Death With Over-Elevens and Adults* (2e). Jessica Kingsley, London.

203 Segal S, Fletcher M and Meekison WG (1986) Survey of bereaved parents. *Can Med Assoc J.* **134**: 38.

204 Woolley MM (1997) The death of a child – the parent's perspective and advice. *J Pediatr Surg.* **32**(1): 73–4.

205 Littlewood JL, Cramer D, Hoekstra J and Humphrey GB (1991) Gender differences in parental coping following their child's death. *Br J Guidance Counsel.* **19**:(2) 139–48.

206 Kohner N and Thomas J (1995) *Grieving After the Death of Your Baby.* The Child Bereavement Trust, Bourne End.

207 Cuisinier M, de Kleine M, Kollee L, Bethlehem G and de Graauw C (1996) Grief following the loss of a newborn twin compared to a singleton. *Acta Paediatr.* **85**(3): 339–43.

208 Wilson AL, Fenton LJ, Stevens DC and Soule DJ (1982) The death of a newborn twin: an analysis of parental bereavement. *Pediatrics.* **70**: 587–91.

209 Rowe J, Clyman R and Green C (1978) Follow up of families who experience a peri-natal death. *Pediatrics.* **62**: 166–9.

210 Lewis E (1979) Inhibition of mourning by pregnancy: psychopathology and management. *BMJ.* **ii**: 27–8.

211 Schweitzer A (1990) *Out of My Life and Thought: An Autobiography* (translated by AB Lemke). Henry Holt, New York.

212 Talbot K (1996) Transcending a devastating loss: the life attitudes of mothers who have experienced the death of their only child. In: DL Infeld and NR Penner (eds) *Bereavement: Client Adaptation and Hospice Services.* Haworth Press, New York, 67–82.

213 Santorum KG (1998) *Letters to Gabriel. The true story of Gabriel Michael Santorum.* CCC of America (Catholic Book Pubishers Assoc), TX.

214 Selzer R (1992) *Raising the Dead.* Viking, New York.

215 Hutchison SMW (1995) Evaluation of bereavement anniversary cards. *J Palliative Care.* **11**(3): 32–4.

216 Fairbairn G (1995) When a baby dies – a father's view. In: D Dickenson and M Johnson (eds) *Death, Dying and Bereavement.* Open University and Sage, London, 290–2.

217 Thuen F (1997) Social support after the loss of an infant child: a long-term perspective. *Scand J Psychol.* **38**(2): 103–10.

218 Pincus L (1981) *Death and The Family: The Importance of Mourning.* Faber, London.

219 Riches G and Dawson P (1996) 'An intimate loneliness': evaluating the impact of a child's death on parental self-identity and marital relationships. *J Fam Ther.* **18**: 1–22.

220 Archer J (1991) The process of grief: a selective review. *J Adv Health Nurs Care.* **1**(2): 9–37.

221 Schank RC (1990) *Tell Me a Story. A New Look at Real and Artificial Memory.* Scribners, New York.

222 Lemmer CM (1991) Parental perceptions of caring following perinatal bereavement. *West J Nurs Res.* **13**(4): 475–93.

223 Sexton PR and Stephen SB (1991) Postpartum mothers' perceptions of nursing interventions for perinatal grief. *Neonatal Network.* **9**(5): 47–51.

224 Gould M (1999) Pressing charges. *Nurs Times.* **95**(18): 12.

225 Klass D (1993) Solace and immortality: bereaved parents' continuing bond with their children. *Death Studies.* **17**(4): 343–68.

226 Rothman BK (1986) *The Tentative Pregnancy: Prenatal Diagnosis and the Future of Motherhood.* Viking, New York.

227 Brody BA (1993) Assessing empirical research in bioethics. *Theor Med.* **14**: 211–9.

228 Kirschbaum MS (1996) Life support decisions for children: what do parents value? *Adv Nurs Sci.* **19**(1): 51–71.

229 Silverman WA (1992) Overtreatment of neonates? A personal retrospective. *Pediatrics.* **90**: 971–6.

230 Lantos JD, Miles SH and Cassel CK (1989) The Linares affair. *Law Med Health Care.* **17**: 308–15.

231 Stahlman MT (1986) Medical ethics and the law. *Pediatr Res.* **20**: 913–14.

232 Brody H (1992) *The Healer's Power.* Yale University Press, New Haven, CT.

233 Lee SK, Penner PL and Cox M (1991) Comparison of the attitudes of health care professionals and parents toward active treatment of very low birth weight infants. *Pediatrics.* **88**: 110–14.

234 Savulescu J (1995) Rational non-interventional paternalism: why doctors ought to make judgments of what is best for their patients. *J Med Ethics.* **21**: 327–31.

235  Charney EB (1990) Parental attitudes toward management of newborns with mye-lomeningocoele. *Dev Med Child Neurol.* **32**: 14–19.

236  American Academy of Pediatrics (1995) Perinatal care at the threshold of viability. *Pediatrics.* **96**(5): 974–6.

237  Forman EN and Ladd RE (1991) *Ethical Dilemmas in Pediatrics: A Case Study Approach.* University of America Press, Lanham, MD.

238  McHaffie HE, Cuttini M, Brölz-Voit G *et al.* (1999) Withholding/withdrawing treatment from neonates: legislation and official guidelines across Europe. *J Med Ethics.* **25**(6): 440–6.

239  Confidential Enquiry into Stillbirths and Deaths in Infancy (CESDI) (1995) *Fourth Annual Report.* CESDI, London.

240  Confidential Enquiry into Stillbirths and Deaths in Infancy (CESDI) (1998) *Fifth Annual Report.* Maternal and Child Health Consortium, London.

241  Confidential Enquiry into Stillbirths and Deaths in Infancy (CESDI) (1999) *Sixth Annual Report.* Maternal and Child Health Consortium, London.

242  Edwards G (1997) CESDI: Confidential Enquiry into Sudden Death in Infants. In: *Neonatal Nurses Yearbook.* CMA Medical Data, Cambridge. 2-17–2-24.

243  Phillips KD (1994) Taking away hope. *BMJ.* **309**: 478.

244  Warnock M (1998) *An Intelligent Person's Guide to Ethics.* Duckworth, London.

245  Nuland SB (1994) *How We Die.* Chatto and Windus, London.

246  McLean S (1992) Law and moral dilemmas affecting life and death. *Proceedings of the Twentieth Colloquy on European Law, Glasgow, 10–12 September 1990.* Council of Europe, Strasbourg.

247  Rest J, Bebeau M and Volker J (1986) An overview of the psychology of morality. In: J Rest (ed.) *Moral Development: Advances in Research and Theory.* Praeger, New York, 1–27.

248  Blum LA (1994) *Moral Perception and Particularity.* Cambridge University Press, New York.

249  McGowan R (1999) Beyond the disorder: one parent's reflection on genetic counselling. *J Med Ethics.* **25**: 195–9.

250  Hope T (1999) Empirical medical ethics. *J Med Ethics.* **25**: 219–20.

# Data on non-respondent families

Information was not available for all parameters, and three mothers were not living with the fathers of their babies.

## Parents (*n* = 22 families)

### Ages

|  | Mothers | Fathers |
|---|---|---|
| Teens | 7 | 1 |
| Early twenties | 3 | 3 |
| Late twenties | 7 | 1 |
| Early thirties | 3 | 4 |
| Late thirties | 1 | 2 |
| Early forties | 1 | 2 |
| Late forties |  |  |
| Fifties |  | 1 |

### Marital status

| | |
|---|---|
| Married | 10 |
| Cohabiting | 8 |
| Living apart | 3 |
| Missing data | 1 |

# Parity

| | |
|---|---|
| Primiparous | 11 |
| Para 1 | 6 |
| Para 2 | 2 |
| Para 3 | 3 |
| Para 4 | 1 |
| Para 5 | 1 |
| Previous obstetric loss | 2 |

# Occupations

Information on occupations was not available for all parents. However, it should be noted that at least 13 mothers and 3 fathers were not in paid employment.

# **Babies** *(n = 33)*
## Gender

| | |
|---|---|
| Male | 10 |
| Female | 13 |

# Gestation

| Number of weeks | Number of babies |
|---|---|
| <24 | 4 |
| 24 | 1 |
| 25–28 | 8 |
| 30–35 | 4 |
| 36–40 | 4 |
| >40 | 2 |

# Weight

| Weight (grams) | Number of babies |
|---|---|
| ≤500 | 3 |
| 501–750 | 6 |
| 751–1000 | 3 |
| 1001–1500 | 4 |
| 1501–2000 | 1 |
| 2001–2500 | 2 |
| 2501–3000 | 2 |
| 3001–3500 | 0 |
| 3501–4000 | 2 |
| 4001–4500 | 0 |

# Diagnosis

| | Number of babies |
|---|---|
| Preterm | 12 |
| Congenital anomalies | 8 |
| Cardiac anomalies | 1 |
| Perinatal asphyxia | 2 |

# Age at time of death

| Age (weeks) | Number of babies |
|---|---|
| 0–4 | 19* |
| 5–8 | 3 |

* Within first week, 15; less than 2 full days, 8.

# Noteworthy differences

- 32% of the non-respondent mothers were teenagers, compared to 8% of the respondents.
- 50% of the non-respondent mothers were primigravidae, compared to 31% of the respondents.
- 59% of the non-respondent mothers did not work outside the home, compared to 19% of the respondents.

# Index